Contemporary Issues in Swahili Ethnography

The term 'Swahili' describes the Muslim peoples of the East African coast, speakers of Kiswahili or closely related languages, who have historically filled roles as middlemen and merchants, the cosmopolitan products of a trading economy between Africa and the Indian Ocean world.

This collection brings together anthropologists working on the greater Swahili world and the issues it confronts, dealing with societies from southern Somalia, northern Mozambique and the Comoro Islands, to Zanzibar and Mafia. The authors discuss a range of contemporary issues such as the shifting roles of Islam on the mainland coast; consumerism, conservation, memory and belonging in Zanzibar; how a Muslim society deals with HIV/AIDS; social change, development and political strategies in the Comoros; and Swahili women in London. The diversity of these themes reflects the diversity of the Swahili world itself: despite a cohesive cultural identity built upon shared practices, religious beliefs and language, the challenges facing Swahili people are multiple and complex.

This book comprises articles originally published in the *Journal of Eastern African Studies* along with some new chapters.

Iain Walker is Research Officer in the Centre for Interdisciplinary Area Studies, Martin Luther University, and Associate at the Max Planck Institute for Social Anthropology in Halle, Germany. He has worked on a variety of themes in the Comoro Islands as well as on migration, disapora, identity and belonging among Comorians and Hadramis in the Western Indian Ocean.

T0383682

Contemporary Issues in Swahili Ethnography

Edited by
Iain Walker

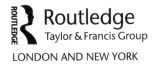

Routledge
Taylor & Francis Group

LONDON AND NEW YORK

First published 2017 by Routledge

2 Park Square, Milton Park, Abingdon, Oxfordshire OX14 4RN
52 Vanderbilt Avenue, New York, NY 10017

Routledge is an imprint of the Taylor & Francis Group, an informa business

First issued in paperback 2018

British Library Cataloguing in Publication Data
A catalogue record for this book is available from the British Library

ISBN: 978-1-138-24101-5 (hbk)
ISBN: 978-0-367-13287-3 (pbk)

Typeset in Times New Roman
by RefineCatch Limited, Bungay, Suffolk

Publisher's Note
The publisher accepts responsibility for any inconsistencies that may have
arisen during the conversion of this book from journal articles to book chapters,
namely the possible inclusion of journal terminology.

Disclaimer
Every effort has been made to contact copyright holders for their permission to
reprint material in this book. The publishers would be grateful to hear from any
copyright holder who is not here acknowledged and will undertake to rectify
any errors or omissions in future editions of this book.

Contents

v

CONTENTS

Citation Information

The following chapters were originally published in the *Journal of Eastern African Studies*, volume 6, issue 4 (2012). When citing this material, please use the original page numbering for each article, as follows:

Chapter 4

One hundred years in Brava: The migration of the 'Umar Bā 'Umar from Hadhramaut to East Africa and back, c. 1890–1990
Alessandra Vianello
Journal of Eastern African Studies, volume 6, issue 4 (November 2012), pp. 655–671

Chapter 5

Reinterpreting revolutionary Zanzibar in the media today: The case of Dira *newspaper*
Marie-Aude Fouéré
Journal of Eastern African Studies, volume 6, issue 4 (November 2012), pp. 672–689

Chapter 6

Medicines of hope? The tough decision for anti-retroviral use for HIV in Zanzibar, Tanzania
Nadine Beckmann
Journal of Eastern African Studies, volume 6, issue 4 (November 2012), pp. 690–708

Chapter 7

Chasing imaginary leopards: science, witchcraft and the politics of conservation in Zanzibar
Martin Walsh and Helle Goldman
Journal of Eastern African Studies, volume 6, issue 4 (November 2012), pp. 727–746

Chapter 8

Constructing translocal socioscapes: consumerism, aesthetics, and visuality in Zanzibar Town
Paola Ivanov
Journal of Eastern African Studies, volume 6, issue 4 (November 2012), pp. 631–654

Chapter 11

Is social capital fungible? The rise and fall of the Sanduk microcredit project in Ngazidja
Iain Walker
Journal of Eastern African Studies, volume 6, issue 4 (November 2012), pp. 709–726

The following chapters were originally published in the *Journal of Eastern African Studies*, volume 7, issue 4 (2013). When citing this material, please use the original page numbering for each article, as follows:

Chapter 2

Transmission of Muslim practices and women's agency in Ibo Island and Pemba (Mozambique)
Francesca Declich
Journal of Eastern African Studies, volume 7, issue 4 (November 2013), pp. 588–606

Chapter 10

Beyond 'Great Marriage': collective involvement, personal achievement and social change in Ngazidja (Comoros)
Sophie Blanchy
Journal of Eastern African Studies, volume 7, issue 4 (November 2013), pp. 569–587

The following chapter was originally published in the *Journal of Eastern African Studies*, volume 9, issue 2 (2015). When citing this material, please use the original page numbering for each article, as follows:

Chapter 9

Integration and identity of Swahili speakers in Britain: case studies of Zanzibari women
Ida Hadjivayanis
Journal of Eastern African Studies, volume 9, issue 2 (2015), pp 231–246

For any permission-related enquiries please visit:
http://www.tandfonline.com/page/help/permissions

Notes on Contributors

Damir Ben Ali is Emeritus Professor of History at the Université des Comores and President of the CNDRS, Moroni, Comoros.

Nadine Beckmann is Senior Lecturer in Social Anthropology, University of Roehampton, UK. She was formerly based at the Institute of Social and Cultural Anthropology, University of Oxford, UK.

Sophie Blanchy is Emeritus Researcher at the Laboratoire d'ethnologie et de sociologie comparative, CNRS – Université de Paris Ouest Nanterre, Nanterre, France.

Pat Caplan is Emeritus Professor at the Department of Anthropology, Goldsmiths, University of London, UK.

Francesca Declich is Associate Professor at the University of Urbino, Italy.

Marie-Aude Fouéré is Lecturer in Social Anthropology at the École des hautes études en sciences sociales (EHESS), Paris, France.

Helle Goldman is Chief Editor of *Polar Research*, the international peer-reviewed journal of the Norwegian Polar Institute, Tromsø, Norway.

Ida Hadjivayanis is a Teaching Fellow at the Department of the Languages and Culture of Africa, School of Oriental and African Studies, University of London, London, UK.

Paola Ivanov is Curator of the Collections from East, Northeast, Central and South Africa, Ethnological Museum, National Museums in Berlin – Prussian Cultural Heritage Foundation.

Alessandra Vianello is an independent researcher and lives in London, UK.

Iain Walker is Research Officer in the Centre for Interdisciplinary Area Studies, Martin Luther University, and Associate at the Max Planck Institute for Social Anthropology, Halle, Germany.

Martin Walsh is the Global Research Adviser in Oxfam GB's Research team. He is a Senior Member of Wolfson College, University of Cambridge, UK.

Introduction: Contemporary issues in Swahili ethnography

Iain Walker

Martin Luther University, Halle, Germany

The contributions to this book emerged from papers presented at the Eighth European Swahili Workshop held in Oxford in September 2010. The origins of these meetings lie in a series of Anglo-French workshops on the Swahili that were held alternately in Paris and London between 1987 and 2001 and which brought together anthropologists from the two countries on a regular basis to exchange ideas. In 2005, in recognition of the fact that a growing number of participants were from elsewhere, the sixth workshop took place in Oslo, and the seventh workshop was held in Urbino, Italy, in 2007. The themes of these workshops have been wide-ranging, varying from social stratification and religion to modernity and the trans-local, and it was in keeping with this breadth that the theme chosen for the Oxford workshop was contemporary issues in Swahili ethnography. It is always difficult to find a theme that is sufficiently broad to provide scope for what is after all a fairly small group of scholars while not being so broad as to have no focus at all. It was gratifying to see that most papers did indeed address contemporary issues, and with some acuity.

The proceedings of these workshops had always been published, either as a special issue of a journal or as an edited volume, and it was intended that the Oxford papers should likewise be published as a collection.[1] Arrangements were made for them to appear as a special issue of the *Journal of Eastern African Studies*, and of the 18 papers, 16 were submitted for publication. Regrettably this special issue did not come to fruition, and several authors either withdrew their submissions or did not pursue publication. However, most remained committed, and a special collection (of six articles) were published in that journal in volume 6, issue 4, 2012; a further two articles appeared in 2013 (7:4), and a final article in 2015 (9:2). It now seems desirable both to group these articles into a single volume and to allow for the publication of some of the papers which were not published. In addition to the original nine, there are two further chapters which appear here for the first time, chapter 3 by Pat Caplan and chapter 12 by Damir Ben Ali.

Research in the Swahili world appears to be on the increase again after a period of quiescence. While it is always difficult to generalise about shifts in research practices, it seems that a general late twentieth century shift in interest from Africa to Asia was accompanied by a belief that the Swahili were perhaps not quite African enough for scholars working on the continent. In the post-colonial moment, working in, or with, a society that appeared liminal may also have seemed politically incorrect: following the Zanzibar revolution, and more generally, the independence of the eastern African states and the accompanying emphasis on African identity, a society that seemed to be at least partly Arab in origin may not have been particularly attractive to young, politically-aware scholars. This has now changed, possibly in part through moving beyond the "who are the Swahili?"

question that long echoed down the corridors of academia and beyond (Topan 2006; cf. Parkin 1994, Eastman 1971). If early (colonial) historians and ethnographers of the coast saw them as outsiders, Arabs, whether Muslim or Jewish, the African nationalist movements of the second half of the twentieth century saw them as African. Definitions were confused by the extension of "Swahili" to stand as a synecdoche for a citizen of Tanzania (Geiger 2005, Eastman 1971). In a sense it does not matter (insofar as definitions of the topic of study are concerned), and as David Parkin (1989) pointed out long ago, the question is not a particularly relevant one. That said, for practical purposes it has been necessary (or perhaps more accurately, desirable) to define "Swahili" as referring to the (largely Bantu-speaking) Islamic societies of coastal East Africa and neighbouring islands, and associated populations, both in East Africa and elsewhere. It is these peoples with whom the papers at the workshop, and in this volume, are concerned.

The chapters in this collection address a number of issues, many of which on closer inspection reveal themselves to be inter-related. For outsiders as well as for scholars who have been working in the region for some time, the most visible issue, if perhaps not the most pressing concern locally, in the Swahili world is the renewed tension between different expressions of Islam and, more generally, the way in which Islamic practice confronts the world. These tensions are particularly acute in a post-9/11 political environment. Islam arrived on the Swahili coast through trading contacts, not through conquest, and has, over the centuries, remained associated with the coast. Although there are Islamic communities (and, of course, individuals) inland, these people are generally exceptions. In contrast, the entire length of the coast the population has historically been predominantly Muslim, from Somalia to Mozambique, as well as on the islands.

Declich's chapter traces the conflicts between orthodoxy and Sufi practitioners in northern Mozambique as the context for a discussion of the roles of women as Sufi leaders. While elements of the tensions between the two groups are familiar the length of the coast, the matrilineal context provides an added dimension to the struggles for power both within and between groups. There is a further aspect to these dynamics as participation in Sufi groups allows for the establishment and reaffirmation of ties between matrilineages. Perhaps unsurprisingly, the exclusion of women from most formal and public roles of leadership allow them to assert their position as community leaders and as custodians of Islamic knowledge and practice in the quotidian. Events linked to the reproduction of the matrilineal kin group – life cycle rituals – depend upon the religious practices of the women of the lineage. However, these responsibilities are increasingly disregarded by a younger generation of women who, enticed both by the reformist Islam of their male coevals and the attractions of a formal education, view Islam as a private matter, eschewing the outmoded practices of their mothers and grandmothers. Individualisation is nothing new, of course.

Differences over the nature of Islamic practices fall along a wider continuum between custom and religion, and similar dialectics between *mila* and *sunna*, old and new, mark both practice and discourse further north on Mafia Island, where Caplan has been conducting fieldwork for half a century. Observing changes in Islamic practice and discourse through the eyes of one man, she relates how the contested ground between *mila* and *sunna* shifts with time, and how, despite rhetoric to the contrary, customary practices remain very much alive even as reformist doctrine grows increasingly influential. Indeed, to separate the two seems a difficult if not impossible task since life is permeated with practices that have meanings that are not easily categorised as "Islamic" or "customary". Caplan's description of the changes in both discourse and practice on Mafia over the years clearly indicate the contingent nature of the changes: the presence of an influential leader, the obligations established by kin links, the desire for an education and to be part of a wider Islamic world, a range of factors shape complex processes of change, and of resistance to change. Both these chapters indicate quite clearly that reducing the current cleavages within Islamic communities to a dualism of the heterodox and the orthodox is simplistic and that there is a continuum along which actors negotiate according to desires, beliefs, constraints and possibilities.

While we have numerous biographies of the Islamic scholars – either the *sada*, descendants of the Prophet, or the *masha'ikh*, the learned classes – who migrated from Hadramawt to East Africa (e.g., Bang 2003, Martin 1971), tales of lower status migrants have generally been subsumed into the general history of migrations along the coast and individual stories lost, if they were ever recorded in the first place. Moving north into Somalia, Vianello relates the history of one of these lesser-known groups who left Hadramawt, the 'Umar Bā 'Umar, who, as a group, were forced to abandon their homes in Ghayl Bā Wazīr following military defeat by the Qu'ayti in the late nineteenth century. Settling in Brava, and later in Dinsor in the Somali interior, they integrated well, as Hadramis are known for doing, a number of them becoming successful in business. However, retaining an "Arab" identity left them vulnerable to accusations of non-belonging in the post-Barre conflicts of the 1990s, and almost the entire clan subsequently returned to Yemen. The persistence of Hadrami/Yemeni identities – in this case over more than a century – is a product both of identity practices internal to the community and of Yemeni nationality law, under which the descendants of migrants enjoy claims to citizenship for several generations.

Zanzibar is the focus of several chapters in this collection. Despite the passage of time, the 1964 revolution remains a topic of conversation in the Isles, and a contested one at that. As Fouéré notes, the suppression of collective memories of the violence during the Karume regime (1964–1972) impeded popular participation in the construction of a national narrative of identity and belonging both at the time and subsequently. Analysing the counter-hegemonic discourse of a group of journalists who, through the pages of the short-lived newspaper *Dira*, challenged the dominant historical narrative of the revolutionary government and it successors, Fouéré observes how one essentialising worldview has been contested by another. Were this the only threat posed by *Dira* this might have been accepted, if not acceptable; but the heir to the revolutionary party, the CCM, remains in power and the contemporary ruling elite are the direct successors (often in a literal genealogical sense) to the leaders of the revolution: any contestation of the revolutionary narrative must therefore necessarily be seen as a contestation of authority of the ruling elite of the early twenty-first century. As a result *Dira* was banned barely a year after its launch.

Competing worldviews, whether Islamic or otherwise, are particularly relevant to perspectives on health. Beckmann's discussion of attitudes to HIV and the variety of treatments available to people who are unwell in Zanzibar is revealing about perspectives on disease, and particularly HIV, both because it is often "invisible" and because sufferers are stigmatised. The treatments chosen depend on a variety of factors, from the prosaic question of cost in a family where there may only be one breadwinner and food is a priority, to the worldview of the patient who may be faced with deciding whether AIDS is caused by a virus, witchcraft or divine punishment. Likewise, leopards, or at least on the face of it. Walsh and Goldman analyse competing discourses of the Zanzibar leopard, generally assumed to be extinct despite constant (and never quite fulfilled) offers to produce one for the inspection of conservationists, academics or collectors. Despite a chronic lack of evidence for the existence of leopards, widely held beliefs that domesticated Zanzibar leopards are used for witchcraft influence the perspectives of "scientists" who continue to accept the possibility of the leopard's continued survival, either by assuming that tales of witches must have some foundation or that the repeated claims to have seen, or know of leopards must have an element of truth to them. Much like Beckmann, Walsh and Goldman's argument is not so much for the internal coherence of different worldviews, or even for the existence of different worldviews, but rather that – and as with the dialectic between *mila* and *sunna* – there is no discrete boundary between worldviews and that there is a false dichotomy between "indigenous" and "scientific" worldviews: after all, is science not simply an "indigenous" Western belief system?

The subjectivity of worldviews is even more in evidence in Ivanov's chapter on aesthetics and consumerism and the role of goods from "outside" the island in the production, and the presentation, of social relations. Ivanov questions the idea that consumerism in Zanzibar, and the consumption of Western goods, is little more than a desire to imitate, suggesting that there is a process of mimetic appropriation of aesthetics at work here, a socially imbued transformation of desire itself into something specifically Zanzibari. Once again, this analysis blurs the lines between the Western and the local, suggesting that such a dichotomy is, in the words of Reinhart Koselleck, an "asymmetrical antonyms". Ivanov focuses particularly on women, and the social meanings that construct and are constructed through the aesthetics of rituals.

Hadjivayanis's chapter also deals with Zanzibari women, but in the UK, and perhaps fittingly discusses the problems confronted by Swahili women whose practices, aesthetic or religious beliefs, are essential in establishing their status both in Zanzibar and among Zanzibaris in the United Kingdom but perhaps viewed with ambivalence by the wider British community. Drawing upon the biographies of three women, Hadjivayanis discusses the different strategies women draw upon to integrate in the UK: all three appear to be embedded in Zanzibar social networks, but, as in Zanzibar, practices, and participation, vary according to the religious beliefs of the women in question. Nevertheless, even despite the increasing adherence to strict Islamic orthodoxy, these women are able to achieve a degree of independence in the UK that might not be available to them in Zanzibar. Once again, the simple dichotomy between Western and Swahili practice breaks down: women appear to have recourse to strict Islamic practice in order to exercise the freedoms on offer to them in Europe.

Although outsiders often see the Comoro Islands as peripheral to the Swahili world, links between the coast and the islands have always been strong. Despite different colonial experiences, a small community of Comorian origin was influential in Zanzibar during the colonial era and more widely Comorian religious leaders were found along the coast as well as inland. Although the Zanzibar revolution saw a decline in contact between the islands, in the post-colonial and post-socialist period, the Comoros have renewed ties with East Africa. Three chapters in this volume consider the islands. Blanchy's text deals with the "great marriage", the principal ritual event in a man's progression through the age system, which confers political power on individuals that undertake it. Although often considered archaic, Blanchy describes how the system has evolved with time, confronting changes brought about by colonisation, the Marxist revolution of the 1970s and large-scale emigration. Despite accusations, often rhetorical, that the system is feudal and irrelevant to the contemporary social and economic problems that the islands, and particularly Ngazidja, face, it seems rather that the system as a whole is able to respond to changing social circumstances and continues to provide a framework that allows customary social structures not only to continue to function but to evolve and contribute to political and economic development.

All-pervasive though the age system may be, there are limits to the role it can play, and to the power that senior elders can, or choose to exercise. Walker's chapter analyses the evolution of a village development bank that was intended to function within the parameters provided by customary structures, with senior powerholders acting as overseers of the bank's operations and customary sanctions being imposed on banks, or their members, that infringed the rules of operation. These customary structures failed, however, for various reasons, one of which being that a bank was expected to be bound by formal legal instruments and many were baffled that the project managers expected the village elders to become involved. Indeed, given the poor track record of development projects in the country, involvement was generally something to avoid since it was more than likely to entail a loss of honour.

The theme of differences and conflicts between worldviews is pursued by Damir Ben Ali, who traces the evolution of the customary Comorian school – the *palashio*, a Koran school with locally specific adaptations – through the pre-colonial period – when the French government attempted to incite Comorians to send their children to French secular schools – to the independent period, and its irregular attempts at reconciling the curricula of the two Islamic schools – the customary and the more formal – with the dictates of the French schools and the requirements of international expectations regarding educational qualifications. The issues have yet to be resolved; perhaps there is no solution, as the various systems remain fundamentally incompatible; training the Comorian child to undertake manual tasks seems irrelevant to many parents who hope to see their child depart for further studies overseas.

As I think this volume makes clear, the theme of contemporary issues has resolved itself as one of an analysis of the interplay between different thought systems, whether they be European, Islamic, "customary" or, indeed, anything else: there are Hindus and, increasingly, Chinese in East Africa, and they too encounter other ways of being in the world. And, as Walsh and Goldman point out, this is a two-way process: if Europeans (for example) assume that Zanzibaris (and "Others") gradually incorporate western beliefs and practices into their worldviews, Europeans equally do likewise. The dialectic between the two remains nebulous and contingent; the Swahili have been negotiating these interfaces for centuries and are likely to continue to do so for some time to come.

Notes

1. See Annex. The proceedings of the Urbino workshop are currently in preparation.

References

Bang, Anne. *Sufis and Scholars of the Sea. Family Networks in East Africa, 1860–1925*. London: Routledge Curzon, 2003.

Eastman, Carol M. "Who Are the Waswahili?" *Africa* 41, 3 (1971): 228–236.

Geiger, Susan. "Engendering and gendering African nationalism: rethinking the case of Tanganyika (Tanzania)". In *In Search of a Nation. Histories of authority and dissidence in Tanzania*, 278–289, edited by Gregory Maddox and James Giblin. Oxford: James Currey, 2005.

Martin, Bradford G. "Notes on some members of the learned classes of Zanzibar and East Africa in the nineteenth century". *African Historical Studies* 4, 3 (1971): 525–545.

Parkin, David. "Swahili Mijikenda: Facing Both Ways In Kenya". *Africa* 59 2 (1989): 161–175.

Parkin, David. "Introduction". In *Continuity and Autonomy in Swahili Communities: inland influences and strategies of self-determination*, edited by David Parkin. Vienna: AFRO-PUB; London: SOAS, 1994.

Topan, Farouk. "From coastal to global: the erosion of the Swahili 'paradox'". In *The Global Worlds of the Swahili. Interfaces of Islam, identity and space in 19th and 20th-century East Africa*, 55–66, edited by Roman Loimeier and Rüdiger Seesemann. Berlin: Lit Verlag, 2006.

Annex: Previous Swahili workshops

1987 London "Social Stratification in Swahili Society." Proceedings published as a special issue of *Africa* (David Parkin & François Constantin, eds, *Africa* 59, 1989).

1989 Paris "Networks and Exchanges in the Coastal Societies of East Africa." Proceedings published as Françoise Le Guennec Coppens & Pat Caplan, eds, *Les Swahili entre Afrique et Arabie*, Karthala, Paris, 1991.

1992 London "Continuity and Autonomy in Swahili Communities: inland influences and strategies of self-determination". Proceedings published as David Parkin, ed., *Continuity and Autonomy in Swahili Communities: inland influences and strategies of self-determination*, Beitrage zu Afirkanstik Band 48, Vienna; SOAS, London, 1994.

1995 Paris "Authority and Power in the Coastal Societies of East Africa." Proceedings published as Françoise Le Guennec Coppens & David Parkin, eds, *Autorité et Pouvoir chez les Swahili*, Karthala, Paris, 1998.

2001 London "The Swahili and Modernity." Proceedings published as Pat Caplan & Farouk Topan, eds, *Swahili Modernities: Culture, politics, and identity on the East Coast of Africa*, Africa World Press, Trenton and Asmara, 2004.

2005 Oslo "Knowledge, Renewal and Religion." Proceedings published as Kjersti Larsen, ed., *Knowledge, Renewal and Religion: Repositioning and changing ideological and material circumstances among the Swahili on the East-African Coast*, The Nordic African Institute, Uppsala, 2009.

2007 Urbino "Past and present of Swahili trans-local connections within and between boundaries" Organizers: Francesca Declich, Kjersti Larsen.

Transmission of Muslim practices and women's agency in Ibo Island and Pemba (Mozambique)

Francesca Declich

Università di Urbino 'Carlo Bo', Dipartimento di Studi Internazionali: Storia, Lingue e Culture, Urbino, Italy; Stanford University, Center for African Studies, Stanford, CA, USA

Ibo and the entire group of the Querimbas Islands have been among the crucial natural harboring areas of the Mozambican northern coast. The main islands have been meeting points for people and traders from many countries within the Indian Ocean and a place where Islam has flourished since at least the 16th century. Nowadays in Ibo, quranic school education is also offered by women teachers who, as well as men, perform Muslim celebrations typical of the locally present brotherhoods. This paper will analyze the present trend in Muslim practices on Ibo Island and Pemba town and the relevant role women played and are playing.

Long-distance travels along the monsoon lines within the countries of the Indian Ocean coast have brought communication and cultural interchanges for centuries along the oriental coast of Africa. Networks of Muslim traders played an important role.[1] However, there are relatively few studies concerning the northern coast of Mozambique, which was the location of a number of ports where traders stopped during their travels to and from what are now Madagascar, Tanzania, Kenya, Somalia, the Comoros and India.[2]

The presence of Muslim traders along the coast did not bring Islamization for most of the population of the present-day hinterland of Northern Mozambique until the early 20th century and perhaps some decades earlier for the Yao language speaker networks and Angoche.

This paper aims to show the importance of women's agency in the process of Islamization in the Ibo Island and Pemba environs in Northern Mozambique. Women have been evidently proactive, and not simply passive, recipients. Women participated in interpreting and constructing the community imagery concerning the new Muslim religion as well as the gender and dependency roles within it. Their segregated spaces used for prayers were also spaces for renegotiation of cultural meanings concerning gender roles. The variety of motivations that have prompted women to join female Muslim groups in the past should be studied as consistently as the motivations for why they join the more recent Islamic revivals.[3] Additionally, older women's group motivation must be compared with those of younger women who choose different religious practices. Until this current generation of women in their 50s and 60s, the Sufi practices have offered a framework in which women had the chance to rise within a religious hierarchy, to become *khalifa*, i.e. leaders of *zikiri* celebrations, to be teachers in the quranic school (*madrasa*) and, in general, to enjoy prestige that the community ascribes to leaders of these activities. In the current reformist trends, women are not offered similar spaces to gain roles of prestige.

The data for this paper have been gathered in Pemba town and on the island of Ibo as examples of the features taken by Muslim practices in the region. Pemba is a large urban centre and port in the region of Cabo Delgado. The population of the oldest part of the town, Paquitequete, has connections to Ibo and a number of its inhabitants have been living in both places, Pemba being the main urban and administrative center close to the island. Ibo in the late 18th century was regarded as the Portuguese trading centre in Mozambique second only to the Island of Mozambique. In 1902 the government district capital of Cabo Delgado was transferred from Ibo to Porto Amélia (now Pemba). During the late Portuguese colonial era Ibo hosted a prison for political prisoners and, thereby, it became unpleasant for civilians.

Despite varying political vicissitudes due to different colonial regimes, the cultural contiguity of this region of Mozambique to the countries lying further north along the Swahili coast is evident. In terms of religious practices the celebrations held by the *turuq* (pl.; *tariqa*, sing.) as well as the other Muslim traditions can be assimilated to those found in neighboring countries of the Swahili coast.

Chains of transmission of religious knowledge

An exhaustive research on the Sufi *khalifa* women and men, as well as the *shaykhs* who operated in Northern Mozambique, has not yet been completed, although an important study has recently been undertaken, focusing in particular on Angoche and the Island of Mozambique.[4] Some brotherhoods, mainly the *qadiriyya*, *shadhiliyya* and *rifa'iyya*, worked in this region of Northern Mozambique through the same operational models used in neighboring countries. Due to the different responses of the recipient people as well as concomitant social, cultural, historical, political, and economic factors, variants appeared in each place. Other variants originate with *shaykhs*, *khalifa*, poets, communities, and individuals who may produce new poetries and introduce local practices leading to local variations. People who progressively join the new religious style interpret and practice in different ways the Muslim religion.

The process of becoming a *khalifa* in this area typically was accompanied by public recognition by the teacher of the student during a large *ziara*. Often diplomas named *ijaza*[5] and/or *silsila* were issued by particularly renowned scholars. The link between those who taught the most renowned *shaykhs* and their brotherhood can usually be traced; however, as the relevant information comes mostly from oral sources, and its content is usually politicized, the resulting genealogies must be studied with the critical eye given to all oral sources, even when these have been transmitted from direct witnesses and have become almost irrefutable oral tradition. In fact, although the *silsila* is a concrete piece of paper certifying the authorities conveyed to the holder,[6] claims of having obtained such certifications were matters of negotiation especially when people had achieved one from faraway places. At the turn of the 20th century *shaykhs* used to collect *ijazas* and *silsila* from several well-known *shaykhs*, sometimes from different brotherhoods and/or founding subsections of brotherhoods, so as to accumulate prestige. It is easier to find this kind of information for male *khalifa* and *shaykhs* than for women, although many women participated in this venture as it is confirmed for the cases of Zanzibar, the Island of Mozambique, Malawi and Somalia.[7] In addition to the more famous *shaykhs*, the constant work of teaching was carried out in the villages by those who learned from the *shaykhs* and regularly organized collective celebrations and *ziara* in the communities. They sometimes became *khalifa* themselves and many of them, especially women, are rarely mentioned in written sources.[8]

In the Querimbas, like in the Comoros, the Muslim religion arrived very early. A crucial factor in the dissemination of the Muslim religion along the coast of Northern Mozambique and its hinterland were the activities of two Sufi brotherhoods, the Shadhiliyya Yashrutiyya in 1897 through Muhammad Ma'arouf Bin Shaykh Ahmad ibn Abu Bakr (1853–1905), and the Qadiriyya in 1905 (or 1904) through Shaykh Issa bin Ahmad who resided in Zanzibar but was originally from the Comoros and a disciple of Shaykh Umar Uways bin Mohammed al-Barawi. The latter had himself disseminated the practice of the *qadiriyya* in East Africa.[9] According to oral sources gathered in 1989, on the Island of Ibo:

> Islam would have gained great momentum at the end of the Nineteenth and the beginning of the Twentieth century … this probably started with the arrival of Yakumbu Abibo. This Pakistani had a quranic school built … which strongly 'contributed to the formation of the local population in the religious domain.'"[10]

Brito Jõao asserts that, following oral sources he gathered in the 1980s, four juridical schools were present on the island: Hanafi, Maliki, Shaf'i, and Hanbali. Present-day sources, however, maintain that only Shaf'i and Hanafi juridical schools are now active, the latter having a mosque that happens to be led by a representative of the Shaf'i group who belongs to the *qadiriyya* brotherhood.[11]

Indeed locally it is recounted that a more in-depth penetration of Islamic practices among common people in the coastal villages facing the Querimbas, and those along the southern coast as far as the mouth of the Lurio River, came with the introduction of the *qadiriyya* brotherhood conveyed by local *shaykhs*. One of these *shaykhs* was Abdul Magid Iasini who operated at least in the 1920s and 1930s[12] and who died in 1940.[13] He started to teach the Muslim religion in the local *qadiriyya* style. In the *madrasa*, as well as in the mosque or through almost private lessons, canticles based on the *deuani qadiriyya* book of hymns, are taught to the pupils. The brotherhood then proposes a yearly *ziara*, named *maulana* Abd al-Qadir al-Jilani, a nighttime pilgrimage dedicated to the founder of the *qadiriyya* in Bagdad. This *ziara* is held the night between the 26th and the 27th day of the seventh month after Ramadan. After the morning prayer, at the end of the *ziara*, the new followers who have been learning the hymns during the year are requested to show their knowledge of the canticles and/or *qassida* they have learned. The more a follower knows, the earlier he/she will be given the level of higher knowledge recognized within the community. Ideally a *khalifa* should memorize all the hymns. Those who are introduced to such knowledge are called, step by step, first *hakibu nu kubai*, then *murshidi*, later *murshidi al qadiriyya*, and finally *khalifa fil qadiriyya*. Men and women can obtain these designations. There is a difference, however, among the *zikiri* performed by the men and the women. The male version is called *zikiri* and starts with a *udhifa*, a special introduction. Women must start their ceremony, the *zauia*, without the *udhifa*.[14] Apart from the *udhifa*, however, the prayer and the hymns are the same. Both are based mainly on the *deuani* book of hymns. Women do not recite the *udhifa* because, for religious dictates, they cannot lead a prayer.[15] The hymns of the *zikiri* are learned in the *madrasa*, or through other lessons given by a *khalifa*.

The *zikiri* ceremony in Pemba can be performed by men either in the mosque or outside the mosque, and for the women it can be performed in the *nsuaburi*. The *nsuaburi* is a female space for prayers and cannot be called "mosque" as it does not have a leader, and women are not allowed to lead a mosque.[16]

After the learning steps mentioned above, a *khalifa* then starts giving his/her own classes to pupils, in this way reproducing the practice and knowledge of this praying tradition, multiplying the believers. Two women *khalifa* interviewed, Moallima[17] from Ibo and Minga[18] from Pemba, recounted the story of their designation as *khalifa*. Moallima, a 70-year-old woman, studied up to five classes in the *madrasa*. She then married but continued her Muslim studies until the local *mwalimu* indicated her as *khalifa* of the *qadiriyya*. She studied in Ibo with a *mwalimu* called Ahmadi Amadi[19] (died in 2002) whom she regards as the highest level of religious authority in Ibo of the time. Ahmadi Amadi came from Nguja (Zanzibar), as she said, and left children in Ibo and in Pemba. Moallima was finally appointed *khalifa* by the *mwalimu* Abdu Rahmani Ahmada during a *ziara* where many *walimu* participated. They came from most of the Muslim centers in between Mocimboa da Praia and Nampula.[20] The Muslim authorities, she asserted, saw that nobody was equal to her for continuing the tradition in Ibo. She enjoys this work because it is work dedicated to God. She teaches a number of individuals and has a *madrasa* for instructing children. She has no former teachers that are living today, therefore she continues her work in order to keep alive the tradition she has studied. It also greatly concerns her that a number of people have started to disregard the *zikiri*, calling it *haramu*, i.e. prohibited. The word *haramu*, here in *kimwani* used for disregarding traditional Muslim practices of the brotherhoods, is much stronger than the word *bidaa* used often in the Swahili world to indicate new moral/religious trends[21] of the religious habits in Kenya[22] and Tanzania.[23]

Although many men have been corrupted by this new belief, she thinks that women now are keeping up the high importance of these ceremonies. "We who were born before, we know the value of these things," she says "it is the young people who do not know. Children go to study and come back saying that the old people know nothing." Three young people went to study in Medina from Ibo and came back with these ideas.

Minga is one among the seven women *khalifa* she knows in Pemba. She asserts that she studied with the *shaykh* called Nttambara, who came from Ngajiza (the Comoros). She is 49 years old and stepped in as the one responsible for the female Muslim celebrations inherited from her maternal grandmother, who was also a *khalifa*. Her family chose to appoint her for this task, among several sisters, after another *khalifa* fell ill in 2002. The family decided and a *ziara* was gathered at the home of the previous *khalifa*. On this occasion the Minga's knowledge of the *qassida* was revealed to the community in the name of her grandmother and she was empowered under the flag of the *qadiriyya*. She teaches regularly to some 25 persons in addition to other people that come and go. Although she likes doing it, she maintains that there is no profit from this activity: she does it because God requests it and the profit will be in the future, in the afterlife. Answering questions about the prayers for Hawa, Fatuma, Khadija, etc. she argues that a good reason for reciting them is to remind women to act like these good female personalities.

Once they are declared *khalifa*, meaning that they know by heart a large number of the verses written in the *deuani* book, the new *khalifa* gather groups of people to recite together. They perform in occasions such as weddings, funerals or taking vows. While spreading Muslim knowledge through this method the *khalifa*, either male or female, well-versed in this activity, are free to develop different rhythms and melodies, following the meanings of the book, once they know the "canonic" number of hymns. This explains why, in nearby places, one can find a number of different hymns more or less regarded by the group of singers as *zikiri* of the *qadiriyya*. A number of *qadiriyya* activists, who have studied with different *khalifa*, may then spread the knowledge of new rhythms and hymns in the same village.

Believers develop strong, emotional attachment to the specific canticles used in worship by their ancestors and the canticles become part of the local tradition.

Zikiri, prayers or what?

On my first visit to Ibo in 2007, a set of hymns sung by a circle of women was performed for me and organized by my guest Mariamo as *zikiri* with no drums involved; on a second visit in 2009 both the *khalifa* Moallima and Mariamo, whom this time I interviewed together with a man linked to the FRELIMO, asserted those they must not be regarded as *zikiri*, but merely as amusement for women. To solve this dilemma, one should consider the FRELIMO government policy of transforming most traditional rituals and dances into folkloric events to be performed as cultural representations on public occasions; the institution named ARPAC (Arquivo do Patrimônio Cultural) is present in most provinces and one of its mandates has been to record traditional dances, giving them legitimacy as folklore. As such some of these songs with religious meanings have been presented in public occasions by groups of women organized as a folkloric dance group, dressing garments made of the same cloth and style as uniforms. It is difficult to establish whether these recitals have really shifted from a strictly religious to a lighter cultural sphere as fostered by the government, and/or to what extent the emergent reformist set of thought is pushing these women to describe them as just amusement for women rather than *zikiri*.[24] Yet the very fact that different perspectives were presented in different contexts by the same woman indicates that a debate is alive; tensions exist on Ibo Island and in Pemba[25] on what constitutes proper Muslim practices[26] and expressing opinions on this is still charged with political meaning.

Concerning tensions on the ways of practicing, leaders of the *qadiriyya* in Pemba explain that drums are not forbidden as such; their use in the mosque is not permitted, though some chanting (i.e. that of *dufo*, typical in Mozambique[27]), is allowed without the use of drums. A dispute about the use of drums in the *maulidi ya dufu* arose in the 1930s and continued through the 1940s in southern Tanzania. The drums called *dufu*, played during recitations of Arabic poetry, coming from the Hadhramaut and Swahili verses known as *maulidi* were condemned as *ngoma*, i.e. drum play, therefore non-Muslim.[28] Disputes about the correct ways to perform religious celebrations occurred in several places in Mozambique, seemingly brought about by Wahhabi-influenced people:[29] a debate between *tawliki* and *sukuti* in Malawi and Northern Mozambique among the Yao about the drumming and the loud chanting used by the *tariqa* at funeral celebrations only ended in 1949,[30] in Angoche from 1968 to 1972[31] a similar discussion was ended by a *fatwa* proclaimed by the respected *shaykh* Momade Saide Mujabo of Mozambique Island, and arguments among the several *turuq* existing on Mozambique Island were settled in 1972 through the mediation of a mufti from the Comoros, brought in by the Portuguese government.[32]

According to some Western-educated Muslims in Pemba the *zikiri*, *maulidi*, and celebrations of the like were strategies the apostles of the early Muslim brotherhoods used to attract people's attention and to introduce them to Islam. Those apostles would have proposed amusing activities peppered with rhythm and melody, the Sufi practice, to be able to penetrate among illiterate people. An educated defender of the *Sufi* practices in Pemba, instead, recounted another reason for the performance of the guttural rhythmical sounds uttered regularly by the majority of the singers to accompany the wording of the hymns as a countermelody. Abd al-Qadir al-Jilani used to participate in performances where people would sing with drums. After following the singers for a while he would propose to accompany the hymns he was teaching with this rhythmical sound, forbidding the use of the drums for praying in the Muslim religion. The very fact that this story is recounted brings to the fore the existing diatribe over the use of singing and dancing as well as playing the drums to pray to God. This concern is echoed throughout Mozambique and further north, in Tanzania and southern Somalia.[33] In this southern part of east Africa, as well as in communities of descendants from East African slaves in southern Somalia, the use of the drums for religious celebrations takes on special relevance. Praying to matrilineal ancestors is common within the Makhuwa communities and implies playing drums while singing and dancing; the prohibition of the early Muslim apostles concerning the use of drums is particularly connected with contrasting these celebrations for ancestors. In certain areas of Northern Mozambique, also Christians have expressed their displeasure over music for the ancestors played with drums, connecting it to an emphasis on learning the new chanting that the church proposed for their prayers.[34] The very act of playing the drums for the practice of "visiting" ancestors and complying with their "requests" cannot be overlooked, considering the harsh tones that the dispute took in this part of Africa.

Reformist trends and national policy towards Islam[35]

The ambiguity of Mariamo and Moallima's declarations shows discomfort towards a much larger problem of discredit that has been placed on Muslim practices in Mozambique, especially in Northern Mozambique. The diffusion of Islam here has not been immune from political influence. The colonial Portuguese policy held an alliance with the Roman Catholic Church towards the construction of the nation. This alliance shared goals of opposing the Muslim religion, or organizing the cooptation of its leaders into the Portuguese colonial project.

As an example, during the 1930s and 1940s Portuguese colonialists in Mozambique held a debate on the policy of the "nationalization of black Islam." The idea was to intervene in the hostile relations between African and Asian Muslims by attempting to channel African Islam into a national benefit, detrimental to Asian/Indian leadership that had easier connections within Indo-British contexts.[36]

The Portuguese officer Pinto Correa advocated ways to "keep Muslim activities in the bosom of 'national' interests" by controlling and institutionalizing the Muslim brother-hoods.[37] Considering the influence of the Muslim religion in the area, the Portuguese local administration supported repairing the Mosque of Mecufi, led by the powerful Muslim *khalifa* Abdul Magid; at the same time, it attempted to foster the building of a mosque on Ibo Island through regular subscriptions collected among the indigenous people which encouraged an assertion of a Portuguese identity on Ibo, in addition to a religious, Muslim identity.[38]

During the same period the legislative *diplômas* 167 and 168, for the authorization of the activities of mosques and *madrasa*,[39] were issued. The administration had the power to grant authorization at its own discretion. However, measures were also being taken to try to replace the practice of the Muslim religion by fostering evangelization through Catholic missions and missionary schools.[40] Locally this kind of policy was perceived as an attempt to impose the knowledge of the Portuguese language through Portuguese schools to the disadvantage of the local languages (Mwani and Makhuwa) and the Arabic script. Indeed, the *madrasa* were seen as challenging national sovereignty because they promoted the Arabic rather than Portuguese language.[41]

New reformist trends came from the wider Arab Muslim environment and became visible in Northern Mozambique from the 1950s. Between 1950 and 1960, the Wahhabi trend of the Muslim religion, regarded as a way to create a pan-Islamic solidarity, and shrouded with anti-colonial narratives, became known through Radio Cairo, which was heard in Northern Mozambique.[42] The Portuguese government realized that changes toward possibly modern Islamic practice were in process and that such changes could be manipulated by radical trends of Wahhabi-influenced people, whose ideals were also anti-colonial. Seeking some form of alliance with the local Sufi Islam then became important to the Portuguese government. The local Muslim leaders, if relegated by both the Catholic Church and the government, would strengthen their anti-colonial positions. The nationalist FRELIMO, founded in June 1962 in neighboring Tanzania, was considered the main enemy to be isolated.

Therefore the early policy of demonizing Muslims ended a few years before the fall of the Portuguese regime.[43] In 1972, after a thorough inquiry about the Muslim world in Mozambique was carried out in the late 1960s, the colonial government decided to attempt alliances with the Sufi leaders.[44] In order to mediate disputes among brotherhoods about correct Muslim practices, in 1972, "the Portuguese brought in the mufti of the Comoros, Sayyid Omar b. Ahmed b. Abu Bakr b. Sumayt al-Alawi, to resolve differences regarding forbidden practices among the eight *tariqa* at Mozambique Island."[45] From previous policy aimed at disenfranchizing all Muslims, the government voted to support a number of *shaykhs* and enlisted their help to publish, in Portuguese, an extract from the *hadiths* by Muhammad ibn Ismail al-Bukhari's. This served to disseminate knowledge of the Portuguese language[46] among the Muslims of the province surrounding Ilha de Mozambique.

The independent government established in 1975 in Mozambique tried to discredit all religious practices they regarded as obscurantist and ideologically backward habits,[47] including beliefs in the ancestors. The socialist revolutionary government, which advocated Marxist-Leninist ideals, refused any alliance with organized religions; abhorring the Portuguese policy in which the colonial state had been supported and legitimized by the Roman Catholic Church, it also built new forms of disrepute on Islam. Under this policy Muslim associations were banned in August 1976, despite the fact that the Sufi anti-colonial leadership had made significant efforts in the achievement of independence.[48] Later, however, in 1983, facing the fact that the despised Sufi groups in Northern Mozambique could be easy ground for the RENAMO and an obvious channel for foreign support to the anti-FRELIMO groups, a national Muslim NGO was officially recognized by the Mozambican government under Samora Machael, the Conselho Islâmico de Moçambique (CISLAMO).[49] This had been established in 1981 in a meeting between the government and *imams* from Maputo which had elected as coordinator (and later first national secretary) Abubacar Musa Ismael, the so-called "Mangira." This man had come back from Saudi Arabia in 1964 having taken a *sharia* course at the University of Medina and had become a vocal advocate of the Wahhabi trend.[50] CISLAMO is not a *Sufi* based organization and "tensions between the *Sufi* leaders of the majority of Muslims in the north and the more radical reformists based in the south have caused the former to split off from CISLAMO and form their own organization, the Congresso Islâmico."[51]

The latter conglomerated several pre-colonial Muslim associations, brotherhoods and groups of Indian Sunni "all sharing an anti-Wahhabi stance."[52]

Nowadays a provincial section of CISLAMO is active in Pemba region and aims, among other things, at organizing sessions to "update" the training of *madrasa* teachers and *shaykhs* of the mosques. Other activities of CISLAMO are community based, social and health projects. In Nampula, for instance, CISLAMO supports a community radio[53] dedicated to broadcasting the Quran, and in the Nyasa region carries out a social project for the prevention of HIV/AIDS. Sections of CISLAMO have organized trainings for Islamic religious leaders and their wives concerning family law, which constituted an open space for debate about the interaction of state and religious law.[54]

There are continuous political tensions between Sufi leaders and the more or less radical reformist trends about what is the proper way to practice the Muslim religion. *Qadiriyya* celebrations are discredited now in this area by a number of people asserting more "modern" ways of being Muslim, including groups of intellectuals in Pemba, Western-educated individuals, who can be described loosely as reformists and may be influenced by early Egyptian-driven Wahhabi trends. Following the pressure of reformist trends and political support, some people began growing ashamed of participating in the *ziara* and the *qadiriyya* because they are publicly discredited; men in particular have abandoned the *qadiriyya* celebrations, although annual *ziara* are still held regularly in Ibo with the participation of people from many villages and towns of Cabo Delgado. Sufi *shaykhs* participate in international networks to counteract and find allies against the negative trend. Yet more formally organized transnational Muslim groups hold specific reformist strategies.

A mission of the African Muslim Agency (AMA) arrived in Pemba town in the mid-1990s, after having settled in Nampula and Quelimani. This is a primarily Kuwait-sponsored non-governmental foundation, created in 1981, which proselytizes a so-called "modern" way of practicing Islam. It is an organization that carries two mandates: the first is the charitable aspect of helping those in need; and the second is a missionary effort, i.e. *da'wa*, which propagates a specific version of Islam.[55] The founder, physician Abdurrahman Hammud Sumayt, affirms having belonged to different Islamic groups including the *Jam'a al-Tablighi*, the Muslim brotherhoods, and the Salafis, and to owing much to all groups, each one having influenced his thinking.[56] According to Chanfi's analysis, the AMA is part of the general Islamist current and since its creation has opened offices and co-sponsored health services, high schools and universities in many West and East African countries.[57] The South African office of this Agency is now involved in Malawi, Mozambique and South Africa with a number of projects including water wells and mosques.[58] Concerning their presence in Pemba, it seems that they initially paid *walimu* to stop the activities of the *qadiriyya*. However some *walimu* became conscious of this harassment and ceased to carry out their wishes. The reformist group supported by the AMA has now made it clear that they do not want to oblige people to change, but only help people to become better Muslims. Sufi leaders, however, see their activities as impositions aimed at undermining the previous social dynamics of Muslim practices based on the *qadiriyya* style led by older people and to which those people are emotionally attached. Moreover, they assert that all Muslims have the same goal, and criticism of the *zikiri* is done only out of a desire to acquire power. One way of fostering these changes in Muslim practices, which occurs in Pemba, is that of paying for diploma studies abroad for young boys unable to otherwise afford study. Supported by scholarships, these young boys are sent to study Muslim religion, law or other subjects. Upon their return, they are happy to assert the prestige of having studied abroad by criticizing the Muslim practices of their elders, presenting themselves as "modern" Muslims and leaders of this new "modern" trend.[59] Indeed the AMA through their scholarships it also fosters the learning of modern sciences in addition to Muslim teachings. As the access to the universities of Maputo or Nampula is difficult and expensive, and only recently private universities have been set up in the area, receiving scholarships to study abroad is a great opportunity. For instance, a lawyer who obtained a scholarship with the AMA studied abroad after studying law in Mozambique and received a specialization in environmental studies that afforded him work in the oil exploration industry. Due to his degrees he was appointed general *shaykh* of Pemba; he now acts for civil cases, transfers legal wedding papers to the civil registry, etc., and, generally speaking, has become a public official, thanks to the religious knowledge and modern education acquired through the AMA.

Today there are various reasons for asserting opposition to the *qadiriyya* celebrations. They follow approximately these lines: young educated people justify their new views by declaring that young people always want to assert new trends rebelling against the old traditions; older Western educated people tend to discredit the system of praying with long hymns dedicated to Abd al-Qadir al-Jilani which raise him almost to a prophet. Others consider the present religious tensions as due to economic interests and argue that: previously, people went to study the Quran in order to become learned, however today those who study abroad are required to return the credit they have acquired from their mentors' scholarship by spreading the new religious discipline they have learned. Another argument opposing the *qadiriyya* celebrations is that hymns and songs were used in a phase of mobilization, to raise interest in the Muslim religion in an animist context, but that now they are outdated.

The tensions between the different trends of religious practices have political implications that come to the fore on different occasions. In 2009, for instance, the dispute on the ending day of the fasting month of Ramadan was one sign of these power tensions. The last day of Ramadan was a cloudy one. Most of the people in Pemba and the surrounding districts could not see the moon and therefore decided to leave this end for the next day, although the person responsible for AMA had declared that the *Id* should be set on Sunday 20 September 2009. The representatives of the *qadiriyya* declared that they had not seen the moon. Nevertheless, at 11 p.m. Nasullullahi Dulla[60] too declared that he had seen the moon, on this cloudy day, and that the *Id* should then start on the 20th. He was a representative in the Islamic Congress of Mozambique, which unites the Muslim brotherhoods, so was therefore considered representative of the *qadiriyya* followers. Most of the people in the districts, the immediate hinterland of the Pemba Bay area, and followers of the *qadiriyya*, did not believe him. They thought AMA supporters had corrupted him. Therefore, they started the *Id* on the day after, Monday 21.

The day of the beginning or ending of Ramadan is often a matter of authority and negotiation between religious leaders. However, the fact that the people's choice to end the fasting month was polarized around the AMA leader and the *qadiriyya* brotherhood leaders highlights the above-mentioned tensions between the two trends. Moreover, the fact that a former student of AMA has been appointed as a general *shaykh* in Pemba shows, in a more general sense, the direction taken by the higher political sectors in the country.

Women's agency and *tariqa*'s celebrations

Despite the several forms of pressure that local Sufi ritual tradition received at different political times, there are groups of concerned women who are active performers of brotherhoods' practices. Both in Pemba and in Ibo, a group of women in their 50s and onwards are leading a number of religious performances or *madrasa*, and are generally active in the organization of religious Muslim activities. They are invested in their *tariqa* roles from their younger years. They understand their roles of teachers and/or *khalifa* as a duty to the community, invested with the collective cause of serving God. They are not the first generation of women in the area to do this. The women's active enthusiasm in embracing the *tariqa* practices and their dissemination has been crucial for the diffusion of the Muslim practice in this area.

I witnessed two kinds of female celebrations in this area.[61] One in Ibo, which resembled the *zikiri* performed elsewhere in East Africa and the Horn,[62] with circles of women chanting litanies of religious meanings in refrains and melodies alternatively by two groups of singers accompanied by guttural rhythmical sounds made by sections of the parties. These specific ones portrayed the behavior of a number of female personalities of the ancient Muslim tradition such as Mariam, Amina and Fatima who were in different occasions related to the life of the Prophet; some describe holy pilgrimages and angels. Those texts are from unknown sources. They could be the production of excellent *khalifa* well versed in poetry and music.[63] The words of the canticles, being sung in a language understandable by all the performers (Swahili and Mwani), creates a performance environment with which singers may identify. These canticles play a didactic role, helping women to memorize the features and characters of the pious women believers should aspire at imitating. Yet, being relatively open poetries, they also offer a space for negotiation of gender meanings.

A second kind of celebration was instead a communal recitation of litanies of the *barzanji* book[64] I attended in Pemba. The *maulidi barzanji* in Pemba is attended and sung by women who are sitting. They only rise up at the end of the celebration.[65] Hymns are sung alternatively by sections of the circle. The female *zauia* performance started with the reading of the *maulidi barzanji* book in Arabic[66] and, towards the end, switched to hymns sung in *kimwani*. The use of the Barzanji book for the *maulidi* prayers of the *qadiri* is common at least in the Comoros where it is part of the daily life Muslim practices.[67] It is also used in Yemen[68] and in Zanzibar[69] where I personally attended a performance of the *maulidi barzanji* on the occasion of a wedding in 2005. The performance recorded in Ibo is more similar to a *zikiri* in which women mark the rhythm of the hymns with guttural sounds used to increase the excitement of the group. These two varieties are certainly not the only ones celebrated in this area.

Some factors may have influenced the initial women's choice of embracing the ceremonial Muslim practices: first, in the Makhuwa matrilineal context, women are crucial to the ritual practices and disseminating new religious practices without women is unthinkable. "Every *mwene* (male chief) has at his side a *pwyiamwene* (female chief) particularly responsible for matters regarding links to the invisible world"[70] and a matrilineage group (*n'loko*) encompasses living, dead and yet to born members. Fertility, well-being, death and future endeavors of the matrilineage members are bound to rituals related to the same matrilineal ancestors. The female-lineage leader of the Makhuwa, the *pwyiamwene*, "was responsible for the relations within the ancestors' and the spirits' world."[71] Women also held a crucial role in reproducing the female initiation rituals. These rituals are believed to ensure fertility and well-being to a woman, to the couple and, eventually, to her matrilineage. Notably, funerals are among the crucial aspects for which matrilineage ceremonies are held. In some continuity with the importance held by the women in this religious sphere, the Muslim female *zikiri* celebration offers a direct role to women as officiating within religious practice and at funerals. Also, the public monosexual settings in which they are performed constitute an important sphere for meetings among women in which a positive feminine identity is represented.[72] The composition of the social group for which the ceremonial services are performed, however, is wider in a Muslim brotherhood than compared with a matrilineage which restricts participants to the lineage; the *tariqa* context, in fact, includes people coming from different social strata and several lineages. Yet, the relationships among the participants in the brotherhoods' celebrations also hold an important function of networking and mutual help, especially at funerals, as reported to an important *shaykh* of the Island of Mozambique.[73] Every individual, whether of slave descent or from free-born families, was able to enjoy this kind of network, beyond family ties.

Nowadays, the women who work in the *madrasa* and as leaders of groups performing the *maulidi barzanji* or *zikiri* groups see their roles as serving the community and in compliance with God's request. While I expected them to enjoy their roles, they rather describe them as hard work they comply with because God selected them. They have been chosen because they were good in the knowledge of religious norms and prayers. They, therefore, keep their role with persistence and stubbornness, and they see it as their path to gain a place in the afterlife. This is a pattern of submission to more general community needs, visible also in the organization of the lineages. Somebody within the lineage is recognized as particularly knowledgeable and smart, and the elders see him/her as bearing the kind of intelligence needed to be responsible for the lineage. When the elders individuate him/her they give him/her training about the lineage history and knowledge of the norms and appoint him/her when the current leader becomes too old.[74] The newly appointed leader then has the duty to take care of the lineage business whenever there is a need for her/his presence. A number of such duties, for instance, concern his/her ritual presence at funerals and initiation rituals.[75]

Women, brotherhoods and the reform

One of the impacts of the reformist movements' activities is that people have now become concerned with the correct way to practice the Muslim religion. Both *khalifa* clarified that they are currently worried about the changes that have occurred in recent decades. Some practices are now regarded as *haramu*, including the performance of the *zikiri* of the *qadiriyya*. The matter at stake here seems not to be the question of whether the *zikiri* can be considered a form of prayer, as occurred in Zanzibar in 1949, but that the *zikiri* should be completely banned. When the boys who are offered scholarships to study in Arabic-speaking countries return, they criticize the traditional Muslim practices of the town in the *qadiriyya* tradition, discrediting them. For this reason, Minga feels that it is much more difficult now to practice the *zikiri*, and many young people abandon them. Formerly, the practice was every Thursday evening, and at weddings and funerals, but presently they are said to perform only on special occasions, *ziara* and Ramadan. Yet, having visited Pemba during Ramadan it was clear to me that *zikiri* are not as commonly performed in Ramadan as the *khalifa* asserts. Apparently, in the old times every wedding or funeral was a good occasion for these celebrations.

In this context, middle-aged and older women, as well *madrasa* teachers are involved in maintaining the tradition of celebrating the *zikiri*, the *maulidi barzanji*, and the instruction of the litanies to new adepts. In contrast, the locally active reformist movements, to a large extent, do not include women as promoters of the new trends. Furthermore, Sufi women are discredited by followers of the AMA. In general, this process not only excludes women from leading and participating in public religious ceremonies, but hampers the process of opening to women an Islamic paradigm which "still focuses upon a fixed center in public space as predominantly defined and inhabited by men."[76] The women's declaration that some *zikiri* performances, which are elsewhere considered religious practices, are "just women's amusement" seems a defensive reaction of the Sufi women to the attacks of the widespread reformist trends, which have become fashionable.

It is useful, at this point, to uncover the position of younger women in the wake of these changes. Noticeably, in some East African contexts, women embrace a constant practice within the *turuq* mainly later in their adulthood.[77] Women decide to follow more regularly the practice when, becoming adult mothers and having raised their children, they have more time to dedicate to other business. Also a fear of death/the afterlife becomes more substantial. Thus, younger women do not perceive the demise of the *zikiri* tradition as a long-term process of eventual female disempowerment in the religious context, nor resist that dissolution because they do not particularly perceive it as a concern of the female community. There is a generational gap in which both the Sufi traditions, as well as the reformist trends, do not offer specific opportunities to young adult women. The AMA instead offers only to a few young boys, not to girls,[78] the chance to study in Arab countries. In addition, the assumption not yet systematically enforced by reformists is that women should not travel but accompanied by brothers or husbands.

In Pemba, during Ramadan in 2010, I met Sahara,[79] a 20-year-old woman with whom I discussed issues concerning the Muslim religion for some days. She seemed a typical young, middle class woman in a context where religious reform does not address her. Her mother was divorced but worked as nurse for development projects, and could support her children. Sahara had a fiancée whom she was going to marry in a few years time; meanwhile, she was striving to find a place to study at university level, but she had been already refused by the Universidade Eduardo Mondlane (UEM), in Maputo. She was then applying to private universities. She agreed to meet with me regularly only if I respected her time for prayers and, indeed, she took her time to do it; she was very disciplined. Although her aunt was a leader of the women's Maulidi *barzanji* she did not look interested in joining the group and was not planning to do so. It did not appeal to her. In fact, she was not interested in being included in a local network of prayer; instead, she wished to enter a university track before marrying. Similarly, she said other friends of hers were pursuing the same objective.

Young girls too do not like to be considered conservative in the social dynamics of young groups, but cannot take a conflictive stand; those who are university students do not find appealing the *zikiri* practices of their grandmothers, and prefer the more "modern" fashion in which the prayer is mostly individual. Those who seek university studies are not interested in being bound by extra ties to their communities through the religious duties of that social network, should they participate in locally organized *zikiri*. Being young women, they are already entangled in ties of neighborhood, lineage and family to which they hold responsibilities and domestic services from which they cannot escape. Rather the individual practice of prayers gives them a sense of discipline and at the same time of independence, still offering them a sense of belonging to the wider community of the practicing Muslims. In other words, practicing the five prayers on their own, rather than seeking a prayer group led by older women in their hometown, helps them to feel freer from kinship and family ties, and look forward to what they will establish once at university or in their future jobs. The educational and promotional role played by their older women relatives, through participation in *zikiri* and similar celebrations, in the public religious sphere does not seem yet attractive to them. They see new and different opportunities being offered to them in the public sphere, through their studies. Also, they imagine they will meet fewer political obstacles in their careers if they do not involve themselves with religious traditions considered obscurantist. In this small urban context they seem to experience a liberating effect "from constraints within the family"[80] by not joining older Sufi Muslim women's groups. Practicing individually seems to give them a personal relationship with spirituality and opens space for new options. This choice, however, is expressed through a visible desire to be disciplined and timely in the five prayer performances, in this way asserting, at least in appearance, agreement to the values of patience, modesty and the other behaviors considered appropriate of Muslim women. This way of asserting agency through piety of the younger women can be read in Mahmood's interpretation of Foucault not as "the meanings they signify to their practitioners, but in the *work they do* in constituting the individual."[81]

In the last decade a number of women anthropologists[82] have worked with groups of reformist women in Egypt, Gambia and Mali and attempted understand the motivations and the rationale underlying the choice of women to embark in activities of reformist movements which, oftentimes, seem to bring women back to Muslim religious behaviors that appear to subordinate them. Some reformist women in Mali and Gambia embrace models of modesty in their way of dressing and disciplines of prayers yet, on the other side, gain in other forms of "negative" freedom.[83] In the Gambia, women activists of the reformist Tablighi movement gain "respect of their husbands and fellow Muslims through their new religious agency" and they "exercise their new piety in what is not so much a contradiction but rather dialectic between submission and religious empowerment."[84] Some women from Mali experience "negative" freedom in terms of freedom from family ties, otherwise impossible unless legitimized by their new, strict religious behavior.[85]

In this area of Mozambique, while traditional *tariqa* practices offered women a path to rise within a religious hierarchy and enjoy positions of prestige, no specific opportunities seem to be offered for women in the new reformist trends. Forms of piety practiced individually, or in the *nsuaburi*, maybe, seem the choice of younger Muslim women. By analyzing and comparing motivations of women from different age groups, in regards to their preferred religious practices, older women, like the *khalifa* interviewed, regard their commitment to Sufi practices as a responsibility to the women of their community; younger women have new kinds of aspirations, in addition to that of forming a family, and see their religious practices more as a connection to a wider religious community which gives support to their individual projects.

Conclusions

As with all religious practices, Muslim religious practices too are negotiated, subject to changes and to political influence. Islamic directions and trends can be fostered through higher policy levels but also need grassroots-based interests either at individual or collective levels. Today in Mozambique, as in the past, reformist trends bring about tensions concerning correct ways to practice the Muslim religion. Part of this dialectic pivot is despising those who should be considered truly knowledgeable as compared with those who should not. After Mozambique's independence, cultural policies were devised to denigrate "non-modern" beliefs; the religions seen as ideologies and the animistic beliefs were regarded as doomed to die. It comes as no surprise that intellectuals today who have a university education, or people who want to be educated and are Muslim, tend to sympathize with reformist movements (not necessarily radical ones) that connect more to science and Western knowledge than with traditional styles of *turuq*.

Since the increase of the brotherhoods activities in Mozambique at the beginning of the 20th century, ordinary women and men have played active roles in the diffusion of Islam; they trained as local *qadiriyya khalifa* and have mobilized the population towards embracing the new religious style. The *madrasa* where Moallima teaches in Ibo is part of this legacy whereby women *khalifa* still play active and leading roles in the reproduction of knowledge within the Muslim religion.

There is no special emphasis on women's active participation in the public sphere in this new phase of reform or in AMA's support to a re-Islamization: women are requested to recite their prayers as much as possible in their private space, although a place still exists for them in the mosque and outside. The public space of the *zauia* ceremony, where woman leaders take on the role of organizers, is looked down upon, and no other powerful role is offered them in this new religious context. Nor are young women offered scholarships by AMA to study abroad. Girls no longer see the role of *khalifa* of the traditional *tariqa* as appealing. *Khalifa* do not consider their role enjoyable, but a serious duty in service of the community in compliance with God's request. Young women do not feel this kind of "spiritual" responsibility towards their village, whereas they hope to gain a Western education. They are striving for new opportunities through their studies outside the village. They then prefer being Muslim by practicing individual prayers[86] or Friday prayers in the *nsuaburi* rather than through the mediation of the local Sufi groups. They feel empowered by the self-discipline acquired through individual daily prayer, than through inclusion in a social network within their home village. Rather than acquiring extra roots in the local network, they want to confront new relations outside.

The present middle-aged and older *khalifa* leaders do not want to abandon their roles, and they retain their *zikiri* group activity. Women still perform *zikiri* at funerals while men have mostly abandoned the habit. In general, the role of the *zikiri* in the Muslim profession of faith is disregarded and *zikiri* are not widely performed to the extent they used to be thirty or forty years ago. In Ibo, as well as in Pemba, male Muslim Sufi religious leaders also count on the older women to keeping the Sufi traditions alive. Older women remain attached to the tradition also to retain leading positions and, to reproduce the only religious tradition they know. In a sense, they reproduce a similar attachment people have for the cult of the ancestors in this area of Mozambique through their strong desire to follow the Muslim celebrations performed by their ancestors. Agency can therefore be traced differently among younger women versus middle-aged and older women, who are especially resistant to the new trends. The latter express concern for their community needs, the former seem to be less interested in their roots, are striving for outside networks and may not wish entanglement in the neighborhood relationships.

Finally, I want to come back to an analysis of the dichotomy between behaviors embraced and portrayed as individual choices by young women, and choices said to be made on behalf of a collective interest by older women. Younger women seem to express an "agency" as individuals while older women appear to be concerned with how their individual acts affect their social context. Strategic and political implication may be at stake, but moral choices comprise a major part. For older women, serving the collective is also preparation for the afterlife. This dichotomy is crucial when analyzing women's agency in the religious Muslim context. Both possible interpretations of agency as "resistance to relations of domination" or as "capacity for action that historically specific relations of subordination enable and create"[87] should be framed either as individual choices justified by individual interest, or as individual choices influenced and motivated by collective endeavors; this is necessary if we are interested in developing an "emergent anthropology of morality,"[88] in giving credit to the moral motivations people expresses through behaviors, and in understanding "morality as one aspect of human condition and social practice."[89]

Acknowledgements

This paper is based on data gathered during repeated fieldwork carried out in Northern Mozambique between 2007 and 2010 under the framework of the Ethnological Mission in Malawi and Mozambique co-financed by the Direzione Generale per la Cooperazione Culturale (DGCC) of the Italian Ministry of Foreign Affairs with grants dedicated to Archeological and Ethnologic Missions for the years 2007, 2008, 2009, 2010 and by the annual Research Funds granted to researchers by the University of Urbino. The project is based at the Dipartamento di Studi Internazionali of the University of Urbino in partnership with the Universidade Eduardo Mondlane (UEM) in Maputo and ARO Moçambique, Pemba Section. The topic for this paper stemmed from the context of an anthropological and historical study addressing memories of slavery and matriliny in Northern Mozambique. The study was geographically focused on Ibo Island, Pemba and Metuge in the region of Cabo Delgado and Lichinga, Metangula, and Cobué in the Nyasa Region. Under this framework, research questions related to matriliny and the practice of Islam in these areas were raised and a few interviews were addressed directly to women *khalifa* in Ibo, women *khalifa* in Pemba, as well as *shaykhs* in Pemba and Ibo mosques. The interviews on this subject were made at different stages in Ibo Island (August 2007, August 2008 and September 2009), Quissanga (September 2009), Pemba (August–September 2009 and August 2010) and Metuge (August 2008). I wish to thank Letizia Tomassone for fruitful discussions; and Pat Caplan, Sophie Blanchy, Sophie Bouffard, Farouk Topan, Kjersti Larsen and other participants at the 8th Swahili Workshop held in Oxford, 21–23 September 2010, where this paper was first presented, for insightful comments.

Notes

1. Bang, *Sufi and Scholars of the Sea*; Penrad, "Shâdhiliyya-Yashrûtiyya en Afrique Orientale."
2. Among the existing studies, see Brito Jõao, *Abdul Kamal*; Lopes Bento, *As Ilhas de Querimba*; and Bonate, "Traditions and Transitions."
3. Schulz, "Renewal and Enlightenment," 93.
4. Bonate, "Traditions and Transitions," 111–112.
5. The *ijaza* in Pemba has been described to me as a sort of holy water made through washing words of the Koran written on wood.
6. Bonate, "Islam in Northern Mozambique," 584, was able to take a picture of one such *silsila* in Pemba.
7. For Zanzibar, see Issa, "Legacy of the Qâdirî Scholars," 353–354, 356; for the Island of Mozambique, see Arnfred, "Tufo Dancing," 45; and Bonate, "Traditions and Transitions," 99–101; for Malawi, see Alpers, "East Central Africa," 313; and for Somalia, see Declich, "Sufi Experience in Rural Somalia"; and Declich, "Sources on Islam Composed."
8. For Mozambique, see Bonate, "Traditions and Transitions," 73–74; for Somalia, see Declich, "Poesia religiosa femminile"; Declich, "Sufi Experience in Rural Somalia"; and Declich, "Sources on Islam Composed"; and for Zanzibar, see Noutio, "Dance that is Not Danced," 199.
9. Bonate, "Islam in Northern Mozambique," 583–584.
10. Brito Jõao, *Abdul Kamal*, 52 (translated from the French by the author).
11. Interview with Abdul Latifu Incacha, Pemba, August 14, 2010.
12. Bonate, "Traditions and Transitions," 85.
13. Brito Jõao, *Abdul Kamal*, 57; Bonate, "Traditions and Transitions," 85.
14. The *wadhifa* is reported in Bonate, "Traditions and Transitions," xi, as "recommendations of principals of *tariqa*." In Pemba this was mentioned as an introduction of the *zikiri*. In Arabic *udhifa* refers also to the call to prayer by a *muezzin*.
15. Interview with Abdul Latifu Incacha, August 2010.
16. Ibid.
17. Moallima Xica Athumani Momadi, Ibo, September 25, 2009.
18. Minga Buanachaque, Pemba, September 22, 2009.
19. The names are here written as the interviewed pronounced them in Mozambique. Concerning the names I found quoted, I have used the simplest English transcription and have used the

Arab form of a name or the Swahili form depending on the possible origins of the individuals mentioned.

20. Mocimboa da Praia is a coastal town of Northern Mozambique; and Nampula is the capital of Cabo Delgado. They are some 800 km apart; mentioning both of them indicates that *shaykhs* came from very distant areas, thus confirming the *ziara* as a very important occasion. Also, Arnfred, "Tufo Dancing," reports these kinds of ceremonies as events where new *khalifas* were announced to the public.
21. I owe this insight to Farouk Topan; Topan, "Swahili as a Religious Language."
22. Kresse, "Debating *maulidi*," 209.
23. Chanfi in Mafia island reports the wahhabites pointed at as *"watu wa bidaa"*; Chanfi, "Pèlerinage maritime de disciples," 411.
24. According to Sophie Bouffard and Sophie Blanchy's assertions at the 8th Swahili Workshop in Oxford, in the Comoros these kinds of performance are commonly shown in television as *sufi* practices.
25. I mention Ibo and Pemba because these are the two places where I was able to discuss these issues. Similar tensions are likely to be crucial also in other coastal areas.
26. This discussion appears to resemble a debate held in Zanzibar in 1949 between Abdallah Salih al-Farsi and Sh Mahmud b. Kombo of Makunduchi who discussed whether the *zikiri* should be considered a form of prayer; Issa, "Legacy of the Qâdirî Scholars," 359.
27. Arnfred, "Tufo Dancing."
28. Becker, "Commoners in the Process of Islamization," 202–203; Issa, "Legacy of the Qâdirî Scholars."
29. Monteiro, "Sobre a actuação da corrente 'Wahhabita'," 90–91.
30. Alpers, "East Central Africa," 312, 313.
31. Monteiro, "Sobre a actuação da corrente 'Wahhabita'," 90–91; Bonate, "Matriliny, Islam and Gender," 145.
32. Alpers, "East Central Africa," 312, 313.
33. A similar opposition to drum-playing was also an issue for the *qadiriyya* and *ahmediyya* brotherhood followers in southern Somalia; Declich, "Identity, Dance and Islam"; Declich, "Poesia religiosa femminile"; Declich, "Sufi Experience in Rural Somalia."
34. Interview in Meparara, Ribáuè district, August 2010.
35. Reform here refers to "attempts to purge Islam from local traditions and to change the way Islam is practiced locally, very often by drawing inspiration from intellectual trends in the Arab and Middle East"; Janson and Schultz, "Introduction: Piety, Responsibility, Subjectivity," 3.
36. For this policy in Northern Mozambique, see Brito Jõao, *Abdul Kamal*, 71.
37. Alpers, "Islam in the Service of Colonialism?" 168; Brito Jõao, *Abdul Kamal*, 72–73.
38. Brito Jõao, *Abdul Kamal*, 72.
39. Ibid., 73
40. Ibid.
41. Monteiro, "Sobre a actuação da corrente," 98–99.
42. Ibid., 90; Alpers, "Islam in the Service of Colonialism?" 170.
43. Alpers, "Islam in the Service of Colonialism?" 177.
44. Ibid., 173–174.
45. Alpers, "East Central Africa," 318.
46. Ibid.
47. Bonate, "Islam in Northern Mozambique," 586.
48. Alpers, "East Central Africa," 318–319.
49. Ibid., 319.
50. Bonate, "Islam in Northern Mozambique," 586; Monteiro, "Sobre a actuação da corrente 'Wahhabita'," 91–92.
51. Alpers, "East Central Africa," 319.
52. Bonate, "Islam in Northern Mozambique 'Wahhabita'" 587.
53. Radio Haq (verdade). See http://www.ionline.pt/dinheiro/jornalistas-encerram-radio-islamica-mocambique-melhores-salarios/.
54. Corradi, "Emerging Challenge for Justice Sector Aid," 303.
55. Chanfi, "Networks of Islamic NGOs," 427.
56. Ibid., 428.
57. Ibid., 428–429.

58. As from web sources (see http://www.africamuslimsagency.co.za/index.php?option=com_con tent&task=view&id=73&Itemid=42 as of September 2, 2010) the South Africa Office has projects for: 132 Ibadat mosques for Mozambique (out of 221 Ibadat mosques divided within Malawi, South Africa and Mozambique); 52 mosques for Mozambique (out of 101 spread in Malawi and Mozambique); and 1157 water wells in Mozambique (out of 1882 projects in Malawi and Mozambique). The agency raises funds among Muslims who want to support this sort of project in Africa.
59. Creating a pool of young people educated out of the country who will foster a new wave of Muslim practices has been also a strategy of several agencies in the Comoros; Blanchy, "Texts Islamiques protecteurs aux Comores," 268.
60. He is a representative supporter of the brotherhood in the Congreso Islâmico, though also a nephew of Dulla Mohamed who is partisan of the AMA.
61. I have videoclips available of both these performances. Both were performed under my request.
62. I refer to the *nabi amaan* performed by *Sufi* women all over Somalia in praise of feminine personalities of the ancient Koranic tradition; Declich, "Poesia religiosa femminile"; Declich, "Sufi Experience in Rural Somalia"; Kapteijns and Ali, "Sittaat: Somali Women's Songs."
63. In the Somali town of Brava, famous poetess Dada Masiti wrote renowned religious poetries; Declich, "Sources on Islam Composed."
64. According to Chanfi, this book of hymns is the main *maulid* text used by shaf'i Muslims, but not only by them; Chanfi, "Passion pour le prophète," 66. Versions of this text had already been published with commentaries by different authors at the beginning of the 20th century; Becker, "Materials for the Understanding of Islam," 51. The author of the *maulidi barzanji* in Pemba is remembered simply as Saidi Na Jafar.
65. A performance called *maulidi barzanji* is common in Zanzibar and is often performed at marriages. This is different from the one witnessed in Pemba: boys and girls rise up and undulate gently almost as if dancing, and tambourines marking the rhythm are part of the celebration.
66. This book of hymns was written by Dja'far b. Hassan b. Abdulkarim al-Barzandji al-Madani (m. 1179/1765).
67. Chanfi, "Passion pour le prophète."
68. Ibid., 69.
69. Issa, "Legacy of the Qâdirî Scholars"; Noutio, "Dance that is Not Danced."
70. Arnfred, *Sexuality and Gender Politics*, 3.
71. Also Arnfred, "Tufo Dancing: Muslim Women's," 200, 47.
72. Arnfred, *Sexuality and Gender Politics*, 28–29.
73. Arnfred, "Tufo Dancing: Muslim Women's," 200, 45.
74. The Queen of Samanga Sadique of the regulado Mazeze in Pemba Metuje, interviewed September 22, 2009, has been appointed according to these criteria.
75. Harrison, "Traditional Power and its Absence," 116.
76. Wadud, *Inside the Gender Jihad*, 8.
77. Declich, "Poesia religiosa femminile."
78. At the 8th Swahili Workshop in Oxford (2010) Pat Caplan referred to have found similarly that in Mafia Island, unlike girls, young boys have been sent to study abroad through Islamic groups.
79. To protect her privacy, this is not the real name of my friend.
80. Schulz, "Renewal and Enlightenment," 111.
81. Mahmood, "Subject of Freedom," 29.
82. Janson, "Guidelines for the Ideal"; Mahmood, "Feminist Theory, Embodiment"; Mahmood, "Subject of Freedom"; Schulz, "Renewal and Enlightenment"; Schulz "Dis/Embodying Authority."
83. Mahmood, "Feminist Theory, Embodiment," 207.
84. Janson, "Guidelines for the Ideal," 164–165.
85. Schulz, "Renewal and Enlightenment," 111.
86. Women's individual relationship with divinity is envisaged in the Quran; Wadud, *Qur'an and Woman*, 34–35.
87. Mahmood, "Feminist Theory, Embodiment," 203.
88. Schulz, "Renewal and Enlightenment," 117.
89. Ibid., 118.

References

Alpers, Edward. "East Central Africa." In *History of Islam in Africa*, edited by Nehemia Levzion and Randal Pouwels, 303–326. Athens, OH: Ohio University Press, 2000.

Alpers, Edward. "Islam in the Service of Colonialism? Portuguese Strategy during the Armed Liberation Struggle in Mozambique." *Lusotopie* VI, no. 1 (1999): 165–184.

Arnfred, Signe. "Tufo Dancing: Muslim Women's Culture in Northern Mozambique." *Lusotopie* XI, no. 1 (2004): 36–65.

Arnfred, Signe. *Sexuality and Gender Politics in Mozambique: Rethinking Gender in Africa*. Woodbridge: James Currey and Nordic African Institute, 2011.

Bang, Anne K. *Sufi and Scholars of the Sea. Family Networks in East Africa, 1860–1925*. London: Routledge/Curzon, 2003.

Becker, C. H. "Materials for the Understanding of Islam in German East Africa." *Tanzania Notes and Record* 68, no. 1 (1968): 31–62. [orig. *Der Islam* II (1911): 1–48]

Becker, Felicitas. "Commoners in the Process of Islamization: Reassessing their Role in the Light of Evidence from Southeastern Tanzania." *Journal of Global History* 3 (2008): 227–249. doi:10.1017/S1740022808002623

Blanchy, Sophie. "Les texts Islamiques protecteurs aux Comores: transmission et usage." In *Coran et talismans. Textes et pratiques magiques en milieu musulman*, edited by Constant Hamès, 267–308. Paris: Khartala, 2007.

Bonate, Lizzat J. K. "Islam in Northern Mozambique: A Historical Overview." *History Compass* 7/8 (2010): 573–593. doi:10.1111/j.1478-0542.2010.00701.x

Bonate, Lizzat J. K. "Matriliny, Islam and Gender in Northern Mozambique." *Journal of Religion in Africa* 2, no. 36 (2006): 139–166. doi:10.1163/157006606777070650

Bonate, Lizzat J. K. "Traditions and Transitions. Islam and Chiefship in Northern Mozambique ca. 1850–1974." PhD diss., University of Cape Town, 2007.

Brito Jõao, Benedito. *Abdul Kamal (1892–1966) et l'histoire du Chiure aux XIXe et XXe siècles. Etude sur la chefferie traditionnelle, les réseaux islamiques et la colonization portugaise*. Paris: Mémoire d'Histoire et Anthropologie pour le Diplome d'EHESS, 1989.

Chanfi, Abdallah Ahmed. "La passion pour le prophète aux Comores er en Afrique de l'Est ou l'épopée du maulid al-barzandji." *Islam et société au Sud du Sahara* 13 (1999): 65–90.

Chanfi, Abdallah Ahmed. "Networks of Islamic NGOs in Sub-Saharan Africa: Bilal Muslim Mission, African Muslim Agency (Direct Aid), and al-Haramayn." *Journal of Eastern African Studies* 3, no. 3 (2009): 426–437. doi:10.1080/17531050903273727

Chanfi, Abdallah Ahmed. "Un pèlerinage maritime de disciples de Shâdhiliyya en Tanzanie." In *Une voie soufi dans le monde: la Shâdhiliyya*, edited by Eric Geoffroy, 399–413. Paris: Maisonneuve er Larose, 2005.

Corradi, Giselle. "An Emerging Challenge for Justice Sector Aid in Africa: Lessons from Mozambique on Legal Pluralism and Human Rights." *Journal of Human Rights Practice* 4, no. 3 (2012): 289–311. doi:10.1093/jhuman/hus018

Declich, F. "Dynamics of Intermingling Gender and Slavery in Somalia at the Turn of the Century, *Northeast African Studies* 10, no. 3 (2003): 45–69. doi:10.1353/nas.0.0024

Declich, F. "Identity, Dance and Islam among People with Bantu Origins in Southern Somalia." In *The Invention of Somalia*, edited by A. J. Ahmed, 191–222. New York, NY: Redsea, 1994.

Declich, F. "Poesia religiosa femminile, *Nabi-amman*, nel contesto rurale della Somalia." *Africa* (Istituto Italo-Africano), 60, no. 1 (1996): 50–79.

Declich, F. "Sources on Islam Composed in the Vernacular: Somali Women's Religious Poetry." In *Islam in East Africa*, edited by B. M. Scarcia Amoretti, 297–320. Rome: Herder, 2001.

Declich, F. "Sufi Experience in Rural Somalia: A Focus on Women." *Social Anthropology*, 3, no. 8 (2000): 1–24. doi:10.1111/j.1469-8676.2000.tb00216.x

Harrison, Graham. "Traditional Power and its Absence in Mecúfi, Mozambique." *Journal of Contemporary African Studies* 20, no. 1 (2002): 107–130. doi:10.1080/02589000120104071

Issa, A. A. "The Legacy of the Qâdirî Scholars in Zanzibar." In *The Global World of the Swahili: Interface of Islam, Identity and Space in 19th and 20th-Century East Africa*, edited by R. Loimeier and R. Seesemann, 343–362. Reihe: Beiträge zur Afrikaforschung, 2006.

Janson, Marloes. "Guidelines for the Ideal Muslim Woman: Gender Ideology and Praxis in the Tabligh Jama'at in the Gambia." In *Gender and Islam in Africa. Rights, Sexuality, and Law*, edited by M. Badran, 147–172. Washington, DC: Stanford University Press and Woodrow Wilson Institute, 2011.

Janson, Marloes, and Dorothea Schultz. "Introduction: Piety, Responsibility, Subjectivity – Changing Moral Economies of Gender Relations in Contemporary Muslim Africa." *Journal for Islamic Studies. Reconfiguring Gender Relations in Muslim Africa* 28 (2008): 2–8.

Kapteijns, L., and M. O. Ali. "Sittaat: Somali Women's Songs for the 'Mothers of the Believers'." In *The Marabout and the Muse. New Approaches to Islam in African Literature*, 124–141. Portsmouth, NH: Heinemann, 1996.

Kresse, K. "Debating *maulidi*: Ambiguities and Transformation of Muslim Identity along the Kenyan Swahili Coast." In *The Global World of the Swahili: Interface of Islam, Identity and Space in 19th and 20th-Century East Africa*, edited by R. Loimeier and R. Seesemann, 209–229. Reihe: Beiträge zur Afrikaforschung, 2006.

Lopes Bento, Carlos. *As Ilhas de Querimba ou de Cabo Delgado. Situação colonial, resistências e mudança (1742–1822)*. Lisbon: Universidade Técnica de Lisboa, Instituto Superior de Ciência Sociais e Políticas, 1993.

Mahmood, Saba. "Feminist Theory, Embodiment, and the Docile Agent: Some Reflections on the Egyptian Islamic Revival." *Cultural Anthropology* 16, no. 2 (May 2001): 202–236.

Mahmood, Saba. "The Subject of Freedom." In *Politics and Piety*, 2–39. Princeton, NJ: Princeton University Press, 2004.

Monteiro, Fernando Amaro. "Sobre a actuação da corrente 'Wahhabita' no Islão Mozambicano: agumas notas relativas ao período 1964–1974." *Africana* 7, no. 12 (1993): 85–111.

Noutio, Hanni. "The dance that is Not Danced, the Song that is Not Sung: Zanzibari Women in the *maulidi* Ritual." In *The Global World of the Swahili: Interface of Islam, Identity and Space in 19th and 20th-Century East Africa*, edited by R. Loimeier and R. Seesemann, 187–208. Reihe: Beiträge zur Afrikaforschung, 2006.

Penrad, Jean-Claude. "La Shâdhiliyya-Yashrûtiyya en Afrique Orientale dans l'océan Indien." In *Une voie soufi dans le monde: la Shâdhiliyya*, edited by Eric Geoffroy, 379–397. Paris: Maisonneuve er Larose, 2005.

Schulz, Dorothea. "Dis/Embodying Authority: Female Radio 'Preachers' and the Ambivalences of Mass-Mediated Speech in Mali." *International Journal of Middle East Studies* 44, no. 1 (2012): 23–43. doi:10.1017/S0020743811001231

Schulz, Dorothea. "Renewal and Enlightenment: Muslim Women's Biographic Narratives of Personal Reform in Mali." *Journal of Religion in Africa* 41, no. 1 (2011): 93–123. doi:10.1163/157006611X556610

Topan, Faoruk. "Swahili as a Religious Language." *Journal of Religion in Africa* 22, no. 4 (1992): 331–349. doi:10.1163/157006692X00040

Wadud, Amina. *Inside the Gender Jihad. Women's Reform in Islam*. Oxford: Oneworld, 2006.

Wadud, Amina. *Qur'an and Woman. Rereading the Sacred Text from a Woman's Perspective*. Oxford: Oxford University Press, 1999.

'It's not Islamic!' Changing views about what it means to be a good Muslim on Mafia Island, Tanzania

Pat Caplan

Department of Anthropology, Goldsmiths, University of London, London, UK

Abstract

The shifting boundaries between '*mila*' (custom) and '*sunna*' (Islamic) practices occupied a number of scholars of Swahili societies in earlier decades. Today, contestation over what it means to be a good Muslim, and what is and is not acceptable practice, is somewhat differently framed by local people. This paper considers the situation on Mafia Island, Tanzania over the past five decades during which the author regularly carried out anthropological fieldwork there. In an attempt to show what changes in views of Islam have meant at the local level, it focuses particularly on one village in northern Mafia and on the life of one man, Mikidadi, who was born in 1953 in northern Mafia Island and died in Dar es Salaam in 2002. It explores some of the influences on his ideas about Islam, ranging from the village Koran school founded by his father to the shifting currents in Dar es Salaam, the city where he lived as an adult. The paper suggests that changes in religious ideas and practice are not uniform on the island or in the village or indeed further afield on the Coast, that customary practice (*mila*) remains significant, and that the religious arena remains one of contestation and negotiation.

Introduction

In 2002, I returned to Kanga village on Mafia Island for my sixth field-trip[1] over a 45-year period. I was accompanied by my younger 'brother' Mikidadi[2], who hailed from Kanga but had been mainly resident in Dar es Salaam for many years. He was to work with me for the duration of my stay on the island.

On occasion, when we wanted a break in the late afternoons, we would go to the beach, some fifteen minutes away across a mangrove swamp and creek, and walk along its length, sometimes talking, sometimes in companionable silence. This was something we had always done when we were both in the village, from the time I first knew Mikidadi as an adolescent boy in 1965.

On one such walk in 2002, I was somewhat taken aback when he began to talk about his funeral. 'I want you to tell them not to have a feast (*karamu*) for me, I absolutely don't want it.' In some surprise and knowing that feasts were always held if not on the occasion of the funeral, then at a later point, I asked why not. 'It's not Islamic'. I probably replied that since I was very much his senior, it was unlikely that I would be around to pass on the message, but sadly, this was not to be the case, because Mikidadi died suddenly at the age of 49 just a few months after I had left the country.

In this paper, I seek to understand first of all, what led Mikidadi to make such a request, and secondly, why, in spite of my several letters to the family elders telling them what

Mikidadi had said to me, they nonetheless did hold a feast for him. This exploration involves not only the life of a particular person, but also an examination of the myriad currents swirling around the East Coast of Tanzania regarding the definition of what constitutes proper Islamic practice and what makes a good Muslim. I focus on Mafia Island, since that is where most of my fieldwork has been conducted, but as will be seen, Mafians receive a wide variety of influences from outside their island, including not only Zanzibar and Dar es Salaam which many of them visit regularly, but also further afield in the Muslim world.

While there has long been a certain tension between *mila* (customary practices) and *sunna* (orthodox practices), my aim here is to record not only the continuing importance of the former to Mafia islanders, but their increasing adherence to the latter as a consequence of increasing religious influences from other parts of the Muslim world, including elsewhere on the East African coast. Yet the purpose is also, perhaps more importantly, to show what these larger shifts and alignments mean for the daily lives of rural residents in a village of northern Mafia.

The changing nature of 'Swahili Islam'[3]

A number of scholars of the East Coast, including myself, have explored local manifestations of Islam, and in particular, the relationship between what is often referred to as '*mila*' (sometimes *desturi* or *ada*) or customary practice, and '*dini*' (sometimes *sheria*, sometimes *sunna*), referring to Islamic practice which is considered more orthodox[4]. In articles published in the 1980s (Caplan 1982, 1983), I noted that the boundary between these two categories was by no means water-tight and that Swahili culture is essentially syncretic, indeed cosmopolitan, in its nature. Topan has also explored this issue in some of his writings, where he shows that *mila* practices have some Islamic authority, and that in its early history, Islam itself was syncretic, borrowing from the existing culture of the Arabian peninsula (Topan 2009).

Some scholars have approached this topic in a somewhat different way, suggesting a contrast between 'African' and 'Middle Eastern' Islam[5]. Seesemann (2006) notes that French scholars also refer to an '*Islam noir*', which is different from Arab Islam, and has resulted from a mixing of traditions. Indeed, Seesemann himself suggests that 'Swahili Islam' is more syncretic and hence more likely than 'Arab Islam' to tolerate local practices such as spirit possession (ibid: 231). As I found in my research this does not, however, preclude a variation in the degree of toleration of local practices. On Mafia there is a long history of voices raised by some against '*bidaa*' (innovations) and '*shiriki*'[6] (polytheism), both terms of opprobrium which are particularly likely to be applied to the spirit possession cults, even as such cults and other *mila* practices have continued. Seesemann's own research on Kenya (ibid: 229–250) suggests that such debates go back many decades spanning much of the 20th century, as can be seen from the writings of coastal scholars such as Alamin Al-Mazrui (Kenya) and Sheikh Adallah Saleh Al-Farsy (Zanzibar).

However, the situation now is perhaps different from previous attempts to impose particular orthodoxies. Today these new tendencies emanate mainly from Iran, Saudi Arabia and the Gulf, and Pakistan. They are backed by large amounts of money for the building of mosques and *madrasa*, welfare projects, and scholarships for young coastal men to study abroad in religious universities. They are part of a globalised Islam which reaches the far corners of the Muslim world not only through mosque sermons and 'missionary' teachers, but also through websites, blogs, books, tracts and other material, and in which an international Swahili diaspora also plays an active part. I do not wish to suggest that people on Mafia passively accept the new orthodoxies; on the contrary there is a great deal of debate, but there is no doubt that the landscape is changing, sometimes quite dramatically.

In the remainder of this chapter, I discuss some of my own observations over a forty-five year period (1965–2010), focusing mainly on the north of Mafia Island, but referring also to the south of the island, Zanzibar and Dar es Salaam where large numbers of Mafians live. Following Marrancini's dictum that anthropologists should be studying not Islam, but *Muslims* (2008), I will use a number of examples from the life of Mikidadi, who aimed to be a good Muslim and actively engaged with the debates around him.

I have divided this long period of acquaintance with Mafia into three periods: firstly the 1960s and 1970s, with the 1979 Islamic revolution in Iran constituting the first watershed; secondly the 1980s and 1990s with increasing influence from first Iran and then Saudi Arabia. The third period is the first decade of the twenty-first century, after the 1998 bombings in Nairobi and Dar es Salaam and the 2001 bombings in New York (9/11), as well as the Mwembechai (1998) and Zanzibar (2001) killings of Muslims in Tanzania[7] which are little known outside the region, but which have come to constitute symbols of the discrimination from which many coastal Muslims feel they suffer.

Changes in Islamic practices in northern Mafia

The 1960s and 1970s

When I first went to work on Mafia in the 1960s, I remember being struck by the rhetorical question sometimes posed by one person to another: '*Wewe ni Mwislamu?*' ('Are you a Muslim?'). It was used as a way of casting aspersions on someone's behaviour, and it reminded me of the phrase I used to hear in my childhood: 'That's not very Christian!' At that time, everyone in northern Mafia did claim to be a believing and practicing Muslim, although the extent to which they practiced varied[8]. For example, in Kanga village, only around a quarter of the adult males in the village went to Friday prayers, and even fewer prayed the requisite five times a day. There were three Koran schools, with around 67 children in them altogether, far from the majority in a village of around one thousand people. Everyone fasted (or claimed to do so) for Ramadhan, and the majority of people, women as well as men, belonged to one or other of the two Qadiriyya Sufi branches in the village, attending the annual ritual (*ziara*) of their Sheikhs[9].

While I quite often heard condemnation of spirit possession and attendance at the *ngoma* rituals from those who considered themselves more pious (see below), no one ever voiced any criticism about the communal rituals which often had both *mila* and *sunna* elements: the annual encirclement of the village (*kuzingua mji*), the observance of the solar New Year's Day (*Siku ya Mwaka*) or the readings of *Maulidi*. The only controversy in the last regard was whether tambourines could be used: the Kanga village Sheikh, who also headed one of the Sufi order branches, forbade their use, and this interdiction was respected in the village during his lifetime. In other villages, tambourines were used, and they began to be used in Kanga after his death.

There were four major rites of passage celebrated in the village: circumcision for boys (*jando*), puberty for girls (*unyago*), marriage and funerals. At that time, most boys were circumcised by a *fundi* (expert – often called '*simba*' – lion) in an elaborate series of *mila* rituals lasting several weeks. However, the end of a *jando* might also incorporate an

Islamic *Maulid* reading. Girls were secluded at first menstruation and many went through the *unyago* ritual, which was designed to teach them how to comport themselves sexually and in marriage; this had no Islamic aspects at all (see Caplan 1976). Weddings had both *mila* and *sunna* elements: the actual ceremony followed the precepts of Islam but surrounding it were rituals of song, dance, exchange of gifts, ritual joking and more, which meant that they generally lasted several days.

Funerals followed Islamic precepts, with burial taking place within 24 hours of death, after ritual washing of the corpse and prayers as well as Koranic readings (*hitima*). Sometimes *dhikiri* (rhythmic chanting and breathing of the kind used in Sufi rituals) would happen. But there were *mila* elements as well, including the payment of *ugongo* fees to cross-cousins[10]. On the third day, the mourners would leave, unless the mortuary feast (*karamu*) was to be held on that day. Otherwise they would return later for the feast, organised by the relatives, which always involved the slaughter of an animal – a bovine for those who could afford it, a goat for those who could not. This was referred to as *sadaka* – a sacrificial offering[11] and would be attended by most people from the village and many from neigbouring villages or even further afield.

There was also a well-developed ancestral cult, with people performing annually a *hitima ya kuwaarehemu wazee* (Koranic reading to remember the ancestors) at gravesites. Ancestors were thought to continue to play a role in the lives of their descendants, and the anger of a forgotten ancestor was one possible explanation for the illness of a child.

Some would also go and pray at the tombs of the few Masharifu[12] in the village, since their blessing, even after death, was thought to be more efficacious than that of ordinary people.

As mentioned above, spirit possession rituals were condemned by the *masheikh* and the mosque leaders not only on the grounds that their practice was a form of *shiriki* (thereby erring from true religion) but also because in both the land spirit cults practiced in northern Mafia (*kitanga*, *mwingo*) and those of the sea spirits (*mkobero*), animals would be sacrificed and their blood drunk by possessed participants, thereby contravening the Islamic prohibition on the consumption of blood[13]. Nonetheless, some Islamic religious leaders were said to secretly 'keep' (*kufuga*) spirits and through their knowledge of religious texts to be more powerful than the shamans (*waganga*). Towards the end of my stay, I learned of several ostensibly pious and orthodox villagers who were reputed to have secretly consulted *waganga* (shamans) for purposes of healing.

One of the Koran schools, then referred to in Swahili as a '*chuo*', had been started by the father of Mikidadi, who at the time of my first visit in the 1960s was a boy of 12 and a pupil in both his father's Koran school as well as the government school. Although this was the largest *chuo* in the village, with some four dozen pupils, it did not provide a living for Mikidadi's father who also fished and, together with his wife, cultivated. The other two *vyuo* were much smaller and their teachers too did other work. The Koran schools taught the children to read and recite the Koran but not to understand it. This meant that they could participate more fully in Islamic rituals and also that they were literate in Swahili, which at that time was still often written using Arabic script (referred to as '*Kiarabu*'). This was very important for the many villagers who had not had access to government schooling, as during this period there was only a small school situated mid-way between Kanga and Bweni villages and teaching only up to Standard Four[14].

During this period I was very struck by the relaxed nature of the Islam that I witnessed and the extent to which it was moderated by *mila* practices which often favoured women (see Caplan 1982). Women did not normally attend Friday mosque, except for a short period in 1966 when a visiting preacher from the mainland said that they should do so and that a curtain could be hung to divide the space. Some of them prayed regularly at home, and some girls attended the Koran schools. But women and men were equal within the Sufi orders, with each of the offices (*shawishi*, *aba*, *mrishidi* and *halifa*) having both a male and female officiant, although the Sheikhs were always male.

This Swahili version of Islam seemed to be symbolized by clothing. Women usually wore two *khanga* over a petticoat and bra, one fastened around the chest falling to mid-calf and the other over the shoulders and sometimes the head. For work, some women wore instead two black cloths known as *kaniki*. When travelling outside the village, and occasionally inside it (especially when attending the clinic) they wore the black *buibui*, at that time a highly flexible garment which might be all-covering, or merely worn over the head and shoulders. Men usually wore a *shuka* (loincloth) over shorts, more occasionally trousers, but *kanzu* (long gowns) were only worn on formal occasions and even then more often by older than younger men. The wearing of *kofia* (embroidered caps) varied, although they were always worn by those attired in *kanzu* (see illustrations 1, 2 and 3).

I have written elsewhere (1975) about how Islam affected the social hierarchy in the village at that time. The very few who claimed Arab or Sharifu status were deemed high-ranking, as was the village Sheikh, whose family originated from Tumbatu Island in Zanzibar. There was also a descent group whose members claimed Comorian ancestry and it was from their ranks that the mosque Imam came[15]. But piety and Koranic knowledge could mitigate low ancestry and earn great respect. Although most of those with higher socio-religious status tended to be slightly wealthier than others, as measured in terms of ownership of coconut trees, virtually all of them were compelled to engage in economic activities such as cultivation.

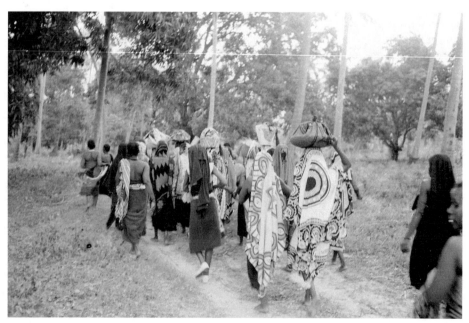

Illustration 1.

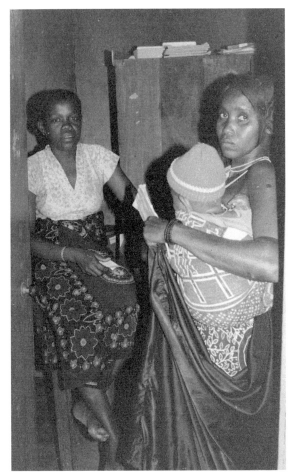

Illustration 2.

People in the villages of northern Mafia were well aware of the significance of other centres of Islamic learning, particularly Zanzibar, which many (especially men) had visited and where some lived for long periods. But they also knew about Egypt, which one man, a shaman of the sea-spirit (*mkobero*) cult who lived in a neighbouring village, had visited. However, after the 1964 Zanzibar Revolution, life became increasingly difficult for Mafian migrants in Zanzibar, and there was less traffic and settlement. Some migrants re-located to Dar or returned back to Mafia. This was also a period when some of the values which had upheld the coastal social hierarchy were challenged in Tanzania by the egalitarian tenets of *ujamaa*[16] both on Mafia and elsewhere, and during its ascendancy fewer people sought to claim (superior) Arab status than had been the case previously.

The 1980s and 1990s

During my visits in this period, I began to discern some changes brought about by the Iranian Revolution. Although the Iranians are Shia and the coastal Swahili are Sunni, the former began to send missionaries and publications to the East Coast. I saw glossy magazines in Swahili in Dar es Salaam, and was told they had come from Iran. This did not

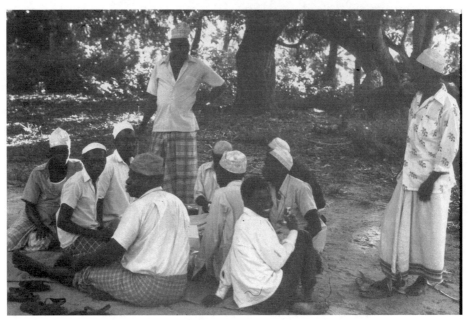

Illustration 3.

result in a switch from a Sunni to a Shia version of Islam, but it did make an impression which was much discussed. During my most recent visit in 2010, I was told that Iran had 'showed us the way' to an 'awakening' (*mwamko*) of a politicized Islam[17].

By the 1980s Mikidadi had completed first his schooling up to Form Four of secondary school (equivalent of GCSE in the UK) followed by two-year training as a forestry officer and was working in Dar for the city council. He joined the Tanzania Youth Muslim Association and eventually became a volunteer Director of Camps. This was a post which I suspected he hoped would lead to a paid job, but although he remained there for three years, it did not. Even so, he came into contact with many new ideas about Islam. On one occasion when we met during this period, perhaps influenced by what is sometimes referred to as the 'new Islam', he had grown a beard but told me that his father did not like it – 'he thinks I am trying to put myself above him' since the beard also suggested seniority. Yet if he did grow a beard for religious reasons, paradoxically he rarely wore a *kofia* at this time, saying that he disliked wearing it because it made his head itchy, but that his father had said he should wear one when he was in the village, as indeed he usually did. I frequently observed such contradictions in compliance with newer practices, as will be seen below.

Mikidadi wanted very much to have a big *madrasa* (the new term for a Koranic school)[18] in Kanga which would teach both religious and secular knowledge at primary and secondary level. He felt that there was no contradiction between these two forms of knowledge, and that such a school would be the most suitable for northern Mafia. He sought funding and managed to raise enough for headed notepaper and for the purchase of a large number of bricks, photos of which he sent to me, but the *madrasa* was not to be built in his lifetime.

While Mikidadi, living in Dar, had clearly been influenced to some extent by some of the new religious currents, at the village level, as far as I could discern, there were few changes in Islamic practice at this time, although some of the *mila* rites of passage were held less frequently than before, such as the boys' circumcision ceremony (see Caplan 1976). One reason was that boys were by this time mostly circumcised in the clinic, but people also said that they could not afford the lengthy rituals which used to be held. This was scarcely surprising, as the 1980s was a period of great economic difficulty in Tanzania and things did not improve much in the following decade, following radical shifts in government policy to a neo-liberal regime and the abandonment of *ujamaa*.

On Mafia clothing did begin to change somewhat in the 1990s and I remember a man complaining to me 'These days women want new things for their wedding trousseau, including, what's that thing called? Yes, that's right, a *shangingi*' (*hijab*)[19] A few women adopted the new form of *buibui* – a coat-like garment. But these were seen as innovations coming from the south of the island or from Zanzibar or Dar es Salaam, and having as much to do with fashion as with propriety. With the increasing availability of consumer goods during this period (in contrast to the previous decade) some people could afford to innovate in clothing. However, it was expensive – I bumped into a woman friend in the district capital and she asked me to buy her the new form of *buibui* – the latest 'must-have' – on the grounds that she was currently single and could not afford it. It was of course recognised that one could not do domestic or cultivation work wearing such a *buibui*, and since the black *kaniki* work clothes had been outlawed by the government during the socialist period[20], the majority of women wore just *khanga* on most occasions, although by this time very often with a dress underneath, rather than simply a petticoat, and used a *khanga* to cover their heads in a rather perfunctory way. Only when travelling outside the village was a covering garment, whether old or new style *buibui*, required.

But the contrast between my photos of the Koran schools in 1985 and 1994 is striking (see illustrations 4.1 and 4.2) – in the former, some adolescent girls wear only a *khanga* tied around their chests, with a second one barely covering their upper torso. By 1994, all the girls in the Koran school were wrapping the second *khanga* tightly around their heads and upper bodies, even as the boys increasingly wore western clothes imported via the

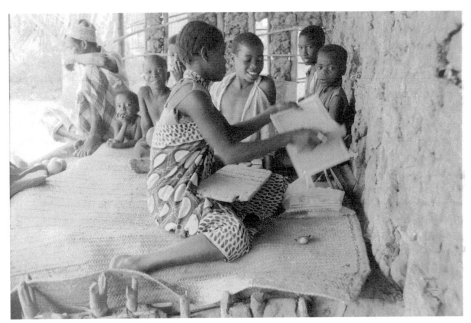

Illustration 4.1.

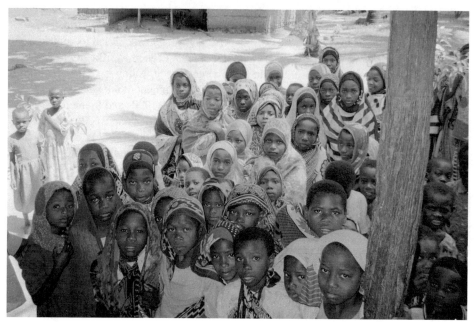

Illustration 4.2.

mitumba[21] trade. Meanwhile men now tended to wear trousers rather than shorts and *shuka* (loin-cloths), while *kanzu* (long gowns) were increasingly only worn by older men. Some men, in spite of the hot climate, would even wear *mitumba* jackets on formal occasions.

The early years of the new millennium

The post 9/11 period has seen yet more profound changes in the nature of commonly accepted Islamic practice on Mafia witnessed in my visits in 2002, 2004 and 2010. However, this is not only because of the repercussions of the bombings in East Africa in 1998 and in the US in 2001. It is also because of a new and growing hostility manifested on occasion between Muslims and Christians on the coast. The 1998 'Mwembechai massacre', when a number of Muslims were killed by police in Dar, is frequently cited by Muslims as evidence of the discrimination they experience. There were further demonstrations in Dar in 2001 to commemorate these killings (see Bruinhorst 2009). In short, by this time, religion had entered politics and was now talked about regularly in Tanzania in a way which was unknown during the Nyerere years.

When I arrived in Dar in the summer of 2002 (less than a year after 9/11) and went to Mikidadi's house, I saw a chalked sign on the door of the annexe 'Osama bin Laden'. I asked Mikidadi about this: 'Oh, that ruffian (*mkorofi*), it was put there by the children'. We did not pursue the topic, but reflecting later I did wonder why, if Mikidadi considered the man to be a 'ruffian', he had allowed the sign to remain, given that he ran his household with a firm hand. Somehow, we never returned to discuss this sensitive topic in any detail[22].

We did however have a number of conversations about Islam during this period. One concerned Islamic punishments – Mikidadi argued that if the *sharia* were to be followed the crime rate would fall. I argued against and we had to agree to disagree, although given that Mikidadi lived in a part of Dar where crime was rampant, I could understand why he wanted something drastic done about it[23].

Mikidadi was the head of the Koran school founded by his father, and when in the village, which he visited regularly from Dar, he would supervise the classes and himself give advanced classes to young men[24]. He explained to me that by this time, although the children were still reading the Koran in Arabic, now the meaning was explained to them, although he, like most coastal Muslims, drew the line at using one of the Swahili translations of the Koran[25]. He told me that the books they used came from various places, but that he did not like the ones emanating from Iran, as he felt they gave too Shi'ite a version of Islam.

It was at this time that we had another conversation about Islam. This concerned animals. The *madrasa* children had chased and tried to kill a monitor lizard. I asked Mikidadi if Islam allowed this. He said 'leave it with me' and a few days later, I noticed a different teacher giving a class to the children. I asked Mikidadi who he was: 'He is more learned than I am, he spent several years in Zanzibar. I asked his opinion and he said he would come to the *madrasa* and talk to the children and explain why it was wrong to persecute God's creatures'. I was struck by the contrast in Mikidadi's sympathy for animals and the harshness of his views on punishment for human crime and felt that in the latter instance, he had been giving the by-now fairly standard line on the *sharia*, and in the former case, had taken the kind of stance I had come to expect from him, indeed from others, during my acquaintance of many years.

Mikidadi's ideas on Islam shifted over time, and were even somewhat contradictory. In some respects, he was liberal, in others, he took a different line. One area which was problematic for him was that of some customary practices (*mila*), which he often referred to as *upuzi* (nonsense). Mikidadi argued that some of these – spirit possession cults, feasts at funerals – should be discarded so that the Swahili could become more fully integrated into the global Islamic community (*umma*). He had always refused to attend *ngoma za shaitani*, telling me he had only ever seen them on the films I had made. But he supported other customary practices such as the Swahili new year's day (*Siku ya Mwaka*) and said that it was important that such traditions should continue. Mikidadi saw no contradiction between Islam and modernity, between a Koranic and a secular education. Nor did he see any contradiction in people, especially women, conforming more closely to the new Islamic dress code, and at the same time receiving the best possible education, both religious and secular.

Observations from 2010

When I arrived on Mafia in 2010, I had immediately noticed further changes in clothing: most women tended to be much more covered up than before. Indeed, when I screened the film which had been shot by the BBC in the village in 1976[26], one woman asked me 'What was the matter with people in those days? Didn't they have any clothes?' In her eyes, a quarter of a century later, the women in the film looked indecently dressed. At a wedding in the village I noticed a proliferation of beards, indeed, one man drew my attention to this, and when I asked him why, he replied that 'we want to look as much like Arabs as possible'. On that occasion, the groom wore an Arab-style *kafiya* (see illustration 5) while the bride (who remained inside) wore a long dress, which was later covered by a black gown and head shawl. On that same visit, I also came across travelling missionaries, who were often sellers of a variety of wares including Islamic tracts, dressed in 'Pakistani' costume[27] (see illustration 6) and invariably with beards. These were members of Answar al Sunna and village people on Mafia referred to them as 'Wasunna'.

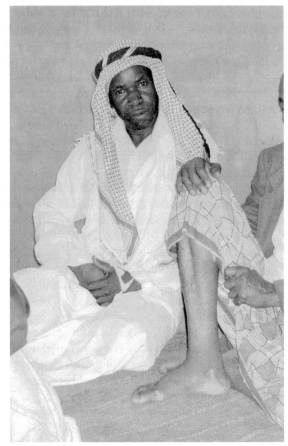

Illustration 5.

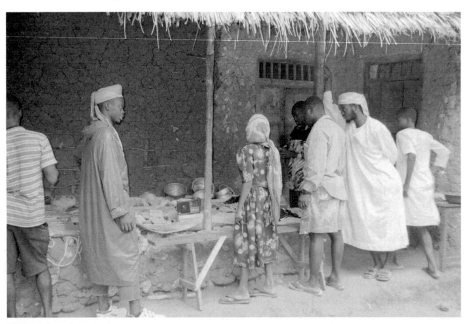

Illustration 6.

I was to hear a number of so-called 'Wasunna'[28] preaching that year at a large meeting in the village. I had been told that such religious meetings were held from time to time 'to remind us of the basics of Islam', which by now included railing against homosexuals and the West. Although there was a large crowed in attendance, including the village Imam who had helped organise the meeting, subsequent conversations suggested that not everyone was convinced by the new teaching.

But even before I got to Mafia in 2010, I had learned that spirit possession rituals had been banned in the neighbouring village of Bweni by the Islamic 'missionaries' sent to the village by one of its sons who had become a very important man on the national scene. A Mafia man I met in Dar told me about this, and others verified it on my arrival in the north of the island: 'Yes, there has been a court case and it has been forbidden'. I remembered the many *kitanga* rituals I had attended in that particular village, and the way in which I had come to understand spirit possession as a way of healing mind and body, of giving explanations for misfortune (see Caplan 1997, 2010). Elsewhere I have argued that spirit possession cults are an integral part of Swahili culture (Caplan 2015) and could not help wondering what would still remain without it.

Some said that even celebratory dances (*ngoma za furaha*) were also forbidden. I remembered the exuberant dancing and singing of both sexes at weddings and other rites of passage, and the young people's dances after the *Siku ya Mwaka* and on other occasions, all of which I had recorded, photographed and filmed on many occasions. Later some people suggested that it was only spirit possession *ngoma* which were forbidden, not ordinary dancing, but there were many criticisms of the disco dances which had begun to be held on the outskirts of the village and where liquor was served[29]. I was only in the north of Mafia briefly, and with a totally different remit[30], so I was not able to investigate further who had campaigned to have *ngoma* forbidden, and why, although I had heard on my previous visits in 2002 and 2004 that a new religious teacher from outside of Mafia had been sent to this village to teach the villagers 'how to be proper Muslims'. On my 2010 visit to this same village where *ngoma* had been banned, there was a new *madrasa* and a new mosque, both large structures, and constructed apparently with money coming from the Middle East (illustration 7), levered by a famous son of the village who had contacts in the Gulf. Not to be outdone, in Kanga, the site of most of my work, plans were afoot to build a new Friday mosque[31].

Here, the bricks so laboriously accumulated by Mikidadi had finally been put to use and a small *madrasa*, which taught only religious knowledge and which had separate rooms for the boys and girls, had recently been built. The girls looked completely different than before, wearing large *hijab* which covered them down to their waists (illustration 9). I asked one of the members of the *madrasa* committee about this: 'Yes about four years ago we decided that this was the right thing for them to wear. We also wanted the boys to wear *kanzu* and *kofia*, but few of them do'. Clearly the parents had complied with the ruling concerning their daughters, but did not deem it necessary for their sons to do so and this was not enforced.

Indeed, by this time most of the women in the village covered their heads at all times, and many wore a *hijab*, rather than a *khanga* to do so. Yet their adoption of a new and much more concealing mode of dress went hand in hand with their greater participation in the public life of the village. Some of the girls in Kanga cycled to the new Bweni secondary school wearing hijabs and all Muslim school girls at both primary and secondary level dressed like this. For the first time, I saw women attending advanced Koranic classes in a *madrasa* in the south of the village and some of these women now held office in the village committees. Women did not yet attend mosque, although it was hoped that when the new Friday mosque had been built, they would do so.

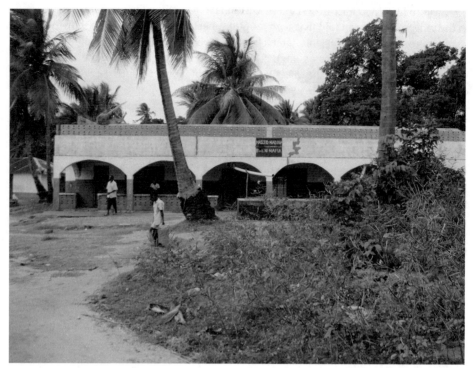

Illustration 7.

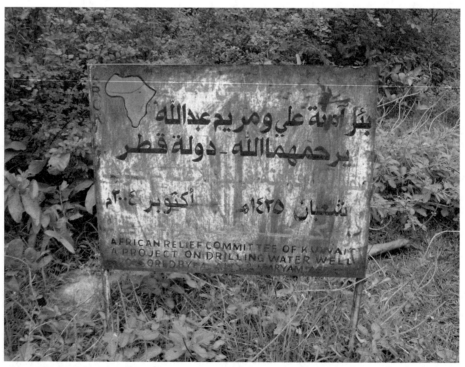

Illustration 8. See endnote 31.

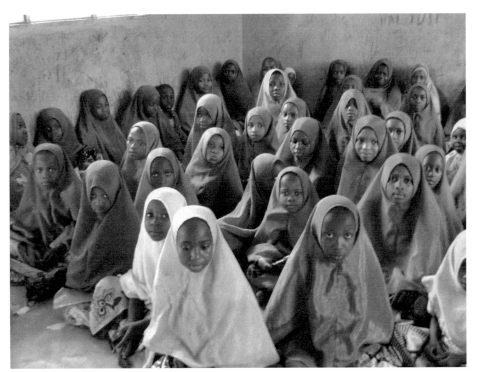

Illustration 9.

It was also clear that in Kanga, more men than before went to mosque on a regular basis, even some whom I had known previously as quite lax in their observance. On only one occasion during the short time I spent in the village on this trip did I get a sense that not everyone went along with the new Islamic practices and teaching mentioned above. A man whom I had known well since his youth stood in front of a *baraza* of other village men and said 'These days it's all like this' (performing one of the Islamic prayer moves); the others laughed.

Yet I was told on several occasions that Islam on Mafia was under threat for a variety of reasons. One was because there were now a number of Christian churches on the island, including in Kanga where some Makonde, originally refugees from the colonial and post-colonial wars in Mozambique, had by this time settled. It was clear that the villagers did not consider these to be Swahili like themselves[32]. It was also frequently pointed out that the senior government servants on the island, who had mostly come from the mainland, were Christians who knew little about Islam or Swahili culture and that this sometimes created problems[33].

All in all, then, things were not what they used to be. My village sister, who had for the last several years been one of the most 'covered' women in the village, would only shake hands with me after she had covered hers with her *khanga*, even though she was clearly delighted to see me. Her son told me not to mind: 'Just because people dress differently, don't think their hearts are not the same'. But a Mafian living in Dar, with whom I discussed changes in religious practice, told me: 'You know, if these people (he meant the Wasunna and similar) had been around when you first came to Mafia, you could not have done your work. They would not have allowed it, they would not have accepted you'. I felt that he was probably right[34].

The changes I have described are uneven. First of all, not all aspects of the newer forms of Islam are followed even by the most religious and secondly, they are not followed or even welcomed by everyone in northern Mafia, as exemplified by the man who satirised ardent prayer. Thirdly, they have penetrated different parts of the island in different ways: for example, when in 2010 I spent a couple of days back on Chole Island in the south of Mafia where I had lived briefly in 2004, I did not see women dressed like some of those in Kanga and Bweni villages.

The same differences can be found in other areas of Tanzania. In a visit to Kilwa in 2010, there was no sign of the kind of *hijab* now worn by some in northern Mafia. However, in a visit to Zanzibar Town the same year, it was common to see a woman wearing not only a *hijab* but also *niqab* (face mask), or, in the local parlance, a *ninja*, and some were also worn by Muslims in Dar. Some people I talked to argued that this gave women freedom to move around and not be harassed, others that most *ninja* wearers were merely making a fashion statement[35].

Mikidadi's feast

Seesemann notes that the Al-Sunna do not only castigate spirit possession – they also preach against extravagant funerals, visiting tombs and the recitation of *maulid*. Was this then why Mikidadi had not wanted a feast? I went to talk to two of the elders of Mikidadi's family, who had been responsible for arranging his funeral and the inheritance of his property, about the feast which had after all been held after his death. I asked why Mikidadi had not wanted it, and why they had held it nonetheless. One of them tried to explain why someone might not want a feast: 'A feast is good and blessed if it is done right, but today that is not always the case. People might feel that they are doing it under pressure, even though they don't have the economic means, so they might even borrow or steal to do it. Or they might do bad things during the feast itself'. This felt to me rather like a rationalisation for Mikidadi's wishes, since he himself had explained it in terms of a feast not being acceptable in Islamic terms. I asked them why they had gone ahead with it, even though I had written to them several times telling them of his express wishes given to me only a few months before he died. They could only explain why they had gone ahead anyway by saying that *of course* a feast must always be held after a funeral. '*Lazima*' – 'it's a necessity', one of the told me. His companion, an Islamic leader in the village who had invited the Wasunna to come and hold the recent meeting, agreed.

I thought about this subsequently and re-read some of my 1960s notes. There I came across a reference to a woman who had died and for whom a funeral without a feast had been held 'because she had no kin', meaning that there was no one to contribute to or organise such an event. Clearly Mikidadi did have kin, and many of them were important people in the village, so it would have been shaming for them not to have organised and contributed to a feast for him, regardless of his own views on the subject. Kinship, I had already learned on Mafia, has its own unassailable obligations and morality.

It is clear that today, many coastal Swahili wish to be viewed as part of a wider Islamic community, and this is symbolized both by adoption of different styles of clothing, greater adherence to Islamic practices such as regular prayer and mosque attendance, and enhanced questioning or criticism of many *mila* practices. It is also shown by the adoption of global Islamic terms for crucial items: *madrasa* has replaced *chuo*, *hijabu* has replaced *shang-ingi*. In other words, 'Arabic' terms, which do not even appear in early Swahili dictionaries like Johnson, have replaced Swahili ones[36]. While Islam in East Africa has always been connected to the global *umma* and been influenced by the shifts in its orientations, the degree to which this has been significant has varied not only historically but also regionally, and even within quite small areas such as Kanga village[37]. What is important to note, however, is that today there is a wider consciousness and discussion of Islamic practice, particularly by some members of the younger generation.

The life of Mikidadi, as lived out in Mafia, Zanzibar and Dar es Salaam, shows how some of the currents discussed above influenced him, while others were rejected. He did not want a feast after his death because 'It's not Islamic', yet the very village elders who were so supportive of the Wasunna went ahead anyway and organised one. This suggests that the relationship between *sharia/sunna* and *mila* remains as complex as it has long been. Expanding religious repertoires encourage constant negotiation or contestation around the meaning of being a good Muslim.

Acknowledgements

I am grateful for comments on this paper to Iain Walker, Lionel Caplan, Ahmad Kipacha and Kai Kresse.

Notes

1. This trip was funded by the British Academy as part of a small research grant. Previous trips had been funded by the Leverhulme and Nuffield Foundations, the BBC, and the University of London.
2. Mikidadi is the subject of a historical biography recently published in Swahili (see Caplan 2014, 2016).
3. I am well aware that this is a highly contested term among scholars and locals, but use it as a convenient shorthand, seeking to show its meaning in various contexts.
4. See, for example, Horton and Middleton 2000: 180 and 187. Middleton 1992: 162–5.
5. Trimingham, for example, distinguishes between 'Islamic culture' and 'traditional culture' (1964: 68–70).
6. *Shirk* (or *shiriki* in Swahili) means challenging the oneness of God which is totally counter to the fundamental tenets of Islam.
7. For an account of the former see Njozi 2000, and for discussions of both see Bruinhorst 2009.
8. There is an account of Islamic practices in northern Mafia as I first observed them in the 1960s in chapter 5 of my 1975 book.
9. The village Sheikh controlled one Sufi branch, but a Sheikh from southern Mafia was the leader of the other branch, and visited the village annually for his *ziara*. For more information on the Sufi orders in East Africa see Nimtz 1980.
10. *Ugongo* is a small sum of money paid to cross-cousins, with whom people on the coast have a ritualised joking relationship.
11. The concept of *sadaka* is discussed by Parkin (1994).
12. The Masharifu are reputed to be descendants of the Prophet Mohammed.
13. See Caplan 1997 for a fuller account of spirit possession on Mafia.
14. By the 1970s, with the push to *ujamaa* (African socialism) following the Arusha Declaration of 1967, many more children went to government schools and '*Kiarabu*' began to decline in use as people used Roman script ('*Kizungu*') more frequently.
15. This tendency to give greater respect to the learning of Islamic teachers coming from outside the island is one which has continued to this day.
16. *Ujamaa* is the term coined by Nyerere to describe what he called 'African socialism'. It was the dominant form of political organisation for approximately a twenty year period between the mid 1960s and the 1980s.

17. This is a complex topic which needs much further exploration than I have room for here. Certainly during my visits in the 1980s and 1990s, people in coastal Tanzania seemed to be very aware of the Iranian Revolution and its aftermath.

18. The earlier Swahili term *chuo* widely used on Mafia had gradually been abandoned in favour of the word *madrasa*, derived from Arabic and widely used in the Muslim world. In previous years, at least in northern Mafia, *madrasa* was used as a term for religious classes for adults, not for children.

19. The Swahili term '*shangingi*' fell into disuse and was replaced by Arab term *hijabu*, again this is the word used throughout the Muslim world.

20. They were criticised as looking 'dirty' although paradoxically people had worn these clothes precisely because they did not show the dirt as much as did *khanga*, and were also very hard-wearing. During the 1960s and beyond, there were campaigns conducted particularly by the TANU Youth League against tight trousers, mini-skirts and traditional Maasai dress. See Ivaska 2004.

21. Bales of second hand clothing brought from the West and hawked around outlying areas such as Mafia by itinerant traders.

22. I was also told by others that many of the dhows in the harbour in Dar es Salaam had 'OBL' on their flags at this time.

23. He wrote before my arrival telling me not to bother to bring him a new watch (my most usual present) 'as I have had them all stolen and now I don't wear one'.

24. By this time, his Arabic was fluent, and he often asked me to bring him Arabic texts from London.

25. For a useful discussion of various translations of the Koran into Swahili, see Lacunza-Balda 1998.

26. This was part of a series of anthropological films screened in 1977 entitled 'Face Values' in which a number of anthropologists, including myself, commented on film footage shot by the BBC in the formers fieldwork locations.

27. This consists of loose trousers which do not cover the ankles, a loose gown coming to mid-calf and a turban.

28. They came from a village in central Mafia and were not wearing 'Pakistani' costume.

29. These 'bars' were run by Christian immigrants to the village, mostly Wamakonde and a few Wanyamwezi. At one such place, there had recently been a fight fuelled by drink and a man was killed: 'Things like that never used to happen here'.

30. In fact I had come to gather additional material for a biography of Mikidadi. See Caplan, 2014, 2015 and 2016.

31. Money for such projects often came from outside, particularly the Gulf states. For example, money had been received from a Gulf-based foundation to construct a borehole outside the clinic (see illustration 8). But unfortunately for the people of Kanga, they had far fewer contacts with potential sponsors than their neighbours in Bweni.

32. Topan (2006) on a discussion of whether Islam is a *sine qua non* for Swahili identity, notes that Christian Swahili numbers are growing, so the only feature left is the Swahili language.

33. For example, when it was proposed to hold an international dance festival, local government officials were initially encouraging to foreign sponsors, whereas Muslim leaders did not want the festival (see Caplan 2011).

34. This view was enhanced by an encounter with an Al-Sunna in Zanzibar who was selling religious literature on a street stall. He refused to sell any to me because I was not a Muslim, although I told him that I had already that day bought literature from several other stalls and that it was for the *madrasa* teacher in the village.

35. More than one person told me 'See, if they are wearing socks and gloves, those are the true believers, but if not, they are just fashionistas!' See Tarlo 2010 for a relevant discussion of Muslim women's clothing in the UK.

36. For example, Johnson's Standard Swahili dictionary (1951) glosses '*hijabu*' as 'neuralgia, swollen glands' and does not even contain a reference to '*madrasa*'.

37. In my first and longest visit between 1965 and 1976, I discovered that there were significant differences between those who claimed to be 'orthodox' and others. See Caplan 1976.

References

Bruinhorst, Gerard van der. "*Siku ya Arafa* and the *Idd el-Hajji*: Knowledge, ritual and renewal in Tanzania." In *Knowledge, Renewal and Religion*, 127–150, edited by K. Larsen. Uppsala: Nordiska Afrikaninstutet, 2009.

Caplan, A. P. *Choice and Constraint in a Swahili Community.* London, New York and Nairobi: International African Institute and Oxford University Press, 1975.

Caplan, P. "Boys' circumcision and girls' puberty rites among the Swahili of Mafia Island Tanzania." *Africa* 46, 1 (1976): 21–33.

Caplan, P. "Gender, Ideology and Modes of Production on the East African coast." In special issue of *Paideuma From Zinj to Zanzibar: History, Trade and Society on the Coast of East Africa*, 29–43, edited by J. de Vere Allen. Stuttgart: Franz Steiner Verlag, 1982.

Caplan, P. "Women's Property, Islamic Law and Cognatic Descent." In *Women and Property, Women as Property*, 23–43, edited by R. Hirschon. London: Croom Helm, 1983.

Caplan P. *African Voices, African Lives: Personal Narratives from a Swahili Village.* London and New York: Routledge, 1997.

Caplan, P. "Bargaining with spirits: Consulting a Swahili diviner." *Utafiti: Journal of the College of Arts and Social Sciences, University of Dar es Salaam* 7, 2 (2010): 18–32.

Caplan, P. "A 'clash of civilizations' on Mafia Island? The story of a dance festival." *Anthropology Today* 27 (2011).

Caplan, P. "Changing Swahili cultures and identities in a globalising world: An approach from anthropology." *Swahili Forum* 20 (2013): 31–47. (http://www.uni-leipzig.de/~afrika/swafo/).

Caplan, P. *Mikidadi wa Mafia: Maisha ya mwanaharakati na familia yake nchini Tanzania* (Mikidadi of Mafia: The life of an activist and his family in Tanzania). Dar es Salaam: Mkuki na Nyota, 2014.

Caplan, P. "The Transcendent Subject? Biography as a medium for writing 'life and times'." In *Extraordinary Encounters: Authenticity and the Interview*, 19–37, edited by Katherine Smith, James Staples and Nigel Rapport. New York and Oxford: Berghahn Publications, 2015.

Chande, A. "Radicalism and Reform in East Africa." In *The History of Islam in Africa*, 349–372, edited by N. Levtzioni and R. L. Pouwels. Ohio: Ohio Universtiy Press, 2000.

Horton M. and J. Middleton. *The Swahili: The Social Landscape of a Mercantile Society*. Oxford: Blackwell, 2000.

Ivaska, A. M. "Anti-mini militants meet modern misses: Urban style, gender and the politics of national culture in 1960s Dar es Salaam, Tanzania." In *Fashioning Africa: Power and the Politics of Dress*, edited by J.M. Allman. Bloomington: Indiana University Press, 2004.

Lacunza-Balda, J. "Aspects du leadership islamique contemporain en Afrique orientale." In *Autorite et Pouvoir chez les Swahili*, edited by F. Le-Guennec-Coppens and D. Parkin. Paris: Karthala, IFRA, 1998.

Loimeier, R. and R. Seesemann (eds.) *The Global Worlds of the Swahili*. Berlin: LIT Verlag, Athens: University of Ohio Press, Oxford: James Currey, Claremont South Africa: David Philip, 2006.

Marrancini, G. *The Anthropology of Islam*. Oxford and New York: Berg, 2008.

Middleton, J. *The World of the Swahili: An African Mercantile Civilization*. New Haven: Yale University Press, 1992.

Nimtz, A. *Islam and Politics in East Africa: The Sufi orders in Tanzania*. Minnesota: University of Minnesota Press, 1980.

Njozi, H. M. *Mwembechai killings, and the political future of Tanzania*. Globallink Communications, 2000.

Parkin, D. "*Sadaka*: Focus on contradictory continuity." In *Continuity and Autonomy in Swahili Communities*, edited by D. Parkin. Wien: Beitrage zur Afraikanstik, London: SOAS, 1994.

Seesemann, R. "African Islam or Islam in Africa?" In *The Global Worlds of the Swahili*, edited by R. Loimeier and R. Seesemann. Berlin: LIT Verlag, 2006.

Tarlo, E. *Visibly Muslim: Bodies of Faith*. Oxford and New York: Berg, 2010.

Topan, F. "From coastal to global: The erosion of the Swahili 'paradox'." In *The Global Worlds of the Swahili*, edited by R. Loimeier and R. Seesemann. Berlin: LIT Verlag, 2006.

Topan, F. "Towards a paradigm of Swahili religious knowledge." In *Knowledge, Renewal and Religion*, edited by K. Larsen. Uppsala: Nordiska Afrikaninstitutet, 2009.

Trimingham, J. S. *Islam in East Africa*. Oxford: Clarendon Press, 1964.

Appendix

List of illustrations

Illustration 1. Women leaving a wedding, 1960s.
Illustration 2. Woman wearing a *buibui* at Kanga clinic, 1985.
Illustration 3. Group of men at a feast, Kanga village, 1976.
Illustration 4.1. Girls and boys together at a Koran school, Kanga, 1985.
Illustration 4.2. Koran school girls, 1994.
Illustration 5. Groom at a wedding, 2002.
Illustration 6. 'Wasunna' wearing 'Pakistani' dress, 2002.
Illustration 7. Friday mosque in Bweni village, 2010.
Illustration 8. Kuwait donation of borehole, 2010.
Illustration 9. Koran school girls, 2010.

One hundred years in Brava: The migration of the ʿUmar Bā ʿUmar from Hadhramaut to East Africa and back, c. 1890–1990

Alessandra Vianello

London NW

Contacts between Arabia and the East African Coast, which have marked the history of the western part of the Indian Ocean since ancient times, have often involved the migration of individuals and groups of people who have contributed to the shaping of the Swahili society. However, details of group migrations from Arabia (even comparatively recent) remain to this day largely unexplored as to their causes, the impact the newcomers had on the East African societies, and their material and cultural contribution to the Swahili coastal centres. It has also never been assessed how long it took an Arab migrant group to become fully integrated into their new socio-economic environment. This paper tries to answer some of these questions by illustrating a migration that took place in the late nineteenth century and involved almost the entire South-Arabian *qabila* of the ʿUmar Bā ʿUmar, originally settled in and around Ghayl Bā Wazīr, some 30 km inland from the ports of Mukalla and Shihr. This group left the Hadhramaut in the 1880s and eventually settled in Brava, a coastal city of Southern Somalia, c. 1890. The first mention of their presence in East Africa is found in the judicial records of Brava, which have been preserved for the period 1893–1900. The events that marked the subsequent period, up to the present, have been reconstructed through personal observations by the author and oral information collected mainly in Brava, which the ʿUmar Bā ʿUmar left when the outbreak of the civil war in Somalia forced them to return to their original home town in the Hadhramaut.

Introduction

Starting from the mid-1970s, archaeological excavations, linguistic studies, and a critical re-appraisal of local chronicles and traditions have led some scholars to emphasise the essentially African origins of the Swahili civilisation and to dismiss the long-held view that the coastal centres of East Africa were "colonies" founded by Arab and Persian migrants.[1] This has resulted in a new evaluation of the role played by the Arabs in their interaction with the Swahili Coast that have marked the history of East Africa: some authors have emphasised the importance of trade connections, which postulate the arrival of individual traders or of small groups of (unrelated) traders on any particular point of the coast,[2] while others have seen the contribution of the Arabs as mainly consisting of "*ideas* rather than people".[3] In my opinion, this latter view stems from the fact that these scholars focused on the migrations of learned men (*masha'ikh*) and of individuals and families who trace their lineage to the Prophet (the *sada* or *sayyids*), whose movements are generally well documented and dated.[4] Although "these holy men were a sizeable contingent among the migrants", it has also been argued that they should be considered "a special sort of migrant".[5] Their proficiency as religious scholars and jurists, and especially the charisma attached to some of them as descendants of Muhammad, made them extremely influential in the centres of the East African Coast, where they often held prestigious positions as *qadis* or advisers to the rulers, and had sometimes a major impact on the spread and consolidation of Islam on the Coast. All these factors make it extremely unlikely that their case might be generalised to reflect that of the *ordinary* sort of migrants.

To my knowledge, if we exclude this learned élite, there has not yet been any detailed record of the migration of groups from the Hadhramaut in any historical period, although several waves of Hadhrami arrivals on the East African Coast – the last taking place at the end of the nineteenth century – have been noted.[6] Group migrations from Arabia that could have occurred in the Middle Ages have been either tentatively suggested,[7] or simply mentioned without details,[8] while the claims to Arab ancestry, advanced by some sections of the Swahili population and by some ruling élites and recorded in local chronicles and oral traditions, have either undergone a critical re-interpretation[9] or have been left unexplored.[10] In any case, the paucity of written sources and the remoteness in time do not allow us to know much about these (actual or supposed) movements and what caused them.

This paper tries to illustrate the events that led the ʿUmar Bā ʿUmar *qabila* to leave their homeland, the Hadhramaut, in or about 1880, and to eventually settle in Brava, on the Benadir Coast of Southern Somalia, c. 1890. The judicial records of the town of Brava, which are still extant for the period 1893–1900, give us a first glimpse of these immigrants as they had just settled in their new environment, and provide details of their economic conditions and of their social standing in the local context.[11] The subsequent period, which saw their gradual integration into the local community, their significant contributions to the economy and the fabric of the city, and the later relocation of some of them in other centres in Somalia, has largely been reconstructed from personal observations and oral information, collected during a twenty-one-year period (1970–1990) through close social interaction with ʿUmar Bā ʿUmar men and women in Brava. After their return to the Hadhramaut, following the outbreak of the civil war in Somalia, yearly visits to Shihr and Ghayl Bā Wazīr enabled the monitoring of their on-going re-adaptation to living conditions in their original homeland.

The ʿUmar Bā ʿUmar in the Hadhramaut

According to their own traditions, the Hadhrami *qabila* of the ʿUmar Bā ʿUmar was originally settled near the inland centre of Ghayl Bin Yamein, an area they left at an unspecified date to move south. By the second half of the nineteenth century they were settled in and around Ghayl Bā Wazīr, a city situated approximately 30 km inland from the two main ports of Shihr and Mukalla and at almost equal distance between these two centres.

In the highly stratified Hadhrami society, historians identify four main classes: the *sada*, whose forefathers (descendants of the Prophet Muhammed through his daughter Fatima) had migrated to the Hadhramaut from present-day Iraq; the *masha'ikh,* learned class indigenous to the Hadhramaut; the *qaba'il,* armed tribes that usually lived outside the towns, and the *masakin/du'afa,* who could not trace their ancestry from a prestigious forefather and, unable to protect themselves, had to establish relations of dependence with other groups.[12] Ghayl Bā Wazīr owes its name to the Bā Wazīr, a group of the *masha'ikh* class, while the 'Umar Bā 'Umar belonged to the *qaba'il* social stratum. The latter considered – and still consider - the Bā Wazīr as "their shaykhs" [13] and formed the armed and fighting branch of the local population, ensuring also the defence of the Bā Wazīr.

Political instability characterised the nineteenth century in the Hadhramaut as the two families of the Kathiri and the Qu'ayti fought for the ultimate control of the region for several decades. The later stages of this contest saw the involvement of all Hadhrami groups (including the *sada*) in a complex and constantly shifting web of alliances.[14] The Kathiri, who hailed from Dhofar, had established a sultanate in the interior of the Hadhramaut as early as the sixteenth century. Starting from the beginning of the eighteenth century, dynastic rivalries and the ensuing constant warfare led them to recruit Yafi'i mercenaries, who moved to the Hadhramaut from their base north-east of Aden. Soon the Yafi'i – of which the Qu'ayti were an off-shoot – had infiltrated and taken control of most centres of the Hadhramaut, starting their bid for power. Later the different branches of the Yafi'i would also fight each other, helped by the constant flow of money, weapons and military aid (in the form of Hadhrami and Indian soldiers), which were sent from India by their supporters.

In the early to mid-nineteenth century many Hadhramis were serving as mercenaries at the courts of Indian princes, among them members of both the Kathiri and the Qu'ayti. Foremost among these Qu'ayti migrants was 'Umar b. 'Awaḍ b. 'Abdallah al-Qu'ayti (died 1882), who had left the Hadhramaut to serve in the armies of Heyderabad. He rose to the rank of *jamadar,* came to enjoy high status at the local court, married a court lady, and amassed a fortune. With the money he sent to the Hadhramaut, his followers were able to buy some strongholds and strengthen their military power, under the leadership of his son 'Awaḍ b. 'Umar, who assumed the title of Sultan. By the mid 1860s the Qu'ayti appeared to have the upper hand, and from the inland areas the fight spread to the coast. First the Kathiri managed to wrest the port of Shihr from the ruling al-Burayk, but their success was short-lived, as in the next year (1867) the Qu'ayti ousted them from this town, which was then the main port of the Hadhramaut. Control of the ports was a vital strategic factor as all supplies of foodstuffs, men, and weapons came by sea. The conquest of Shihr gave the Qu'ayti the key to the supremacy on the whole southern Yemeni coast and promoted closer ties between them and the enemies of the 'Umar Bā 'Umar (who backed the Kathiri), in the triangle Shihr–Ghayl Bā Wazīr–Mukalla. The loss of the port of Shihr and the consequent political and economic isolation left the 'Umar Bā 'Umar in a weak position and obliged them to sign a pact with the Qu'ayti.

On Thursday, the 27 Rabi' al-Awwal 1286 H./8 July 1869, the elders of the 'Umar Bā 'Umar signed an agreement with the Qu'ayti sultan and his brothers.[15] Nine shaykhs of the Bā Wazīr acted as witnesses, the pact being put down in writing by Sālim b. 'Abd al-Hādi Bā Wazīr. The signatories were the heads of the Bin Shayba, Ba'ūd, Miya, Al-Ghallas, Dawla, Bā Bakar, Bin Bishir and Mardūf families, some of whose members would be living in Brava a few years later.[16] With this agreement, the 'Umar Bā 'Umar engaged not to help the enemies of the Qu'ayti and to consider the Sultan's interests as their own, while their lands were incorporated into the Qu'ayti

Sultanate. A Qu'ayti representative was installed at Ghayl, but peaceful relations were soon shattered, as 'Abdallah bin 'Ali al-'Ulqi (then serving as a *jamadar* in Heyderabad) attempted to revive the alliance between the Kathiri and the 'Umar Bā 'Umar with a view to expelling the Qu'ayti from the coast. In 1291 H/1874 AD a coalition of Kathiri, Kasadi, and 'Awāliq, backed by the 'Umar Bā 'Umar, confronted the Qu'ayti in a decisive battle, which ended in an overwhelming Qu'ayti victory.

In 1292 H/1875 AD the Qu'ayti army, 1600 men strong and composed of Yafi'i, Indians and slaves, moved towards Ghayl Bā Wazīr. Ghayl prepared for defence, amassing 'Umar Bā 'Umar, Badwi and Kathiri, under the command of two Kathiri leaders. The 'Umar Bā 'Umar had already evacuated their women and children from Ghayl, sending many of them to Sayhut and Raydat and a few others to a nearby fortress of the 'Awāliq. The Qu'aytis' siege of Ghayl lasted only two days; on the third day the battle raged both within the town and in the surrounding countryside, with widespread hand-to-hand fighting with swords and daggers. Many 'Umar Bā 'Umar were killed and some of their sub-clans (like the Dār Ghallas al-Ḥisn) were completely wiped out. After the victory, the Qu'aytis established themselves in Ghayl, where the Bā Wazīr shaykhs maintained a state of neutrality. The 'Umar Bā 'Umar survivors fled with their allies, and some took shelter in the 'Awāliq fortress. However, the Qu'ayti followed them there and laid siege to it for two months, until it surrendered.

The following years were marked by the British involvement in the contest: they sided with the Qu'ayti, helping them conquer the port of Mukalla (1881) and oust the ruling Kasadi family, and they made an agreement with the Kathiri, which allowed the latter to retain a limited power-base in the interior, but took away from them the ports, thus rendering them dependent on the Qu'ayti for all their supplies. British support was formalised in a treaty of friendship they signed with the Qu'ayti in 1881, which was followed by a Protectorate agreement in 1888.

After their defeat, the loss of lives and property, and the imprisonment of most surviving fighters, the 'Umar Bā 'Umar still refused to submit. Eventually the Qu'ayti Sultan 'Awaḍ b. 'Umar gave them the option either to remain in his territories as subjects (*ra'āyā*)[17] or to leave his dominion. Most decided to leave for East Africa, while a couple of families went to Indonesia[18] and a few moved to other regions of Yemen (Lahaj and Abyan). The only material remains of the 'Umar Bā 'Umar's presence in Ghayl are nowadays the ruined fortress of Ḥusn 'Abūd, built by 'Abūd b. Sālim on a site that has been almost totally covered by modern buildings, and the domed tomb of his father Sālim b. 'Alī.

The 'Umar Bā 'Umar in East Africa

While it is recorded that the Kasadi ruler and his followers left Mukalla for Zanzibar on a British ship in 1881,[19] we do not know much about the journey of the 'Umar Bā 'Umar from Hadhramaut to East Africa, both with regard to their means of transport and to their choice of destination. Probably they left in little family groups, on local dhows. Zanzibar beckoned, as the largest and most important centre of East Africa: so many people from Hadhramaut had already settled there that the term *washihiri* had locally become common to indicate all South-Arabian labourers. Some 'Umar Bā 'Umar were already serving the sultans of Zanzibar in a military capacity, a natural choice for people who had a tradition of armed service.[20] Some of these soldiers were manning the Zanzibari garrisons along the East African Coast: at Brava, in particular, the garrison numbered 150 to 170 *askaris*, mainly Hadhrami and Baluchi.[21] We have definite proof that some 'Umar Bā 'Umar went first to Zanzibar and only at a later date moved to Brava,[22] probably after they had received some positive information about that centre from kinsmen and/or other Hadhramis already living there.[23]

At the time of the 'Umar Bā 'Umar's arrival, Brava was still part of the Zanzibar dominion and the seat of a Zanzibari governor. However, like the other city-ports of the Benadir, the town enjoyed a large autonomy and a local council was responsible for conducting all internal affairs. The approximately 5000 people then living in Brava were a mixture of Somalis of the Tunni clan (itself divided into five sub-clans) and of people of Arab ancestry (the Hatimi and the Barawis or Bida), who formed together the "seven tribes" (*toddoba tol*) represented in the council. The local population included also the Naziri and the Mahadali, two groups of *sada* whose forebears had settled in Brava in the seventeenth century, and some 500 slaves.[24] Brava's economy was based, on the one hand, on trade with Zanzibar and the Swahili coast, and on the other on its connections with the interior of Somalia, to which the Somali sector of the urban community greatly contributed, as the Tunni clan that lived in the city formed also the bulk of the population of the surrounding region. The rural Tunni were holders of agricultural land and semi-sedentary pastoralists, and sent to Brava the products of the interior (live cattle, hides and skins, maize and sesame), for consumption and export.[25] In 1893 the Sultan of Zanzibar granted the administration of the Benadir Coast to Italy, and the Italian government, in its turn, entrusted it to a private Italian trading company, which left in place both the Zanzibari administrative set-up (governor, garrison, and customs master) and the local council. Until 1905, when the Italian government eventually took over, the Italian presence in Brava was limited to one man, the Resident.

The 'Umar Bā 'Umar immigrants consisted of a few old men and of a number of women, but mostly of people who had been too young to participate in the fights of the 1870s in their homeland (some were still under age).[26] A total of 39, including four women, are mentioned in Brava Court's Records (see Appendix 1). However, this comparatively small number could be misleading: those who were under age would not often appear in court, and it is very probable that, unlike the Bravanese female population, the 'Umar Bā 'Umar women were not used to take recourse to the judicial authorities to claim or secure their rights. In any case, they had little or no property to sell, donate or bequeath; in fact, the records concern almost exclusively their marriages or deaths.[27] If, however, we supplement these data with family records, and with the records kept by the *qadis* after 1900,[28] we can confidently state that women formed a significant part of the 'Umar Bā 'Umar immigrants. It is also evident from the *qadis'* records that nuclear family groups were largely represented, as mothers, sisters, wives, brothers, and uncles are mentioned.[29]

In Brava, the 'Umar Bā 'Umar settled in an environment very different from their homeland. The peace prevailing in the town afforded them perfect security; the cost of basic necessities was affordable; food was in plentiful supply, milk, goats and cattle being brought daily from the countryside, and fish being part of the local staple diet. Also the climate was much less harsh than in the Hadhramaut. They seem to have established good relations with the Zanzibari authorities (the governor and the members of the military garrison) and to have been readily accepted, if not exactly welcomed, by the urban population, despite the many traits that marked them immediately as aliens. Their scruffy and unkempt appearance distinguished them from the well-groomed Bravanese, as the 'Umar Bā 'Umar must have looked then much as Révoil described some men from Mukalla in the early 1880s:

> They have smooth hair, which they keep very long and tie with a camel-hair string. Their legs are naked and they go bare-chested; at their waist they wear a simple *futa*, supported by a large belt. To this belt are suspended all kinds of daggers and the various accessories of their long muskets.[30]

At that time Bravanese men favoured the long *haanzu* (Swahili *kanzu*) rather than the now ubiquitous sarong-like *chiguwo*, they routinely shaved their head and wore skullcaps and well-wound turbans. The newcomers, on the contrary, covered their heads, if at all, with a loosely wrapped *ileemba*, a strip of cloth that did not conceal their long hair, and sometimes wore a shawl to cover their chest.[31] In the privacy of their homes, their women wore the *tafgora*, the distinctive dress still prevalent nowadays in the countryside of coastal Hadhramaut, a colourful garment that reached just above the ankles in front and had a long train in the back.[32] The 'Umar Bā 'Umar prized the possession of firearms and weapons in general, and this was another characteristic that differentiated them from the other town-dwellers. All foreign travellers' reports about Brava stressed the fact that at that time the local population – unlike the Somalis of Mogadishu and Merka – went unarmed and men "carried only a stick".[33] On the contrary, there is evidence that the 'Umar Bā 'Umar brought their weapons with them: in a court case dated 30 June 1894, two brothers pledged as security, in addition to other possessions, a golden dagger, a silver dagger, three silver knives, two muskets (one of which inlaid with silver), two silver-inlaid pistols, and two silver-inlaid daggers.[34] It is interesting to note that, while Somalis from the countryside were obliged to leave all weapons at the town gate when entering Brava, the new immigrants were apparently allowed to keep theirs.

Brava male population had then a high rate of literacy in Arabic,[35] whereas the 'Umar Bā 'Umar were mostly illiterate or, at best, semi-literate. Some had acquired a smattering of Swahili during their recent stay in East Africa, but they must certainly have felt isolated, as the local Bantu vernacular – called Chimbalazi or Chimiini – and the other Swahili dialects are not mutually intelligible.[36] Like their Bravanese fellow-citizens, the 'Umar Bā 'Umar were Sunni Muslims and followers of the Shafi'i school of Islam. They took over a small mosque, called the Alwiyah Mosque, then located near the city walls in the area of the main town gate.[37] Later they established a pious endowment (*waqf*) consisting of some shops, for the upkeep of this mosque. At the turn of the twentieth century, Brava was experiencing a vibrant religious revival: the arrival of European colonial powers on the East African Coast had triggered the reaction of the local *'ulamā*, affiliated to the Qadiriyya and Idrisiyya *tariqas*, who perceived the foreigners as a threat to Islam and started a campaign to re-affirm and spread the Islamic tenets among all sections of the population. This campaign took the form of a large production of religious-didactic poetry in the local vernacular, targeting in particular women and the lower classes, who did not know Arabic.[38] The 'Umar Bā 'Umar's low cultural level and initial marginalisation did not allow them to contribute significantly to the town intellectual life: they are only recorded with introducing in Brava the *maulid* of al-Dayba'i, which they favoured instead of the more common Barzanji.[39]

The *qadis'* records show that by 1900 six 'Umar Bā 'Umar had married Arab women, while three others had Bravanese wives.[40] Intermarriage with local women would become more and more common in the following years, so much so that by the third generation only a handful of 'Umar Bā 'Umar could boast an entirely Arab ancestry. However, despite their status of newcomers and their weak economic position, the 'Umar Bā 'Umar considered themselves as belonging to a more prestigious social class than the local inhabitants (except the *sada* or *mashariifu*) and did not give their women in marriage to Bravanese.[41]

The 'Umar Bā 'Umar started their new life in Brava as small shop-keepers, living in the local wattle-and-daub huts ('*arīsh*) they partly used also for their trading activities.[42] Here they sold dry foodstuffs (maize, sesame, sorghum), general household goods, and some cloth.[43] Before 1900, only one of them, 'Abdallah b. Saʿīd b. 'Abdallah al-Baʿūd, had rented a stone house that later, after the owner's death, he bought from his heirs.[44] By the early twentieth century some of the 'Umar Bā 'Umar had acquired a few slaves and employed them in their shops.[45] Although Hadhramis are generally well known for their mercantile abilities, there is no record that the 'Umar Bā 'Umar had ever had connections with trade in their homeland, where their occupations had been mainly farming and military service, but once they settled in Brava, we find them all trying their hand at trading. In this they followed the local trend, as most Bravanese at that time filled the role of brokers and middlemen, supplying foreign trading houses with goods originating from the interior of Somalia. As newcomers, however, and possessing little or no initial capital, the 'Umar Bā 'Umar could not at first compete successfully with the town merchants, and their trading activities were in general very modest. From these humble beginnings, their fortunes soared after the First World War and reached their peak in the early 1930s. The consolidation of the Italian colonial rule played in their favour, as the Italians favoured the Arab sector of the urban population in the Benadir. Some of the 'Umar Bā 'Umar extended their business activities to Mogadishu, although they still kept their family homes in Brava, where they also opened larger shops. They also established privileged connections with the Arab *nakhudas* and soon had all but in name a kind of monopoly on the importation of dates from the Arabian Gulf. The advent of motorised transport in the 1920s saw them starting regular connections by lorry with several centres in the interior of Somalia (see infra).

The most visible – and quite spectacular – contribution of the 'Umar Bā 'Umar to Brava concerns the fabric of the town. As soon as their economic conditions rose from mere subsistence level to that of leading merchants, they started building on a grand scale, leaving a legacy of palatial houses that testify to their prestige and wealth. At least a dozen of these were very large, consisting of two or three storeys, and accommodated the different branches of the Shiddād, 'Abūd, Dawla, and Yislam families. These houses are quite eclectic in style and appear to blend different architectural traditions, without showing particular affinities with Hadhrami buildings.[46] Their exterior is often embellished with fancy crenellations, while the rooms, ornamented with plastered niches and filled with heavy pieces of furniture of Indian manufacture, show many similarities with the interior of contemporary houses of the wealthier Zanzibaris. Most of these houses were erected in the Biruni quarter, where many plots of lands were still available for building in the early twentieth century, but a few others stand in all other areas of Brava. It is worthwhile to note that traditionally Brava had no separate quarters for the different clans that made up its urban population. Living alongside local people promoted the creation of strong neighbouring ties, which certainly contributed significantly to the 'Umar Bā 'Umar's integration into the local community.

One of the most enthusiastic builders and arguably the man who epitomises the 'Umar Bā 'Umar's success story in Brava is 'Abūd b. Musā'ad. The first time he is mentioned in the *qadis'* Register, in 1893, he had borrowed some money from a freedwoman[47] and we learn from the records that he was living with his brother Aḥmad in a simple hut.[48] In 1900 he married the daughter of his kinsman Shiddād b. 'Abdallah, and went on to marry into the leading family of the Tunni Da'faradhi clan, establishing close relations with all other Tunni groups. He started trading with a small borrowed capital,[49] which he put to good use, opening a shop in Brava and building up little by little an extensive network of business connections that ensured the success of his import–export activities. By the early 1930s, he had built three large stone houses in Brava, one of which was taken over and enlarged by the Italian colonial authorities and to this day is known popularly as "the Resident's House". 'Abūd resided by preference in a villa that had been built in Brava by two of the first Italian settlers and that he had bought from their heirs.[50] In Mogadishu, he owned a house in the area then called "Villaggio Arabo" (now part of the Shibis quarter) as well as another two-storied house in the Hamar Weyn quarter, with a residential upper floor and a shop on the ground floor. His charitable works on behalf of the community included a public well he built in Brava and a string of other wells along the coast south of Brava, which are still used by the local herders. Eventually he earned a knighthood, which was bestowed on him by the King of Italy for his important contributions to the newly built Garesa Museum of Mogadishu.[51]

None of the 'Umar Bā 'Umar of the first generation went ever back to Arabia. However, some of them left Brava and settled elsewhere in Somalia. Yisir b. 'Abūd and a couple of other 'Umar Bā 'Umar families moved from Brava to Merka, where some of their offspring continued to live until 1990. Some others settled in the Lower Juba area, in and near the centres of Jamama and Jilib. Manṣūr b. 'Abūd spent his life in Brava, but his son 'Umar extended his business activities to the Upper Juba region and in the late 1920s started a family in Dinsor. Until a tarmac road linking Mogadishu to Baidhabo was built in the early 1970s, the most direct route from Brava to the Upper Juba followed a dirt track which ran due west from the coast, crossing the Shabelle river at Havai and passing through the village of Yak Bravai before reaching Dinsor. Although it often became impassable during the rainy season, Bravanese and 'Umar Bā 'Umar traders plied it regularly to transport goods by lorry to and from the Upper Juba centres. Dinsor being at a distance of only 80 km from Baardheere, they extended their trade to this town and beyond, along the Juba river, to Bo'ale and Saakow. By the late 1920s some 'Umar Bā 'Umar (as well as other traders from Brava) had settled permanently in Dinsor, opening their shops and eventually acquiring also some farmland. They received cloth, sugar, dates, coffee, etc. from the coast and sent to Brava clarified butter and red sorghum, the staple commodity of the area. 'Umar Manṣūr 'Abūd married into the local Somali clan of the Dabarre and soon had a very large family, which he lodged in an extensive fenced compound on the outskirts of Dinsor.[52] While he was a Chimiini-speaker and went back to Brava in his old age, his children spent their lives in Dinsor, adopting the local Maay dialect as their first language. 'Umar himself and most of his male offspring practised polygamy on a grand scale, always keeping three or four wives at a time and divorcing frequently. As a result, each of them had many children, often more than twenty. Intermarriage with members of the 'Umar Bā 'Umar living on the coast was rare: the group in Dinsor almost invariably favoured endogamous marriages or marriages into the Dabarre clan.

The 'Umar Bā 'Umar's generally prosperous conditions experienced a dramatic downturn at the onset of the Second World War and during the following period of British military administration in Somalia. Unlike the Italians, the British favoured openly the Somali element of the urban population rather than the Arabs, and during the riots that erupted in Mogadishu in January 1948 the shops of the 'Umar Bā 'Umar were looted. The war and the subsequent unsettled political situation had also an adverse effect on the dhow trade from Arabia and the Gulf. After the death of the elders who had amassed some respectable fortunes, their heirs started squabbling for their shares of the inheritance, and this added to the economic decline of the second-generation 'Umar Bā 'Umar, a decline that hit Brava in general (most Bravanese merchants, and in particular the *mashariifu*, experienced similar reverses).

The third-generation 'Umar Bā 'Umar who grew up in Brava after the Second World War were all Chimiini speakers and for many of them, who had Bravanese mothers, Chimiini was their first language, although knowledge of Arabic did not disappear.[53] Bravanese in general attributed particular importance to a good education of their young, which they traditionally saw as a sound knowledge of Islam and written Arabic. Children of both sexes attended Koranic schools and boys could then complete their education in the schools attached to some mosques or at the houses of the local *'ulamā*. Starting from the 1950s, they also attended state schools and acquired a fair to good knowledge of Italian.[54] On the contrary, education was never a central issue for the 'Umar Bā 'Umar: even those who were well off appear not to have urged their children to study, but to have let them follow their particular inclination. As a result, they produced a few religious scholars,[55] and a few others went on to complete their education to secondary or university level, but most were not well educated and some are illiterate to this day. In any case, their access to the civil service after Somalia became independent was restricted by the fact that both during the colonial period and in post-colonial times they were labelled as "Arabs" on their identity documents and were not considered Somali nationals. Being mostly self-employed, only very few applied for Somali naturalisation. Third-generation 'Umar Bā 'Umar had become, however, indistinguishable from other Bravanese, as far as language, dress, and general appearance and behaviour are concerned. Even some of their given names show the influence of Brava's religious culture, as they, like their Bravanese fellow-citizens, adopted personal names that were connected to Brava's particular reverence for some Islamic saints, in particular Jeylaani (from Shaykh 'Abdulqādir al-Jilānī, the founder of the Qadiriyya brotherhood) and Rufai, from Shaykh Aḥmad ar-Rifā'ī.

Economic conditions improved slightly in the late 1970s, a period when several young men from Brava went to work in Saudi Arabia and the Gulf, and with their remittances were able to give financial help to their families. During the Siyad Barre regime only very few 'Umar Bā 'Umar kept any ties with Yemen: a mere handful worked in Aden, although this town was no longer a commercial centre of major importance after the end of British colonial rule.

The return of the ʿUmar Bā ʿUmar to Yemen

After the onset of the civil war in December 1990, the ʿUmar Bā ʿUmar at first tried to hold on in Somalia, both in Brava and Dinsor. However, 1991 saw Brava won, lost and re-captured by Hawiya and Darood fighters in swift succession, and each of these changes brought about pillage and killings, although the town did not suffer the extensive destruction of Mogadishu. By November 1991 over 90% of the ʿUmar Bā ʿUmar, together with a large number of other Bravanese, had left Brava for Kenya, some by road and others by sea, on dhows and smaller boats. Some rich merchants of Bravanese extraction, who had settled long before in Mombasa, welcomed the newcomers, acting as sponsors for them *vis-à-vis* the Kenyan authorities and putting a former school with its extensive grounds at the refugees' disposal.[56]

Meanwhile the Yemeni government had been alerted to the plight of the ʿUmar Bā ʿUmar and acted very swiftly to rescue them, organising an air-lift in the first months of 1992 (February to April). Seven aircraft took them from Mombasa to Yemen, four flights landing at Aden and three at Riyan Airport, on the Hadhramaut coast. Each aircraft had a seating capacity of 130 passengers, but many young children were not allotted individual seats and travelled sitting on the lap of adults.[57] The total number of people evacuated from Mombasa can therefore be estimated at approximately 1000. Most of these were ʿUmar Bā ʿUmar from Brava, but there was also a small number of Ḥamūmi who had fled the area of Jilib and Jamama (Lower Juba region).[58] Some of these refugees, but by no means all, had still in their possession some documents, such as old Yemeni passports of their fathers, to prove their origins; the Yemeni government recognised all of them as citizens, although their forefathers had left the country 100 years before. Unlike the Somali asylum seekers, they were not confined to refugee camps, but were allowed to settle anywhere in Yemen, and some at first chose to live in Aden and Taʿizz.[59] In 1993, a large and then unoccupied area immediately west of Shihr was selected by the local authorities to resettle those who wished to live in the Hadhramaut, and small plots of land (12×12 metres) were allocated to each family. Here at first the refugees built some rough and cheap dwellings with corrugated iron sheets and plywood partitions; later, little by little, they started building more permanent houses with bricks, sometimes hiring local masons, but more often tackling this manual work themselves and even, in some cases, making their own bricks. In the Ghayl Bā Wazīr area, the ʿUmar Bā ʿUmar were recognised as the original rightful owners of some date plantations and other plots of land, and several settled there, while a few families went to live in nearby Mukalla.

The 1992 airlift had taken to Yemen only the ʿUmar Bā ʿUmar originating from Brava. Those from Dinsor migrated later, starting from 1993, and unlike the first group, they did not arrive all together, but in small numbers, most of them making a long overland journey from Dinsor to the northern Somali port of Boosaaso, then travelling by dhow to Mukalla.[60] The elders of this group go still back to Somalia every year, bringing in some more of their relatives. These later immigrants from Dinsor were also allotted plots of land in the same area of Shihr, and have now been living as neighbours of their kinsfolk from Brava for some years, the group from Dinsor being by now the larger. The fact that all the ʿUmar Bā ʿUmar coming from Somalia have been settled together in a separate area of Shihr has not afforded them the opportunity of living alongside local people and therefore of establishing with the latter the kind of close neighbouring ties that would certainly have promoted a speedier assimilation. Differences between the two 'Umar Bā 'Umar groups are also still very noticeable. The adults speak their respective languages – Chimiini and the Somali Maay dialect – although it was noticeable that those coming from Brava were more familiar with Arabic. However, the younger ones of both groups, who are all enrolled in the local schools, have now Arabic as their first language. As a result, Chimiini is fast disappearing;[61] Maay seems to hold better, as the women who are still coming out from Dinsor have a scanty knowledge of Arabic. It is also apparent that those formerly living in Brava have preserved some traditions (for example dances and wedding ceremonies) that go back unchanged to the nineteenth century, while those hailing from Dinsor have become much more "Somalised" in the course of time. On the other hand, the influence of the Bravanese outlook, which upholds peaceful living as a virtue, has sapped the warlike attitude that was formerly one of the characteristics of the 'Umar Bā 'Umar, whereas this is still very much in evidence in the group from Dinsor. Another important division, which appeared in recent years, is based on religious practices. While the 'Umar Bā 'Umar hailing from Brava are keeping alive the old Sufi traditions of the East African coast, celebrating the *Maulid* and seeking the intercession of the Prophet and the *awliyas*, fundamentalist preachers (who also distribute food and monetary aid) have launched a successful proselytising campaign among those hailing from Dinsor. As a result, the two groups do not worship together and the little mosque that was built in the settlement is practically monopolised by the Dinsor group, the others preferring to attend religious services downtown.

The favourable attitude of the Yemeni Government towards these returning citizens did not extend to providing financial assistance to see them through the initial stages of their new life.[62] Conditions are harsh in the Hadhramaut, especially for newcomers, as regularly paid jobs are very hard to find. Most 'Umar Bā 'Umar men are now working as drivers of taxis and private buses, some have opened small shops, and a mere handful have found employment in the local fish canning industries. In general, they are all back to subsistence level, as their forefathers were when they first settled in Brava. Following Brava's traditions, 'Umar Bā 'Umar women now living in Shihr strive to supplement their household economy with some financially rewarding domestic activities, some teaching the Qur'an to groups of young children, others making sweetmeats, biscuits and cooked food to be sold in the town's shops and market stalls. Despite the economic difficulties the 'Umar Bā 'Umar are experiencing at present, their self-confidence has been boosted by the Yemeni Government granting them full citizenship rights. After spending almost 20 years in Yemen, and in view of the unsettled situation still prevailing in Somalia, they now consider unrealistic any hope of returning to East Africa and look forward to a better future in their original homeland.

Conclusions

Three main reasons have been invoked for migrations from Arabia to East Africa, viz. political troubles and threatened subjection at home, religious persecution of minorities, or trade interests and connections with the Swahili Coast. An area like the Hadhramaut, poor in resources, has seen demographic pressure push many of its inhabitants to migrate since the Middle Ages. Scholars have stressed that this has been a constant factor in its history. In the case of the 'Umar Bā 'Umar, neither trade nor religious persecutions can be invoked. Rather, they were compelled to migrate by their situation of political subjection following their defeat by the Qu'ayti, coupled with the harsh economic conditions that derived from the general political instability of the area.

Two factors should be taken into consideration when assessing the overall impact the 'Umar Bā 'Umar had on Brava: the historical period during which their migration took place, and the comparatively short time they lived in East Africa. A few years after their arrival, Brava came under full colonial rule and lost the autonomy it had enjoyed while being part of the Sultanate of Zanzibar. The local council, formerly responsible for political and administrative decisions, was abolished in the first decade of the twentieth century. Had their migration occurred at the time when the coastal centres of East Africa were flourishing as fully autonomous city-states, the 'Umar Bā 'Umar's swift rise in economic status would very probably have resulted in their acquisition of political influence through their inclusion in the council of elders of Brava.[63] And if their stay in Brava had lasted for some centuries instead of a mere one hundred years, they would have eventually coalesced into the Bida, the largest group of Bravanese of Arab descent, which was itself a federation of people whose forebears had belonged to various *qabilas* (Wa'ili, Amawi, Qahtani, etc.) and had migrated from Southern Arabia at different times. Instead, owing to the short time span the 'Umar Bā 'Umar were in Brava, their integration into the local community did not develop into a complete assimilation.

Their cultural impact on Brava was not as significant as the mark that Arab migrants of the learned classes left elsewhere on the East African Coast. Culturally, the local inhabitants of Brava were much more sophisticated and had a much better knowledge of Islam than the newcomers. The few distinctive cultural traits that the 'Umar Bā 'Umar still maintained in the twentieth century were not adopted by their fellow-citizens. The case of the 'Umar Bā 'Umar seems to disprove the theory that the contribution of Arabs to the East African Coast consisted mainly "of *ideas* rather than *people*". This holds true only for particular migrants in particular historical periods. It is in the field of material culture that the 'Umar Bā 'Umar left their permanent mark on Brava. Their rise in economic and social status appears to be outstanding, if compared to the experience of others who migrated from coastal Hadhramaut roughly in the same period (the so-called *washihiri*), most of whom never rose above the status of labourers.

The 'Umar Bā 'Umar's integration in Brava was completed within three generations. The means through which it was achieved – socially, linguistically, culturally and economically – were the frequent intermarriages with local women, common business interests and partnerships with local traders, and neighbouring relations with people of different ethnic background, which in Brava formed an important part of social life. The Swahili world owes its existence to people of many different ethnic backgrounds. Belonging to it is not so much a question of descent, rather it is connected to the belonging, and the feeling that one belongs, to a certain place, and to the adoption of a set of cultural, social and religious values and behaviour patterns. The 'Umar Bā 'Umar of the third generation saw themselves as Bravanese first, and had never thought or wished to go back to the Hadhramaut, as they considered Brava to be their home town.

The need to adjust one's life to a foreign environment is a main issue for many people at the present time, when the urge to move to other countries has been triggered by a variety of causes, from disruptions caused by civil war, to oppression of minorities, to the hope of finding a haven where it is possible to better one's education and economic standard, avoiding the uncertainties that plague life at home. Re-adaptation concerns many different facets of life, from acquiring competence in a foreign language, to the minutiae of everyday routine in alien surroundings, to the available choice of jobs, housing, and food, and the adoption of different fashions in dress. Life for a resettled community is never easy, but the ʿUmar BāʿUmar have proved to be particularly flexible and resilient, twice meeting the challenge to re-adapt quickly, first in their East African environment, then, 100 years later, in the Hadhramaut.

Notes

1. The old view is exemplified by Reginald Coupland's *East Africa and its Invaders*, which mentions an "Arab and Persian colonisation of the Coast" and "a chain of Arab colonies" (Coupland, *East Africa and its Invaders*, 24, 28). This view has been rejected by Allen, "Swahili Culture Reconsidered"; Pouwels, "Medieval Foundations of East African Islam"; Nurse and Spear, *The Swahili*.
2. Pouwels, "Eastern Africa and the Indian Ocean". Farsy's biography of Ahmad b. Sumayt (Farsy, *The Shafiʾi Ulama of East Africa*, 148) mentions that his father, Sayyid Abū Bakr b. Abdallah (born in Shibam, Hadhramaut – died at Itsandaa, Comoro Islands, in 1874), had migrated to East Africa because of business (he was the owner of several dhows).
3. Pouwels, "Medieval Foundations of East African Islam", 201. Pouwels' italics.
4. See, for example, the biography of Ahmad b. Sumayt (I) in Farsy, *The Shafiʾi Ulama of East Africa*, 148 ff. Martin, "Arab Migrations to East Africa", 380 ff., provides details of the migrations of several sharifs (descendants of the Prophet Muhammad through his daughter Fatima, also called *sada* in Yemen, *washarifu* in Swahili, and *mashariifu* in Brava): the sons of Abu Bakr b. Salim and Ahmad b. Harun Jamal al-Layl to Pate and Lamu, and the descendants of Ahmar al-Uyun to Mogadishu.
5. Both quotations are from Martin, "Arab Migrations to East Africa", 371, 367.
6. Martin, in "Notes on Some Members of the Learned Classes", 527, mentions "another wave coming at the end of the nineteenth century", but adds that "[t]o decide how and when these Hadramis or Washihiri came to East Africa is a matter for future research."
7. Pouwels, "Tenth Century Settlement of the East African Coast". According to Pouwels, the journey to East Africa of the "Seven Brothers of Al-Ahsa", recorded in the Chronicle of Kilwa, provides several clues that suggest the possibility of a Qarmatian migration.
8. Martin, "Notes on Some Members of the Learned Classes", 527. "Some information is already at hand which suggests that the period from the 14th to the early 17th century was an epoch of migration from the Hadramawt."
9. Tolmacheva, "'They Came From Damascus in Syria'".
10. This is the case of the Hatimis' claim to have come to East Africa from Andalusia, which is also mentioned in the "History of Pate" (Freeman-Grenville, *The East African Coast*, 258).
11. Vianello and Kassim, *Servants of the Sharia*.
12. Arai (*Arabs Who Traversed the Indian Ocean*, 16, 17) with further bibliographic references.
13. Interview with Abū Bakr Musāʿad ʿAbūd, Shihr, 15 November 2007.
14. For details of this struggle, see Hartwig, "Expansion, State Foundation and Reform."
15. I am indebted to Musāʿad ʿAbdallah ʿAbūd, who made available to me his unpublished research (2004), for the details of this agreement and for the account of the subsequent battle at Ghayl Bā Wazīr.
16. They were ʿAbūd Sālim Mardūf, Abū Bakr b. Aḥmad b. ʿUmar b. Musāʿad, ʿAli b. Muḥammad b. ʿAli b. Shiddād, Saʿīd b. ʿAbdallah b. Muḥammad b. Shiddād al-Baʿūd, ʿUmar b. Aḥmad b. Ḥisni, Muḥammad b. ʿAbdallah b. ʿUmar Bā Bakar, ʿAbdallah b. Saʿīd b. ʿUmar Shiddād, Aḥmad b. Sālim b. Saʿīd b. Muḥammad Shiddād, and Sālim b. ʿAbdallah b. Saʿīd b. Muḥammad Shiddād.
17. This status involved the obligations already included in the agreement of 1869, i.e. the transfer of land property to the Sultan, the prohibition for the ʿUmar Bā ʿUmar to follow

policies and contract alliances that were contrary to the Sultan's interests, and the payment of taxes.

18. Some descendants of these migrants went to Shihr in the early 1980s to enquire whether any of their kinfolks were still living in the area (interview with 'Attās Sālim 'Abūd, Shihr, 18 December 1998).

19. Martin, "Muslim Politics and Resistance to Colonial Rule", 482.

20. The judicial records of Brava mention several times a 'Umar b. Muḥammad 'Umar Bā 'Umar who was serving as *shawush* of the local Zanzibari garrison (Vianello and Kassim, *Servants of the Sharia*, 1091, case QR 500.1, and *passim*). It is almost certain that he started his military career in Zanzibar.

21. Révoil, *Voyage au Cap des Aromates*, 55; Robecchi Bricchetti, *Somalia e Benadir*, 78.

22. According to family tradition, 'Abūd b. Musā'ad and his brother Aḥmad spent some years in Zanzibar before moving to Brava (interviews with Muḥammad 'Abūd Musā'ad, Shihr, October 2004).

23. The judicial records mention as living in Brava some 10 individuals of the Al-Burayk clan, a couple of Kathiri, one Kasadi, two Bā Wazīr, over ten Ḥamūmi (a *qabila* settled just north of Ghayl Bā Wazīr), and a number of individuals belonging to several smaller Hadhrami clans. See Vianello and Kassim, *Servants of the Sharia*, 2129–2185 (Index of Names).

24. The first reliable estimate of the population of Brava was made in 1907 by the then Italian Resident Giovanni Piazza, who assessed it at 5062 (Piazza, "La Regione di Brava nel Benadir", 20). Slavery was not officially abolished in the Benadir until 1904.

25. For details of the economy of Brava at the turn of the twentieth century, see Vianello and Kassim, *Servants of the Sharia*, 45–49, with bibliographic references.

26. One of the oldest must have been Yislam b. Ḥamad, whose death was recorded on 21 Safar 1317/30 June 1899 (Vianello and Kassim, *Servants of the Sharia*, 1245). Cases QR 74.1 and 75.1 concern Abūd and Umar, the sons of the late Saīd b. Abūd, who were still minors in 1893 (Vianello and Kassim, *Servants of the Sharia*, 217, 219).

27. See, for example, Vianello and Kassim, *Servants of the Sharia*, 827, case QR 371.1. The *qadis* of Brava acted also as registrars and notary public and, in addition to civil suits, recorded also marriages, divorces and deaths, as well as contracts, acknowledgments of debts, donations, etc.

28. Records of Brava civil court covering the period 1900–1905 were extant until 1990, but were subsequently lost (probably destroyed) during the civil war. The author had access to them in the 1980s.

29. For instance, Aḥmad bin Sālim had migrated to Brava with his wife, mother, and two sisters (Vianello and Kassim, *Servants of the Sharia*, 1233, case QR 568.2). Abūd b. Musāad was in Brava with his mother Aliya (not mentioned in the judicial records), his brother Aḥmad, and two uncles, Yisir and Manṣūr, with their respective families. Another uncle, Saīd, died in Brava leaving two underage sons.

30. Révoil, *Voyage au Cap des Aromates*, 21.

31. The Bravanese used to make fun of them, as evidenced by the ditty "Marabu Benga Benga – ka chishaali ka chileemba".

32. In the 1970s some old 'Umar Bā 'Umar women could still be seen wearing the *tafgora* in Brava.

33. Révoil, *Voyage au Cap des Aromates*, 56. Also all Italian travellers and officials remarked upon the peace reigning in Brava at the turn of the twentieth century.

34. Vianello and Kassim, *Servants of the Sharia*, 217.

35. Piazza, "La Regione di Brava nel Benadir", 23.

36. Although Chimiini has been classified among the Northern Swahili Dialects (Nurse, "A Linguistic Reconsideration of Swahili Origins"), lexical and morphological borrowings from Somali, as well as some archaic Bantu features still present in the language set it apart from all other Swahili dialects.

37. Guillain did not include this mosque in his list of the 14 mosques existing In Brava in 1846 (Guillain, *Documents sur l'histoire*, 167–168), therefore it must have been quite recent. According to popular tradition, its name originates from a young *sharifa* called Alwīya, who died at sea while travelling from Hadhramaut to East Africa and was buried in Brava (interview with Sharif Mardadi, London, 23 August 2008).

38. Vianello, "The Poetic Heritage of Brava", 5–10, with further bibliography.
39. Shaykh 'Abd al-Raḥman b. Muḥammad b. 'Umar b. Yusuf b. 'Ali al-Dayba'i (866–944 H.) was an Islamic scholar of Zabid, Yemen. The *maulid* composed by Jafar b. Ḥasan b.Abd al-Karīm b. al-Sayyid Muḥammad b. Abd al- Rasūl al-Barzanjī (born in Medina in 1128 H.) was the best known in Brava and in East Africa in general.
40. Sa'īd b. Muḥammad Bin Shayba, Sālim b. 'Umar, and Musā'ad b. Sālim b. Aḥmad married Bravanese women, while Sālim b. 'Ali, Sālim b. Mardūf, Aḥmad b. Sālim, Muḥammad b. Sālim, Aḥmad b. Muḥammad Bā Bakar, and Manṣūr b. Ja'far had Arab wives. In 1900 many of the young 'Umar Bā 'Umar were still unmarried.
41. The Shafi'ite principle that a woman should not be given in marriage to a man of lower status created in Brava a social hierarchy, which was based on each group's self-assessment of its social prestige and not on its actual power, influence, or economic conditions. This hierarchy was reflected in the refusal by certain groups to give their women in marriage to men of other groups they considered as inferior.
42. It was apparently common for such small shops to be set up in huts, even by affluent merchants. Other Arab shopkeepers' huts are recorded, see Vianello and Kassim, *Servants of the Sharia*, cases 258.1 and 296.1.
43. The most detailed description of the contents of a shop kept by an Arab is found in QR 391.1 (Vianello and Kassim, *Servants of the Sharia*, 867). Other records show that the Umar Bā Umar dealt in *marekani* cloth (QR 411.2), sesame (QR 45.1), butter (QR 291.1), ambergris (QR 76.1), teak wood (QR 411.1) and goats (QR 577.1).
44. Vianello ad Kassim, *Servants of the Sharia*, 579, case QR 252.1.
45. Robecchi Bricchetti, *Lettere Illustrate alla Societa' Antischiavistica d'Italia*, 193, 194. These were Muḥammad b. Sālim, Shiddād b. Abdallah, and Abdallah b. Saīd al-Baūḍ.
46. The plans and architectural features of some of these buildings are given in Molon and Vianello, "Architettura Domestica a Brava". For a comparison with traditional Hadhrami buildings, see Damluji, *A Yemen Reality*.
47. Vianello and Kassim, *Servants of the Sharia*, 101 (QR 16.1).
48. Vianello and Kassim, *Servants of the Sharia*, 217 (QR 74.1).
49. Vianello and Kassim, *Servants of the Sharia*, 219 (QR 75.1).
50. The builders and original owners of this villa were Messrs. Bricchi and Zoni, who had been granted a large farmland concession near the Shebelle river where they had tried to grow caoutchouc. This house, known in Brava as "Daar Zoni", is already mentioned in Piazza, "La Regione di Brava nel Benadir", 19. It was demolished in the late 1970s and Brava Town Hall now stands on its site.
51. See Museo della Garesa – Catalogo, *passim*.
52. Interviews with Aḥmad 'Umar Manṣūr and 'Abūd Musā'ad 'Abūd, London, May 2007.
53. Their parents, the second generation 'Umar Bā 'Umar, still used to speak their Hadhrami dialect among themselves. They had, however, acquired a good knowledge of both Chimiini and Somali, although few of them had received a regular education.
54. Until 1968, Italian was the language of learning in state schools in Southern Somalia at all levels of education.
55. In particular Muḥammad b.'Abdallah b. Muḥammad Shiddād and his son Ḥasan.
56. Later they offered some of their agricultural land just outside Mombasa, where a permanent refugee camp for Bravanese was set up. The former St. Anne's school and the later Bravanese refugee camp are also mentioned in Pérouse de Montclos 1999.
57. Interview with 'Attās Sālim 'Abūd, Shihr, 18 December 1998. 'Attās was directly involved in listing the 'Umar Bā 'Umar present in Mombasa who later boarded the flights to Yemen.
58. The few 'Umar Bā 'Umar families who found themselves stranded in Mogadishu and Merka reached Yemen later and by other routes.
59. Interview with 'Abdallah b. Sālim 'Umar Bā 'Umar, Ta'izz, 23 November 1998.
60. The port of Mukalla faces directly the Somali port of Boosaaso across the sea and the crossing by dhow lasts approximately 24 hours. Dhows used to ply regularly this route before its recent disruption by Somali pirates.
61. This is the case also in the Bravanese communities in Europe and the United States. Chimiini is now considered an endangered language.
62. Food rations were, however, distributed for some time by Islamic relief agencies.

63. Unlike other coastal cities, where eventually sultans replaced the councils of elders, Brava was always ruled by a local council.

References

Allen, J. deVere. "Swahili Culture Reconsidered: Some Historical Implications of the Material Culture of the Northern Kenya Coast in the Eighteenth and Nineteenth Centuries." *Azania* IX (1974): 105–38.

Arai, K. *Arabs who traversed the Indian Ocean: the History of the Al-Attas family in Hadramawt and South-East Asia.* PhD dissertation, University of Michigan, 2004.

Coupland, R. *East Africa and Its Invaders.* New York: Russell & Russell, 1965 (reprint).

Damluji, S.S. *A Yemen Reality – Architecture Sculptured in Mud and Stone.* Reading: Garnet Publishing, 1991.

Farsy, Shaykh A.S. *The Shafi'i Ulama of East Africa, ca. 1830–1970 – A Hagiographic Account.* Translated, edited and annotated by Randall L. Pouwels. Madison: African Studies Program, University of Wisconsin, 1989.

Freeman-Grenville, G.S.P., ed. *The East African Coast: Select Documents.* London: Rex Collings, 1975.

Guillain, Ch. *Documents sur l'histoire, la géographie et le commerce de l'Afrique Orientale* (3 volumes). Paris: Arthus Bertrand, 1856.

Hartwig, F. "Expansion, State Foundation and Reform: The Contest for Power in Hadhramaut in the Nineteenth Century." In *Hadhrami Traders, Scholars and Statesmen in the Indian Ocean, 1750s–1960s,* ed. U. Freitag and W.G. Clarence-Smith, 35–50. Leiden: Brill, 1997.

Martin, B.G. "Muslim Politics and Resistance to Colonial Rule: Shaykh Uways b. Muhammad al-Barawi and the Qadiriya Brotherhood in East Africa." *The Journal of African History* 10, no. 3 (1969): 471–86.

Martin, B.G. "Notes on some members of the learned classes of Zanzibar and East Africa in the 19th century." *African Historical Studies* 4, no. 3 (1971): 525–45.

Martin, B.G. "Arab Migrations to East Africa in Medieval Times." *International Journal of African Historical Studies* 7, no. 3 (1974): 367–90.

Molon, M. and A.Vianello. "Architettura domestica a Brava tra la fine dell'Ottocento e i primi del Novecento." *Quaderni del Dipartimento di Progettazione dell'Architettura,* Politecnico di Milano 8 (1988): 45–56.

Nurse, D. "A linguistic reconsideration of Swahili origins". *Azania* XVIII (1983): 127–50.

Nurse, D. and Th. Spear. *The Swahili: Reconstructing the History and Language of an African Society, 800–1500.* Philadelphia: University of Pennsylvania Press, 1985.

Pérouse de Montclos, M.-A. "Exodus and Reconstruction of Identities: Somali 'Minority Refugees' in Mombasa". Accessed in English at www.somref.org. Previously published (in French) in *Autrepart,* no. 11. Paris: IRD, 1999: 27–46.

Piazza, G. "La regione di Brava nel Benadir." *Bollettino della Societa' Italiana di Esplorazioni Geografiche e Commerciali* Fasc. I e II (Jan.–Feb. 1909): 7–29.

Pouwels, R.L. "Tenth century settlement of the East African Coast: The Case for Qarmatian/ Isma'ili Connections." *Azania* IX (1974): 65–74.

Pouwels, R.L. "The Medieval Foundations of East African Islam." *International Journal of African Historical Studies,* vol. 11, no. 2 (1978): 201–26.

Pouwels, R.L. "Eastern Africa and the Indian Ocean to 1800: Reviewing Relations in Historical Perspective." *International Journal of African Historical Studies* 35, no. 2/3 (2002): 385–425.

Regio Governo della Somalia. *Museo della Garesa – Catalogo.* Mogadiscio: Regia Stamperia della Colonia, 1934.

Révoil, G. *Voyage au Cap des Aromates.* Paris: A. Dentu, 1880.

Robecchi Bricchetti, L. *Somalia e Benadir.* Milano: Aliprandi, 1899.

Robecchi Bricchetti, L. *Lettere Illustrate alla Societa' Antischiavistica d'Italia.* Milano: La Poligrafica, 1904.

Tolmacheva, M. "'They came from Damascus in Syria': A Note on Traditional Lamu Historiography." *International Journal of African Historical Studies* 12, no. 2 (1979): 259–69.

Vianello, A. "The Poetic Heritage of Brava: An Introduction." *Halabuur* 3, nos. 1 and 2 (2008): 5–10.

Vianello, A. and M.M. Kassim, eds. *Servants of the Sharia: The Civil Register of the Qadis' Court of Brava 1893–1900.* (2 volumes). Leiden: Brill, 2006.

Appendix 1

'Umar Bā 'Umar mentioned in the Civil Register of the Qadis' Court of Brava

'Abdallah bin Saʿīd bin Muḥammad (Baʿūd)
'Abdallah bin Shiddād bin 'Abdallah
'Abūd bin Musāʿad b. 'Abūd b. Sālim (Mardūf)
'Abūd bin Saʿīd bin 'Abūd b. Sālim (Mardūf)
'Abūd bin Sālim
Aḥmad bin Sālim (Dawla)
Aḥmad bin Sālim (Mardūf)
Aḥmad bin Musāʿad (Mardūf)
Aḥmad bin Muḥammad (Bā Bakar)
Fatima bint Yisir bin 'Abūd (Mardūf)
Ḥamad bin Muḥammad
Khalisa bint Sālim (Mardūf)
Manṣūr bin 'Abūd b. Sālim (Mardūf)
Manṣūr bin Jaʿfar
Muḥammad bin Musāʿad bin Bishir
Muḥammad bin Sālim (Baʿūd)
Muḥammad bin Sālim (Dawla)
Musāʿad bin Sālim b. Aḥmad (Mardūf)
Nūra bint Sālim
Saʿīd Bā Ḥamad
Saʿīd bin 'Abūd b. Sālim (Mardūf)
Saʿīd bin 'Ali b. Sālim
Saʿīd bin Muḥammad bin Shayba
Saʿīd bin Sālim b. 'Ali b. Saʿīd b. Muḥammad
Saʿīd bin Sālim bin 'Ali (Baʿūd)
Saʿīd bin Sālim
Sālim bin 'Ali
Sālim bin 'Ali bin Sālim b. 'Umar b. Muḥammad
Sālim bin Saʿīd (Baʿūd)
Sālim bin Saʿīd bin Sālim
Sālim bin 'Umar
Shiddād bin 'Abdallah
Tislam bint Saʿd bin Khamis (client of the Mardūf)
'Umar bin 'Abdallah
'Umar bin Muḥammad (*shawush*)
'Umar bin Saʿīd bin 'Abūd b. Sālim (Mardūf)
'Umar bin Sālim (Mardūf)
Yisir bin 'Abud bin Sālim b. 'Abūd (Mardūf)
Yislam bin Ḥamad bin 'Abdallah

Reinterpreting revolutionary Zanzibar in the media today: The case of *Dira* newspaper

Marie-Aude Fouéré

Institut Français de Recherche en Afrique, Nairobi, Kenya

For years, the official narrative of the Zanzibari nation imposed a specific conception of identity and citizenship built on a racial understanding of the Isles' history and the silencing of collective memories of violence perpetrated by the 1964–1972 regime. The democratization process of the mid-1990s allowed for the emergence of a critical public sphere which contributed to the public circulation of alternative national imaginaries and the resurfacing of clandestine collective memories. This paper explores the role of the press in the production and circulation of alternative narratives of the 1964 Revolution and its aftermath by focusing on a newspaper called *Dira*. It shows how issues raised by the newspaper's memory entrepreneurs engage with collective representations of belonging and the nation in Zanzibar.

Introduction

In the history of Zanzibar, the Revolution of 1964[1] and its early aftermath constitute a central episode that has shaped contemporary representations of belonging and nationhood until today.[2] In contemporary Zanzibar, there is not a single memory narrative, but on the contrary multifaceted and competing narratives of the murky revolutionary past which are linked to a socially contested present.[3] The Revolution and the 1964–1972 years[4] are recalled and given meaning in ways that reflect social status, ethnic or racial identities, generational belonging and political affiliations. Also depending on everyday situations of remembrance (family discussions, street corner talks, political gatherings, etc.) themselves linked to larger socioeconomic configurations, narratives of the revolutionary event and the following decade of authoritarianism are characterized by plurality, transformation and intertwining over time and in the present.[5] Among the variety of existing narratives, the official version deployed by the state has held a dominant position in the public space. Indeed, until the mid-1990s, state control over the production, transmission and circulation of ideas combined with the use of repressive measures aimed at imposing silence on competing memory narratives made it possible for the regime to gain monopoly on representations of the past, though this did not deter the clandestine transmission of unofficial memories within networks of kin and acquaintances. This official discourse was characterized by recurring racial binary tropes putting the

"Arabs" against the "Africans", to refer to identity categories locally in use, that presented a clear-cut and unambiguous version of the past and its meaning for the present, with the explicit objective to foster national unity in the frame of the nation-building project, and with the implicit strategy to discursively build state hegemony, that is, bind citizens to obedience, and enhance the legitimacy of the men in power.

Yet, as the mid-1990s democratization process and the rise of the media opened new avenues for political competition and the constitution of a critical public sphere, the position of the regime to produce overwhelming versions of the past came to be questioned. The present article focuses on one such competing narrative produced in print and publicized with the declared intention to undermine the official historical version of the Revolution of 1964 and its aftermath. Published from 2002 to 2003 in the pages of an independent Zanzibari newspaper in Swahili called *Dira* ("vision" in Swahili), this rewriting of the past significantly contributed to publicly voiced memories of the revolutionary period and used them as a political resource to meet contemporary needs. *Dira* is one among various media through which, since 1964, politically engaged Zanzibari figures have challenged the contentious state narrative of revolutionary times, attempted to discredit the men who seized power by force and the ideology that they brandished to justify their action, as well as proposed alternative conceptions of identity and belonging, or more generally of the Zanzibari *patria* – the moral community worthy of political defence.[6] Although the historical narrative that unfolded in *Dira* cannot be said to be more original or authentic than others – it intersected earlier homespun versions of history and, like all other narratives, saw the past from a partisan vantage point, portraying the stances of the interest groups of their authors rather than meeting the standards of academic historiography – it was unique for several reasons. It was a collective initiative, albeit strongly relying upon one man only, *Dira*'s Chief Editor, in the face of a variety of individual essays of rewriting of history in the form of patriotic pamphlets, autobiographies or literary works;[7] it involved home-grown patriotic intellectuals from the post-revolutionary generation, while other similar initiatives had mostly been taken by direct victims of the Revolution, that is, people of the revolutionary generation who fled the country in 1964 and afterwards, and lived in exile in the Arabian Peninsula or in Europe;[8] finally, being published in the form of a newspaper and written in Swahili, it reached a large audience and had a high popularity from the town to the village, among the youth and the elders, whereas previous pieces of works – often written in English – had remained rather confidential, circulating within narrow circles of politically engaged urban individuals. *Dira*'s impact was all the more significant as the Isles had not had, since independence, any privately owned and independent written media;[9] the mainland publications available in the Isles had not been not able to bridge the gap on information of local interest for Zanzibaris[10] and the government gazette *Zanzibar Leo* has, until today, rarely given room to dissenting voices. Consequently, this publication, in its intention and with regard to its authors' commitment, can be placed in the filiation of the nationalist newspapers of the pre-independence period, *Mwongozi* in the first place[11], with their politicization as "partisan pamphleteering" [12] and their "war of words"[13] – a legacy which the journalists of *Dira* consciously embraced, and which the educated readership was aware of.

This article engages with the question of history writing, imaginaries of belonging and political struggles in Zanzibar by focusing on the case of *Dira* newspaper as a medium of selective representations of identity and the Zanzibari *patria*. Being a piece of anthropology about present-day historically informed patriotic discourses, this article does not aim at digging into the history of the Revolution, as a classical work of historiography would, to unravel the revolutionary intrigue in the hope of discovering the "truth" of what happened. Rather, it explores both how homespun historical narratives constitute a bricolage that conjoins individual and collective memories, earlier secondary sources and a socially pervasive racial thinking, and how they mediate and shape contemporary conceptions of autochthony and allochthony, of belonging and citizenship in their relation to political legitimacy and sovereignty. In that sense, it embraces Garth Myers' argument that "how the story [of the Revolution of 1964] is told has become as interesting and enlightening as a recounting of what actually happened".[14] The article first presents a short sociology of the newspaper's team of journalists. It then explores what is said about the past in locating it within the bulk of confrontational narratives of the revolutionary times and how this departs from the stances of the official narrative, showing that representations of belonging and citizenship are infused by pre-revolutionary nostalgia and nativist conceptions of authenticity and auto-chthony. It finally gives insight into *Dira*'s audience and reception among Zanzibaris, highlighting how the memory- and history-scape sketched by *Dira*'s educated homespun-history entrepreneurs engaged with contemporary political debates and contests between the party in power, *Chama Cha Mapinduzi* (CCM, Party of the Revolution), and the Civic United Front (CUF) opposition party – hence its eventual banning by the state. Similar to pre-independence newspapers, *Dira* contributed to (re)inventing Zanzibari nationhood, but it did so by deploying the rhetoric of coastal chauvinism and cultural distinctiveness that has long shaped Zanzibaris' political subjectivities.

Dira the troublemaker

The weekly newspaper *Dira* was started at the end of 2002 by a team of journalists and intellectuals registered as the Zanzibar International Media Company (ZIMCO). The publication project slowly matured out of informal discussions held at Masomo bookshop, the then meeting point of intellectuals and personalities of the Isles' media scene and political life who informally gathered together there on Sunday mornings to discuss the state of affairs in Zanzibar. It actually came to birth under the impulse of journalists from Tanzania mainland who handed its concrete realisation to Zanzibaris thanks to the financial support of Ismail Jussa, then an emerging CUF politician, and Zanzibaris from abroad. The original team gathered an experienced journalist, the late Ali Mohamed Nabwa, a veteran of the revolution who was made Chief Editor; Ismail Jussa Ladhu, then CUF's director of Foreign Affairs and International Cooperation[15]; a civil servant, Hamza Zuber Rijal, who used to own a Muslim newspaper called *Maarifa* ("knowledge" in Swahili) dealing with Muslim history and religion; locally renowned professional journalists, namely Ally Saleh – known in Zanzibar for his outspoken stand, he has been the BBC Swahili correspondent in Zanzibar for years as well as a regular correspondent for various mainland newspapers, a book translator and a poet – and Salim Said Salim, an experienced Zanzibari journalist of the same generation as Ali Nabwa who was trained in China; and finally, joining the newspaper shortly after its launching, fierce emerging journalists who did not fear to express critical opinions and exhibit their pride in Zanzibari cultural uniqueness, such as Mohammed Ghassany (educated in Germany, he used to write for the former weekly mainland-based *Rai*, a newspaper that was owned by renowned journalist Jenerali Ulimwengu and was highly esteemed by the educated upper-middle class), Jabir Suleiman, who does not mince his words against the wheeling and dealing of both the Zanzibari and the Mainland political elite in the page of *Mwanahalisi* today, and Salma Said, now correspondent for the mainland newspapers *The Citizen* and *Mwananchi*, and a reporter for the Deutsche Welle Germany-based radio. Although *Dira*'s members were not registered in any political party, except for Ismail Jussa, they were known for their critical stand against CCM and their sympathy for CUF[16].

Different generations of outspoken personalities of the media scene in Zanzibar were therefore represented in *Dira*'s team. Their commitment to challenge the conformity of the media landscape is linked to how their historical experience – or *times* – shaped their political subjectivities[17]. Although *Dira* members were variously informed by their times, undergoing a process of subjectivation, in the Foucauldian sense, through a generational experience of the local socioeconomic and political situation that shaped their representations of politics and orientated their political practices, they all shared a common disillusion and frustration which, from 1964 on, has accompanied every new generation eager for change. Ali Nabwa and Salim Said Salim were grown men at the time of the revolution and followed step by step the history of Zanzibar in the making. They belong to a generation of enthusiastic educated Zanzibaris whose understanding of history and expectations for change were shaped by a cosmopolitan, pan-Africanist, nationalist and Marxist identity, but who witnessed the decay of anti-colonial and anti-capitalist ideologies of liberation in the face of the rise of authoritarianism[18]. Ally Saleh and Hamza Rijal, who are today in their fifties, were young kids when the revolution took place but still have vivid memories of the pre-revolutionary atmosphere.[19] They matured in the early years following the Revolution, a period marked by socialist-borrowed rhetoric of nation-building (the *kujenga taifa* Swahili watchword), the promotion of a revolutionary ethos and discipline which supposed that citizens should commit themselves for the construction of a new society, and the deployment of concrete modernizing endeavours intended to bring development for all.[20] Yet, as the authoritarian character of the Karume decade appeared in full light, and that economic deterioration affected each and every Zanzibari, the post-revolutionary period soon buried popular "expectation of modernity".[21] People in their fifties today bear witness to the deception, disillusionment and frustration of a generation deluded with false and unrealized promises of modernity and development. As for the younger journalists, in their early forties, they were born shortly after the Revolution. Their childhood and adolescence took place in an economically prostrate Zanzibar. They reached their twenties at the end of the 1980s or early 1990s, a time when structural adjustment programmes introduced the liberalization of the economy, offering a new modernizing rhetoric when democratization was a promise of greater freedom of expression and circulation, and when multiparty competition, reintro-duced in 1992, condensed hopes for a better society based on greater political morality, economic justice and social justice. This context appealed to a youth aspiring to social and economic upward mobility and success but led, again, to disillusion: socioeconomic disparities increased, the first-past-the-post system and repeated electoral frauds, not to mention cases of intimidation and violence, have prevented adequate expression and representation of the opposition, even exacer-bating tensions and divisions among Zanzibaris, and between Zanzibar and the mainland.[22] *Dira*'s conception of the post-revolutionary era, considered as the origin of Zanzibar's predicament, reflects this collective embittered disenchantment and accounts for their commitment to remedy it by speaking out openly against the political elite. In interviews, former members of *Dira* justified the need to create a newspaper on the ground that, contrary to what happened in Tanzania mainland where a vibrant private press developed,[23] the Zanzibari media landscape was characterized by the absence of freedom of expression and tight control of the state. The newspaper clearly aimed to be an avenue for plural and alternative opinions that could not be expressed elsewhere, and for tackling sensitive issues specific to the situation in Zanzibar. According to Ismail Jussa, it was well known that Ali Nabwa was a "troublemaker" (*mchokozi*), and this is exactly why he was chosen to lead *Dira*. Opening up public debates about the past was, as we will see now, a means to expand the boundaries of public expression and concretely challenge the legitimacy of the elite in power.

Recasting revolutionary times

To produce a historical narrative that would undermine the official history deployed by the state was, from the start, a declared objective of the newspaper. Two topics that are central to the state meta-narrative were continuously given new light and new meanings: the Revolution of 1964 and its aftermath;[24] the Union between Zanzibar and Tanganyika that gave birth to the United Republic of Tanzania in April 1964. The very first issue of the newspaper set the tone. It opened with an article by Ali Nabwa entitled "Nyerere si Malaika" (Nyerere is not an Angel) which, based on the author's personal memories, interpretations of past events and re-readings of the words and actions of Tanzania's first president, Julius Nyerere, was aimed at dismantling Nyerere's contemporary official image. Departing from the state-built eulogistic imagery that figures Nyerere as a national hero who placed morality and justice above pragmatic considerations and *realpolitik*, and who sacrificed his personal interest for the common good,[25] the article portrays Nyerere as a condescending, disloyal and self-interested man who resorted to all sorts of backroom deals, intrigues and sly machinations to reach and keep power, cunningly manoeuvred to get rid of popular politicians who got in his light, and stabbed even faithful companions in the back. Nabwa notably explains in great detail what he presents as Nyerere's biased perceptions of the history and culture of the islands that, to Nabwa, had extremely severe long-term consequences on Zanzibar future. Nyerere is indeed said to have regarded Zanzibar as a racially divided society between Arabs and Africans bearing the marks of the nineteenth century all-Arab inhumane slave trade and slavery, and the pervasive social, economic and political domination over black Africans by Arabs which should be buried; Nyerere would also have considered Zanzibar as a place where the Arab-Islamic-referenced cosmopolitan Swahili cultural specificities which took shape and flourished over the centuries contributed to diffuse[26], among Zanzibaris, collective attitudes of distinction from the African continent. For Nyerere, in Nabwa's narrative, such a distinct Zanzibari ethos needed to give way to a black African- and mainland-centred culture, hence his alleged plotting of the Revolution.

The article also intends to reveal the role Nyerere played in manoeuvring for the Union between the two sovereign nations of Zanzibar and Tanganyika. Under the pressure of the anti-Communist United States who feared that Zanzibar might become their 'Cuba of Africa'[27] and for fear of the increasing popularity of Abdulrahman Babu, the pro-Communist leader of the deceased Umma Party, that threatened Karume's rule, Nyerere is said to have plotted the Union. He would have intrigued to impose it without seeking any popular mandate neither the consent of the political elite.[28] The article defends the idea that the Union was meant not only to control the political destiny of the Isles, but to destroy the economy and culture of a place that, not so long before, as Ali Nabwa reminds the reader, Nyerere wanted to "tow out into the middle of the Indian Ocean".[29] As for Karume, it is said that he disregarded the shaky legal and political foundations of the Union, even more its potential detrimental long-term consequences, and agreed to it as a means of getting rid of real or perceived threats to his power.[30] In revising both the mainland and Zanzibari official narratives about the Union as a profitable institutional tool for both state parties, *Dira*'s journalists did not produce a radically new political interpretation. Earlier or contemporary patriotic literature on Zanzibar as well as academic works have interrogated the legality of the treaty of Union and pointed to its flaws and detrimental impact on the Isles[31]. However, what *Dira* did was to use the theme of the Union to openly advocate for sovereign self-rule for the Isles. In doing so, it both resonated with popular concerns about the current political and economic strains and shortcomings attributed to the Union, but also provided a narrative tool to compete with official interpretations of the Union as a structure that all Tanzanians would have benefited from.

For *Dira*'s chief editor, depicting what, to his view, was Nyerere's biased understanding of the past and the present of Zanzibar, and listing the many inappropriate and harmful political actions that, according to him, ensued, do not merely equate with symbolically attacking the one-and-only icon of the mainland for the sake of it. More than anything, it constituted a pretext to challenge the hegemonic state narrative of the revolutionary episode. Indeed, Nyerere's racially-oriented nationalism is equated with "racial nationalism", as the historian Jonathon Glassman has termed it,[32] that is, a conception of nationhood and belonging built upon racial dichotomies that planted its roots at the end of the 1950s in Zanzibar and constituted the ideological ferment of the revolution.[33] Revolutionaries justified their action on the grounds that an alien Arab oligarchy, aided by privileged minority groups such as Comorians and Indians,[34] ruled for centuries the true "African" owners of the Isles, exploiting and oppressing them.[35] In the state rhetoric of the early 1960s, the category "African" therefore encompasses Shirazis, or the indigenous populations of Unguja and Pemba, and the later-arrived populations from the mainland – hence the name of the political party which claimed to represent all Africans, the Afro-Shirazi Party (ASP). Race was used as the criterion of identity and citizenship. The overthrow of the first independent government of Zanzibar was labelled an "African Revolution" by the new men in power, for it was said to have been carried out by the African majority and for its benefits, and to be the result of a popular mass movement which expelled an alien illegitimate power. Combined with a superficial socialist leaning, racial revenge and justice constituted the trope upon which the state rhetorically built its legitimacy and introduced institutional and economic measures from 1964. When ASP merged with TANU (*Tanganyika African National Union*, the single party in the mainland) in 1977 to form CCM, a "Tanzanianization" of the revolution occurred, that is, as Garth Myers puts it, the intensification of the "African-ness of the revolutionary script, conceiving the revolution as African liberation and blocking out non-black understandings of identity on the islands".[36] Earlier more flexible conceptions of African-ness displayed by the ASP elite and Karume himself, who both and sometimes contradictorily defended the superiority of blackness while recognizing the historical specificities of blood mixing in Zanzibar totally disappeared from official discourses in the late 1960s. Karume even attempted to ban the use of the ethnic designation of "Shirazi" to refer to Zanzibar's indigenous populations, for it was said to be a colonial fabrication, and rather impose the ethnonym "African".[37]

Imagining an exclusionary *patria*

The provocative "Nyerere si Malaika" paved the way for a radical revision of this hegemonic racially-grounded revolutionary ideology. Feuilleton articles unrolled over a year of newspaper issues, such as Nabwa's biography "Siku moja itakuwa kweli" (One day it will be true), not yet published as a book, "Mapinduzi ni matokeo ya ubinafsi" (The Revolution is the product of individualism) and "Siku 100 za kuundwa Muungano wa Tanzania" (The hundred days that made the Union of Tanzania), to cite only a few of Nabwa's pieces. Most articles of the team, notably those by Ally Saleh and Mohammed Ghassany, developed a similar competing narrative aimed at contesting the hegemonic ideology upon which the political elite had legitimized its exercise of power for decades. In spite of variations between the journalists, a common interpretation of the history and culture stands out from *Dira*'s pages. It is characterized by the rejection of simple dichotomies between the exploitative rich Stone Town-based Arabs and the wretched ex-slave Africans of mainland origin. Quoting recognized academic historiography, but also earlier secondary sources published by "civilizational" nationalists from the former Zanzibar Nationalist Party (ZNP), to borrow from Jonathon Glassman's categories of nationalist ideologies,[38] articles give way to increased subtleties in depicting the sociological components of the pre-revolutionary society and the causal factors of the revolution. The nature and scope of slavery, of Arab rule, and of the Revolution is thus radically revised. The responsibility of Arab and Swahili merchants in the slave trade and slavery is put into perspective by highlighting that the latter were one link only among others in the chain of the wide-scale international economic system based on human exploitation that existed at that time; and its oppressive and humiliating aspects are counterbalanced by arguments that emphasize the significant proportion of inter-marriages and the continuous social incorporation of slaves in Zanzibari society. The Omani Arab sultanate that ruled Zanzibar in the nineteenth century is not regarded as a colonial oppressor, as it is in state history; rather, it is equated with strong nostalgic tones with an era of true independence characterized by social harmony, economic prosperity and political prestige – this nostalgia for the pre-revolutionary period often relates to narratives about the urban development of Stone Town, early cosmopolitanism and openness to the world.[39] Last, the revolution is not associated with liberation but is considered an illegitimate "invasion" (*mavamizi*) of mainland foreigners who built a new, and detrimental, "colonial" power in Zanzibar.[40]

Rather than race or ethnicity, it is culture which, in *Dira*'s imaginaries of the Zanzibari nation,[41] is promoted as a legitimate marker of Zanzibari identity and political sovereignty. Culture is seen as ways of doing and ways of thinking developed over the centuries and rooted in religious practices (Islam), norms of sociability (from hospitality and friendliness to politeness and etiquette), island-based yet urban and cosmopolitan way of life, and Swahili language correctness. However, in such cultural nationalism which promotes *ustaarabu* (civility), cosmopolitanism and blood-mixing, culture is politicized in the sense that it is used as a criterion for belonging and citizenship as well as for political rights and privileges. If the Zanzibari community imagined by *Dira*'s literati seems to break away from narrow racialist and racist definitions of national identity that have prevailed in official discourses, it nevertheless resorts to an essentialized notion – culture – as a basis for inclusion and exclusion in the Zanzibari *patria*. Thought of as the product of age-old processes, Zanzibari culture could not easily be learned or appropriated – it is constructed as distinct, incommensurable and un-appropriable.[42] Mainlanders remain the "insider outsiders", for whatever their efforts they remain deprived of the adequate Zanzibari culture and *washenzi* (barbarians, uncivilized). The identification assigned to them locally as *Wazanzibara* (*bara* meaning mainland Tanzania in Swahili), an oxymoron built upon an evident dichotomy with *Wazanzibari*, points to their non-belonging. Given that culture is conceived as the criteria for inclusion in the political community, mainland "outsiders" are also deprived of the right to have a say in the political future of the Isles. In this island chauvinist narrative of nationhood, the flattened-out citizenry that the national government sought to create, at least rhetorically, is replaced with parochial politics underpinned by cultural discrimination and political disenfranchisement.

Resurfacing clandestine memories

For a year, *Dira* kept on producing dissenting historical narratives based on the re-reading of past events that have left their mark on the Isles' society. It also resurfaced and publicized personal and family remembrances in relation to the wave of arrests, imprisonments, tortures and assassinations that took place during eight years of autocratic rule under the authority of Abeid Amani Karume and the Committee of 14,[43] until the latter was assassinated in April 1972. Using Myers' typology of memory narratives, it could be said that *Dira* strove to voice, and therefore introduce in the public sphere, the "excluded scripts" of revolutionary Zanzibar, that is, the hidden and silenced personal stories of thousands of ordinary citizens.[44] By prohibiting dissenting comments, complaints or criticisms from the public sphere, the state monopoly of the production of what could be, and could not be, openly said of Karume and his rule has contributed to limiting the recalling of the arbitrary power of the regime within the sphere of family, close friends and former prisoners.[45] With regard to the many imprisonments and assassinations that took place from 1964, very few initiatives have yet taken place to request explanations, public repentance or compensations, be they symbolic or strictly financial. The call made in 1988 by Shaaban Mloo, a CUF founder who became its first Principal Secretary from 1992 to 2000, to incite the government to break the wall of silence and open its archives has remained unanswered.[46] The state has kept stubbornly silent.[47] However, as mentioned above, significant written productions have emerged from the diaspora, particularly from the Arab Peninsula (Oman and Dubai) where thousands of people of Arab origin and ZNP partisans took refuge after fleeing the revolution and during the following years.[48] The latest books and pamphlets make use of a harsher language than the Isles-based political opposition presenting the revolution as an illegitimate "invasion" – in the same way as *Dira* did – sometimes even an "ethnic cleansing", if not "genocide", to denounce the deliberate and selective dimension of the massacres.

From the start, *Dira* made it clear that it would come back to the hidden side of revolutionary Zanzibar by digging up personal, family and group memories. In "Nyerere si Malaika", Ali Nabwa hinted at the disappearing of important figures of the Zanzibari political and intellectual scene: "Until today, the fate of Saleh Sadalah and Hanga is not known, in the same as the fate of Othman Shariff, Mdungi Ussi, Jaha Ubwa, Jimy Ringo…and the list continues".[49] In the pages of the newspaper, the fate of these men was depicted through the eyes of common Zanzibaris, in the first place actors, victims and witnesses of this period, or their descendants. Three family memories were given greater visibility: those of Aboud Nadhif Abdallah, Ali Mzee Mbalia and Muhammed Pandu Yussuf. The first family memory to be published (18–24 July 2003) concerns Aboud Nadhif Abdallah, Principal Secretary in the Ministry of Trade and Industry from 1964 to 1969. Aboud Nadhif Abdallah belonged to the lettered of the Isles who frequented the best schools of Zanzibar before being trained abroad. His son, Ibrahim Aboud Nadhif, recalled in an interview the conditions of arrest of his father that his mother passed on to him and his siblings.[50] The head of state security (or Central Intelligence Directorate) today remembered for his unfailing loyalty to the cruel rulers in power, Hassan Mandera, came in person to arrest Aboud under the pretext that he had refused to return to the post he had been dismissed from some months before. Aboud was imprisoned and never seen again. Interestingly, Aboud Nadhif Abdallah's son, Ibrahim, was not only a regular and enthusiastic reader of *Dira* but knew Ali Nabwa and the other journalists personally. He asserted that he was the one who approached Nabwa with a draft of the article he wanted to have published, knowing that *Dira* was the only media that would accept it. The second memory story, published in the 3–9 October 2003 issue under the title "Alijiuwa kuepuka mateso" (He committed suicide to escape pains/torture), was taken from a prior but not widely circulated publication of 1994. The article tells how Ali Mzee Mbalia, a young man in his mid-twenties, committed suicide after he was arrested and tortured simply because he refused to help a female friend of his to abort, arguing that the father should be the one to take his responsibility. Ali's plight was that it was none other than Brigadier Yusuf Himid – a member of the Committee of 14 who took part in the first Cabinet of the Revolutionary Government in 1964 before being commander of a brigade of the Tanzania's People's Defense Forces – who had made the girl pregnant. This personal story of an anonymous young man illustrates how an arbitrary and extremely violent power could crash down on anyone, even for a peccadillo. The last personal story came in the 31 October–6 November issue. Entitled "Yuko Wapi Muhammad Pandu Yussuf?" (Where is Muhammad Pandu Yussuf?), the article tells about the arrest and disappearance of a Customs Officer through the eyes of his second son, Talib. Today a fisherman in his forties but only aged four at the time of the event, Talib remembers the men who came to his village to cart off his father Muhammad at night, half-dressed with a T-Shirt and a *kikoi* loincloth. According to what Talib told me in an interview, the family has never known the reason that led to the arrest of this respected ASP member and civil servant.

The publication of these three family stories constituted an act of subversion in contemporary Zanzibar. Indeed, they unveiled various facets of the autocratic power that was in place in Zanzibar from 1964–1972. It was a power that silenced well-educated Zanzibaris by kidnapping them and imprisoning them for years until they died, for fear they might raise their voice and foster a radical opposition against the state. It was a power that operated in secret so as to avoid open and massive rebellion and resistance. It was, finally, a power that leaders would confiscate for their personal benefit, not hesitating to use it for trivial matters. Moreover, as sad or scandalous as they might be, these stories embody the hundreds similar events which occurred during this period, targeting people of various backgrounds and origins. In other words, they represented the murky past of the Isles as a whole. It was how *Dira's* journalists and the families that came to them to recall the stories of their fathers, brothers and sons gave sense to their actions. In an interview, Ibrahim Aboud Nadhif, son of Aboud Nadhif Abdallah, told me he hoped that the mediatization of his painful family story would make other families speak out and similar tragic stories resurface publicly, so as to lead, in the end, to a large-scale public debate on the revolutionary decade in Zanzibar. Public repentance, if not individual financial compensations, were on the horizon of this man who mentioned the work of Truth and Reconciliation commissions in various countries to assert his claims.

Dira did not publish in detail stories of high-ranking politicians who also met with tragic fates, such as the renowned Kassim Hanga, Othman Shariff or Abdulaziz Twala, all ex-members of the ASP who occupied various major positions in the government: Kassim Hanga was the deputy general secretary of the ASP before becoming the vice-president of the People's Republic of Zanzibar, and then occupying different posts in the Union ministries; Othman Shariff was made Minister of Education and Culture in the first Revolutionary Council of the People's Republic of Zanzibar, then ambassador of the United Republic of Tanzania in Washington after April 1964; last, Abdulaziz Twala was Minister of Finance. The three men were considered dangerous by the new state, first of all by Karume himself who feared lettered politicians and civil servants able to articulate critical political views and mobilize the population for alternative government options. Many among this intelligentsia "disappeared" during the Karume years and rumours keep on circulating about how Hanga, Sheriff and Twala were murdered in 1971.[51] Yet, by the end of 2003, *Dira* published photos of the three men together with about 10 photos of other prominent political figures who had disappeared from 1964 to 1972. The article briefly retold the stories of these men and denounced the silence of the government on what happened to them. Touching upon the fate of these renowned political figures in the Isles could not pass unnoticed.

Dira's readership was aware of the potential disruption that could ensue from the emergence of competing narratives of a traumatic past in a society where many families bear the marks of this turbulent period, either as victims or as perpetrators, and in some cases as both. The elite feared that the public circulation of alternative historical narratives of the revolution and the Union lead to a general state of confusion, if not unrest. They even more feared it since, beyond the state ideological rhetoric of the social revolutionary for the masses, many among the contemporary political and socioeconomic elite are the children or the grandchildren of the stalwarts of the early revolutionary period in a state where nepotism rather than democratic processes rules – the Karume family being the first beneficiary of this state of affairs. During *Dira's* lifetime, in 2002–2003, the incumbent President of Zanzibar, Amani Karume, was the son of the first president Abeid Karume; another of Abeid Karume's sons, Ali Karume, was Ambassador in Italy – his name appeared in *Dira's* articles accusing him of having raped Arab young girls during his teenage-hood; and other members of the Karume family hold strategic economic positions and sustain clientelist networks. Delving into the dark past was, consequently, not writing about another country, as the saying goes, but about contemporary politics in Zanzibar. It meant questioning the legitimacy of the current political elite to rule in a situation where the state-citizens moral contract has been abandoned. In view of this, it is less surprising to observe that, although academic historiography about the Karume's decade generally devotes a few sentences to the dark side of the regime, there has been no major work that has yet focused on it only or depicted it in depth.[52] Official biographies of Karume or political declarations, speeches and notes referring to him have always consisted in hagiographic and laudatory productions.[53] The past must remain untouchable if the status quo of the present is to be maintained. That *Dira* was writing about the present through an exploration of the past also explains why attacking the state narrative about the Union amounted to undermining the concrete mechanism through which the elite has been able to retain power until today.[54] The newspaper did not simply go too far in its accusation against the authoritarian nature of the first regime: it jeopardized the very foundations upon which the revolutionary heirs have remained in power.

The life and death of *Dira*

The popular success of the newspaper is widely depicted. The assertion that the pages of *Dira* would never be used to wrap doughnuts ("*Dira halitafungiwa maandazi*") – a common practice among street food sellers – was mentioned several times over the course of the research to highlight the gazette's popularity. Many common people interviewed insisted that they had stored copies of *Dira* at home, pointing with their finger to the place in the house, a room or an attic, where the newspapers were kept. Journalists explained that *Dira* first had a print run of about 1400 copies (among them about 1000 sold) at the end of 2002 but gained a circulation of 10,000 sold copies in Zanzibar and 2000 on the Mainland in 2003.[55] The following anecdote was also recalled several times to illustrate the newspaper's great popularity: one Friday, the boat transporting newspapers from Dar es Salaam to Zanzibar arrived late.[56] At Masomo bookshop where, until today, newspapers are delivered in the late morning then directly sold or dispatched to other bookshops and street-sellers, a crowd of people gathered impatiently waiting for the newspaper to be delivered. They almost stormed the shop when *Dira* arrived in the late afternoon that day. Groups of people were seen sitting together at coffee stands or other popular gathering points, reading and commenting on a copy of the newspaper.[57] Although collective reading is a common practice in all Sub-Saharan African countries, it is said that it had never been seen before at such a level in Zanzibar, and was never seen again after the ban on *Dira*. The success of the newspaper is also reflected by the fact that numerous anonymous or non-anonymous articles were sent for publication to the Editor's desk by common citizens, sometimes from abroad, or by politicians of various statuses. Ibrahim Hussein, a former Umma Party sympathizer who spent 8 years in prison after the treason trial that followed the assassination of President Karume, and who later left the Isles, contributed with articles about the Union. Biographies of important Muslim figures and life stories of the lettered of the Isles were written by the well-known late Maalim Idris Saleh. Some CCM politicians, anonymously or not, even sent articles denouncing the party's internal affairs. As explained by *Dira*'s journalists, it is the ever-increasing participation of citizens that kept the newspaper alive as the team could not have carried forward the newspaper single-handedly.

The success of *Dira* was explained in the pages of the newspaper on the ground that it was the first Zanzibari post-revolutionary newspaper that expressed the voices of the common people. As a journalist put it: "*Dira* is the voice of the people and not the Master's voice",[58] the latter being embodied by the state-owned *Zanzibar Leo*. All CUF sympathizers and many non-partisan Zanzibaris interviewed expressed a similar idea, saying that *Dira* was a "popular platform" (*jukwaa la jamii*) or a "breathing space" and underlying how they now missed the newspaper – no similar newspaper has yet re-appeared. Many also perceived *Dira* as an informative gazette that taught silenced or distorted history. Many interlocutors, from the lettered to the less educated, insisted that the newspaper contributed to enlighten citizens and give them the means to think by themselves with adequate information in hand – a credo that ran through the pages of the weekly. However, more than its informative quality or troublemaking character, it is the resonance between the journalists' political subjectivities and a collective moral economy based on expected reciprocal rights and prerogatives between the state and citizens that accounts for the popularity of the newspaper. *Dira* made waves because it brought to the open the abandonment of the implicit moral contract binding the state and citizens.

Yet, among many CCM grassroots members or sympathizers, *Dira* is not remembered with nostalgia at all. For example, the CCM stalwarts sitting at the *maskani* called Kizota in Darajani area recall the newspaper as a sheer rag that published wrong and calumnious news with the intention to foster division between political parties and among the population. In their words, *uchokozi* (troublemaking, provocation) is not positively connoted nor associated with freedom of speech, legitimate opposition, even less expression of truth. On the contrary, when discussing *Dira*'s objectives, the term *uchokozi* was made part of a lexical field about divisions and discord which included terms recurrently used to depict the endless political battlefield in the Isles, such as *chokochoko* (provocation), *migogoro* (dispute), *mgongano* (dispute), *kugawa* (to divide) and, encompassing all others and extremely pejorative, *fitna* (dissension, intrigue). *Dira* was not only accused of fuelling existing tensions, if not violence, but also of presenting a biased and distorted version of history. As an active Kizota CCM supporter said, people should leave the past with the past, as painful as it might be; and considering that it is the role of a state to maintain stability and security, the banning of *Dira* was said to be the only means to prevent the politics of hatred that the newspaper was fuelling from badly affecting society.

The team of *Dira* did not have to wait long for state reaction. The first significant attack against the newspaper personally targeted the Chief Editor. Of Comorian origins, Nabwa was suddenly and arbitrarily declared a non-citizen, just a few years after he was officially granted Zanzibari citizenship.[59] The second attack was radical: it consisted in banning the newspaper. Only one year after its birth, in December 2003, *Dira* was closed by the Government on the allegation that it violated "professional ethics" by publishing slanders and false assertions against the government[60], therefore fomenting hatred within society. On 3 December 2003, the Media Council of Tanzania circulated a brief to counter accusations that this national body for the surveillance of the national media would be involved in a conspiracy with the Government of Zanzibar in order to ban *Dira*. The brief quoted the official complaints of the Government of Zanzibar: "*Dira* was carrying out a campaign of incitement by publishing stories aimed at undermining peace and security by selectively digging up parts of the Zanzibar history, notably the 1964

Revolution; *Dira* was unethical in that it omitted to balance controversial stories; *Dira* was engaging in incitement by challenging the legality of the Government and President Amani Karume".[61] *Dira* was undeniably perceived as a threat by the national authorities. It was finally dead and buried in December 2003, its oration being made by Zanzibar's Deputy Chief Minister and Minister for Information, Culture and Sports, Ali Juma Shamhuna who declared that *"Gazeti la* Dira *siyo tu kwamba limefungiwa. Kwa hakika hili limezikwa kabisa"* (It is not as if *Dira* newspaper had just been closed. With certainty it is completely buried.).

Conclusion

Dira illustrates the role of print culture in constituting public spheres and nationalisms, a phenomenon that was not confined to Europe[62] but also concerned the rest of the world, notably the Indian Ocean world.[63] Similarly to pre-independence newspapers, this weekly contributed to (re)inventing Zanzibari nationhood. It did so, however, by following in the footsteps of earlier Zanzibari nationalists who, for years, had deployed the rhetoric of coastal chauvinism and cultural nativist distinctiveness that shaped the political subjectivities of Zanzibaris. *Dira*'s nationalist entrepreneurship developed its homespun historiography by delving into the most polarizing period in Zanzibar, the Revolution of 1964 and the authoritarian decade that followed. Journalists committed themselves to both rewriting the history of the period and voice vivid family memories of violence, therefore working to "reconstitute the revolution as a 'chosen trauma' in the current political drama".[64] *Dira*'s civic and political agendas were made explicit, namely, to expand the boundaries of the public sphere and challenge the elite in power, heirs of the leaders of the Revolution. Even though the commitment of these architects of renewed patriotism did not translate into an actual shift in power from CCM to CUF, the fact that they used ideas that were consonant with ordinary citizens, which were drawn from a repertoire of pervasive social and cultural motifs, and were adapted to fit issues of concern at that time, explains the gazette's high popularity and impact on ordinary imaginaries of the nation. Despite the fact that the page of *Dira* was turned when the newspaper was banned, and that no other similar newspaper took its place, the early post-revolution history is still well alive in Zanzibar as a political tool, if not increasingly significant in the current political debates and discussions about the Union at all levels of society.

Notes

1. The violent overthrow of the constitutional monarchy of Zanzibar on 11–12 January 1964, one month only after independence from the British protectorate powers, is referred to as a "Revolution" in state terminology and in academic historiography. This article will show and explain why this qualification is contested today.
2. Fieldwork was partly funded by the *Institut Français de Recherche en Afrique* (IFRA), Nairobi, Kenya. It was conducted from November 2008 to January 2009, and in summer 2009. I wish to thank Professor Abdul Sheriff for his comments on the first version of this paper, as well as Ally Saleh and Ismail Jussa, both former members of *Dira*, for their critical reading of the text and additional inputs. My sincere thanks also go to William C. Bissell for his insightful comments and to the two anonymous reviewers of the journal.
3. Although this article focuses on historical narratives and political discourses, we argue that discourse analysis only makes sense if it is related to contemporary forms of economic processes and the exercise of power, or in other words, if it is part of a political economy of

contemporary Zanzibar, similarly to Frederick Cooper's book of reference, *From Slaves to Squatters* on nineteenth/early twentieth century Zanzibari society.

4. The years from 1965 to 1972 correspond to the period of authoritarianism under President Abeid Karume, assassinated on 7 April 1972. A gradual relaxation of power occurred in spite of the maintaining of arbitrary rule and enduring control over the freedom of expression until today.
5. Burgess, "Memories, Myth and Meanings"; Fouéré, "Sortie de clandestinité"; Loimeier, "Memories of Revolution"; Myers, "Narrative Representations".
6. I borrow the term *patria* from Lonsdale, "Writing Competitive Patriotisms", that relates to the concept of "moral ethnicity" as a shared ethos of the legitimate and the illegitimate, the just and the unjust, shaping communal representations and orientating practices (Lonsdale, "The Moral Economy").
7. Myers, "Narrative Representations".
8. See, for example, Babakerim, *The Aftermath*; Fairooz, *Ukweli ni huu*; Ghassany, *Kwaheri Ukoloni*; Muhsin, *Conflicts and Harmony*.
9. If we except, from 1992, *Jukwaa* (Plateform) and *Maarifa* (Knowledge, that took its name after a well-known weekly published from 1952 to 1964), but none of them were critical to the government.
10. The Zanzibar Newspaper Act of 1988 empowers the President to suspend or ban 'foreign' publications considered as a threat to the Isles' peace and unity, hence high control over publications from the mainland.
11. The first issue of the weekly *Mwongozi* (The Leader) came off the presses in 1941. It ceased publication after the revolution when the Editor, Ahmed S. Kharusi, fled the country. The paper was an open supporter of the Arab Association and gained a regular circulation of 1000 copies. See Sturmer, *The Media History* and Hamdani, "Zanzibar Newspapers".
12. Lofchie, *Zanzibar*, 210.
13. Glassman, *War of Words*.
14. Myers, "Narrative representations", 430.
15. Ismail Jussa was elected member of the House of Representatives for the Stone Town constituency in the 2010 general election.
16. Mohamed Ghassany openly joined CUF in late 2009. He actively contributed to the party's activities after the rapprochement (*maridhiano*) between President Karume and opposition leader Seif Shariff Hamad in November 2009, most notably during the referendum campaign for the formation of a government of national unity in July 2010. He suspended his activities when he started working for Deutsche Welle in Germany in September 2010.
17. For the significance of historical experience more than race or ethnic identity in shaping generational identity and political positions in Zanzibar, see Burgess, "An Imagined Generation".
18. See Burgess, "An Imagined Generation".
19. During an interview, one journalist recalled writing the name of the ZPPP/ZNP party – at that time perceived by a majority of Zanzibaris as the anti-African party of the Arab elite – in the sand in his schoolyard when he was a child; because of this, he was beaten by his schoolmates. ZPPP means the Zanzibar and Pemba People's Party and ZNP the Zanzibar Nationalist Party.
20. Burgess, "Cinema, Bell Bottoms, and Miniskirts"; Burgess, "The Young Pioneers".
21. Ferguson, *Expectation of modernity* – the phrase refers to hopes for a society built upon political morality, economic justice and social equity that pre-independence nationalist mobilisations had raised among citizens.
22. Cameron, "Narratives of Democracy"; Rawlence, "Briefing"; Bakari, *The Democratization Process*.
23. Stürmer, *The Media History*.
24. See among others Clayton, *The Zanzibar Revolution*; Lofchie, *Zanzibar: Background to a Revolution*; Martin, *Zanzibar: Tradition and Revolution*.
25. About the production of Nyerere as a political icon since his death in 1999, see Askew, "Sung and Unsung"; Fouéré, "Tanzanie".
26. See Caplan and Topan, *Swahili Modernities*.

27. About the fear of the growing influence of Communism in Zanzibar in the context of the Cold War, see Wilson, *US Foreign Policy*; Speller, "An African Cuba?"; Petterson, *An American's Cold War Tale*; and the recently-opened CIA archives by Hunter, *Zanzibar: The Hundred Days Revolution*.
28. For a detailed presentation of the driving forces that led to the formation of the Union, which are only sketched out here, see, for example, Shivji, *Pan-Africanism*, 69–99.
29. *Dira*, "Nyerere si Malaika (part III)", 20–26 December 2002, p. 4. The oft-quoted sentence "If I could tow that island out into the middle of the Indian Ocean, I'll do it", which first appeared in Smith, *Nyerere of Tanzania*, p. 90, appears in publications arguing that Zanzibar was a burden to Nyerere.
30. See Shivji, *Pan-Africanism*, 123, who asserts that "official historiography repeats *ad nauseam* that Karume was a Union enthusiast. Nothing could be further from the truth. If there was one thing that Zanzibaris venerate Karume for, in spite of his despotic rule, it is Karume's Zanzibariness and his dogged resistance to get integrated into the Union and lose Zanzibar autonomy."
31. Bailey, *The Union of Tanganyika and Zanzibar*; Shivji, *The Legal Foundations of the Union*; Othman and Peter, *Zanzibar and the Union Question*. Since the formation of the Government of National Unity in Zanzibar in October 2010, the Union issue has come to the front again and various political actors are advocating for a complete revision of the Union treaty.
32. Glassman, *War of Words*.
33. In this paragraph presenting racial nationalism which emerged during the period called the "time of politics" (*zama za siasa*) from 1957–1963 and was reproduced after 1964, I use the recent historiography on revolutionary Zanzibar and competing nationalisms, most notably Glassman, *War of Words*; Shivji, *Pan-Africanism*; Myers, "Revolutionary Zanzibar"), some of which Nabwa explicitly uses – he quotes his references – and conflates with his own personal memory. I do not present here the extensively studied 1957–1963 period.
34. The last census before the Revolution, in 1948, gives the racial distribution of the population, counting 264,059 inhabitants: 16.9% Arabs, 5.8% Indians, 1.1% Comorians, and 75.7% Africans (24% from the mainland; 74% native, that is, Shirazis). See Lofchie, *Zanzibar*, 71.
35. Sheriff, "Race and Class."
36. Myers, "Narrative representations", 438. Mapuri's book, *The 1964 Revolution*, published in 1996, is said to exemplify this new trend that articulates autochthony, blackness, African-ness and political legitimacy.
37. See Amory, "The politics of identity", 116, who reminds us that Karume had some 18,000 Zanzibaris sign declarations saying: "I am not Shirazi, and I don't even know the meaning of Shirazi identity."
38. Glassman, *War of Words*.
39. Bissell, "Engaging Colonial Nostalgia"; Presthold, *Domesticating*.
40. The term appears in most of the patriotic literature on Zanzibar. The latest title in date is Harith Ghassany's *Kwaheri Ukoloni* that, compiling personal accounts of the planning of the Revolution, asserts that the Revolution was neither a popular uprising nor a state overthrow led by Zanzibaris but a coup organized by the mainland top leaders. It argues that the end of colonialism (the first part of the book title, *Kwaheri Ukoloni*, meaning "goodbye colonialism") ironically did not equate with independence, but with the end of independence (the second part of the title, *Kwaheri Uhuru*, meaning "goodbye freedom").
41. Anderson, *Imagined Community*.
42. Such a reified conception of culture obviously goes against today's academic conceptions of culture and identity as changing, multivalent and malleable, as Laura Fair's *Pastimes & Politics* skilfully demonstrates in the case of Zanzibar.
43. The Committee of 14, gathering instigators and leaders of the 1964 Revolution, was the decisional power within the Revolutionary Council formed in 31 January 1964.
44. Myers, "Revolutionary Zanzibar".

45. An early exception is Kharusi, *Africa's First Cuba*, 41–44, that provides accounts of massacres of Arabs perpetrated by mainlanders, but this account is partial as this partisan piece of work is characterized by its pro-Arab and anti-mainlander stances.
46. Crozon, "Zanzibar en Tanzanie", 226.
47. Only Bakari, *The Democratisation Process*, 109, mentions in endnote 29 that Karume's successor, Aboud Jumbe, hinted at the fact that the "disappeared" were no longer alive: "The first time the authorities confessed that those who had mysteriously disappeared had been killed was in 1975 when Sheikh Aboud Jumbe told the ITV's 'World in Action', who had visited Zanzibar and interviewed him, that: 'They [Hanga, Othman Shariff, Twala, Muhammed Humud, Juma Maringo, Mdungi Ussi, Saleh Sadalah, Abdul Madhifu (sic)] have not vanished.' '...they have paid the price of revolution'...'They are dead, yes'."
48. Thousands of people of foreign origin (Arabs most of them, but also Comorians and Indians) fled the island – or were expelled – to escape the uncontrolled killings and the arbitrary decisions, endless humiliations and repressive measures against the supposedly "non-African" populations.
49. Nabwa, "Nyerere si Malaika-III", 4: "*Hadi leo khatima ya Saleh Sadalah na Hanga haijulikani, kama isivyojulikana khatima ya Othman Shariff, Mdungi Ussi, Jaha Ubwa, Jimy Ringo...na orodha inaendelea.*"
50. For a detailed presentation of the life story of the Nadhifs, see Fouéré, "Sortie de clandestinité".
51. See Fouéré, "Sortie de clandestinité", 109–110; Shivji, *Pan-Africanism*, 118; Crozon, "Zanzibar en Tanzanie", 232–235.
52. However, a greater attention to the authoritarian rule under Karume is noticeable in recent works. See, for example, Shivji, *Pan-Africanism*, 106–117.
53. For example, Mwanjisi, *Ndugu Abeid Amani Karume*.
54. Cameron, "Narratives of Democracy"; Rawlence, "Briefing."
55. Figures vary according to interlocutors.
56. The newspaper was edited and laid-out in the tiny *Dira* office in Stone Town but sent to Dar es Salaam for printing – one member of the team, usually the Sales Manager Salim Said Salim, being in charge of bringing a burned CD of the coming issue by plane. Printed issues reached the Isles every Friday.
57. Personal communication, Prof. Abdul Sheriff, 27 July 2010.
58. "*Dira ni sauti ya watu badala ya kuwa sauti ya bwana* (Master's voice)", *Dira*, 31 October–6 November 2003 (by Hasnul N.A. Riyamy, p. 2). He goes on: "*Kuja kwa Dira kumeleta muamko mpya (...). Muamko huo umeletwa na ukweli kwamba* Dira *husema kile ambacho jamii inataka kisemwe; kile ambacho jamii ilikifutika moyoni mwao; kile ambacho watawala hawakutaka kiwekwe bayana*" ("The coming of *Dira* brought a new awakening (...). This awakening has come from the truth that Dira says this that the people want to be said; this that the people buried in their hearts; this that the leaders do not want to be said openly").
59. Not only has much ink been spilled over the issue of Ali Nabwa's citizenship in the pages of *Dira*, but the attack against Nabwa was reminiscent of the endless persecution of the Comorian community since 1964. See, for example, Mohamed, "Les Comoriens de Zanzibar".
60. In its last issue, *Dira* published the letter from the Department of Information which stated that the newspaper would be banned on the ground that its articles published "*taarifa potofu, masengenya na kejeli*" (distorted news, slander and calumnies), *Dira*, 21–27 November 2003, p. 9, issue 51.
61. MCT (by its Executive Secretary Anthony Ngaiza), "A brief on the position of the Media Council of Tanzania", 3 December 2003, p. 2.
62. Anderson, *Imagined Communities*; Gellner, *Nations and Nationalism*.
63. See special issue on "Print Culture, Nationalisms and Publics of the Indian Ocean", *Africa* 81, no. 1 (2011).
64. Glassman, *War of Words*, 296.

References

Amory, Deborah Peters. "The Politics of Identity on Zanzibar." PhD diss., Stanford University, 1994.

Anderson, Benedict. *Imagined Communities: Reflections on the Origin and Spread of Nationalism*. London: Verso, 1983.

Askew, Kelly. "Sung and Unsung: Musical Reflections on Tanzanian Postsocialisms." *Africa* 76, no. 1 (2006): 15–43.

Babakerim. *The Aftermath of Zanzibar Revolution*. Muscat Printing Press (self-published), 1994.

Bailey, Martin. *The Union of Tanganyika and Zanzibar: A Study in Political Integration*. Syracuse, NY: Syracuse University Press, 1973.

Bakari, Mohammed A. *The Democratization Process in Zanzibar: A Retarded Transition*. Hamburg: Institut für Afrika-Kunde, 2001.

al-Barwani, Sauda A., R. Feindt, L. Gerhardt, L. Harding, and L. Wimmelbücker. *Unser Leben vor der Revolution und danach – Maisha yetu kabla ya Mapinduzi na baadaye. Autobiographische Dokumentartexte sansibarischer Zeitzeugen*. Köln: Köppe Verlag, 2003.

Bissell, William C. "Engaging Colonial Nostalgia." *Cultural Anthropology* 20, no. 2 (2005): 215–48.

Burgess, Thomas G. "Cinema, Bell Bottoms, and Miniskirts: Struggles over Youth and Citizenship in Revolutionary Zanzibar." *International Journal of African Historical Studies* 35, no. 2–3 (2002): 287–314.

Burgess, Thomas G. "An Imagined Generation: Umma Youth in Nationalist Zanzibar." In *In Search of a Nation. Histories of Authority and Dissidence in Tanzania*, ed. Gregory H. Maddox, and James L. Giblin, 216–49. Oxford: James Currey Ltd, 2005.

Burgess, Thomas G. "The Young Pioneers and Rituals of Citizenship in Revolutionary Zanzibar." *Africa Today* 51, no. 3 (2005): 3–29.

Burgess, Thomas G. "Memories, Myth and Meanings of the Zanzibari Revolution." In *War and Peace in Africa*, ed. Toyin Falola, and Raphael C. Njoku, 429–50. Durham: Carolina Academic Press, 2010.

Cameron, Greg. "Narratives of Democracy and Dominance in Zanzibar." In *Knowledge, Renewal and Religion. Repositioning and Changing Ideological and Material Circumstances among the Swahili on the East African Coast*, ed. Kjersti Larsen, 151–76. Uppsala: Nordiska Afrikainstitutet, 2009.

Caplan, Pat, and Farouk Topan, ed. *Swahili Modernities: Culture, Politics and Identity on the East Coast of Africa*. Trento, NJ: Africa World Press, 2004.

Clayton, Anthony. *The Zanzibar Revolution and its Aftermath*. London: C. Hurst & Company, 1981.

Cooper, Frederick *From Slaves to Squatters. Plantation Labor and Agriculture in Zanzibar and Coastal Kenya, 1980–1925*. New Haven & London: Yale University Press, 1987.

Crozon, Ariel. "Zanzibar en Tanzanie. Essai d'histoire politique." PhD in Political Science, Université de Pau et de l'Adour, 1992.

Fair, Laura. *Pastimes and Politics. Culture, Community and Identity in Post-Abolition Urban Zanzibar, 1890–1945*. Oxford: James Currey, 2001.

Fairooz, Amani T. *Ukweli ni huu. Kuusuta uwongo*. Dubai, 1995.

Ferguson, James. *Expectations of Modernity. Myths and Meanings of Urban Life on the Zambian Copperbelt*. Berkeley & Los Angeles: University of California, 1999.

Fouéré, Marie-Aude. "Tanzanie: La nation à l'épreuve du postsocialisme." *Politique Africaine* 121 (2011): 69–85.

Fouéré, Marie-Aude. "Sortie de clandestinité des années sombres à Zanzibar (1964-1975)." *Cahiers d'études Africaines* 197 (2010): 95–122.

Gellner, Ersnt. *Nations and Nationalism*. Oxford: Blackwell, 1983.

Ghassany, Harith. *Kwaheri Ukoloni, kwaheri Uhuru! Zanzibar na Mapinduzi Afrabia*. Anno Domini, 2010.

Glassman, Jonathon. "Sorting out the tribes; the creation of racial identities in colonial Zanzibar's newspaper wars." *Journal of African History* 41 (2000): 395–428.

Glassman, Jonathon. "Slower Than a Massacre: The Multiple Sources of Racial Thought in Colonial Africa." *The American Historical Review* 109, no. 3 (2004): 720–54.

Glassman, Jonathon. *War of Words, War of Stones. Racial Thought and Violence in Colonial Zanzibar*. Bloomington and Indianapolis: Indiana University Press, 2011.

Hamdani, Mariam. "Zanzibar Newspapers, 1902 to 1974." Diploma thesis, Tanzania School of Journalism, 1981.

Hunter, Helen-Louise. *Zanzibar. The Hundred Days Revolution*. Santa Barbara: ABC-CLIO, 2010.

Kharusi, Ahmed S. *Zanzibar: Africa's First Cuba. A Case Study of the New Colonialism*. Richmond: Zanzibar Organisation, 1967.

Lofchie, Michael F. *Zanzibar: Background to Revolution*. Princeton: Princeton University Press, 1965.

Loimeier, R. "Memories of Revolution: Zur Deutungsgeschischte einer Revolution (Sansibar 1964)." *Afrika Spectrum* 41, no. 2 (2006): 175–97.

Lonsdale, John. "Writing Competitive Patriotisms in Eastern Africa." In *Recasting the Past. History Writing and Political Work in Modern Africa*, ed. Derek R. Peterson, and Giacomo Macola. Athens, OH: Ohio University Press, 2009.

Lonsdale, John. "The Moral Economy of Mau Mau." In *Unhappy Valley: Conflict in Kenya and Africa*, ed. Bruce Berman, and John Lonsdale, 265–504. London: James Currey, 1992.

Mapuri, Omar. *The 1964 Revolution: Achievements and Prospects*. Dar es Salaam: Tema Publishers, 1996.

Martin, Esmond B. *Zanzibar: Tradition and Revolution*. London: Hamish Hamilton, 1978.

Mohamed, Toibibou A. "Les Comoriens de Zanzibar durant la 'Révolution Okello' (1964–1972). La xénophobie de la République." *Journal des Africanistes* 76 (2006) 2: 137–54.

Muhsin, Ali. *Conflicts and Harmony in Zanzibar, Memoirs*. Dubai, 2002.

Mwanjisi, Rungwe K. *Ndugu Abeid Amani Karume*. Nairobi: EAPH, 1967.

Myers, Garth A. "Narrative Representations of Revolutionary Zanzibar." *Journal of Historical Geography* 26, no. 3 (2000): 429–48.

Nabwa, Ali. *From the Gallows to the Firing Squad. A True Life Drama*. (n/p), 2003.

Othman, Haroub, and Chris M. Peter. *Zanzibar and the Union Question*. Zanzibar: Zanzibar Legal Services Centre, 2006.

Petterson, Don. *An American's Cold War Tale. Revolution in Zanzibar*. Boulder, Colorado: Westview Press, 2002.

Presthold, Jeremy. *Domesticating the World: African Consumerism and the Genealogies of Globalization*. Berkeley: University of California Press, 2008.

Rawlence, Ben. "Briefing: The Zanzibar Election." *African Affairs* 104, no. 416 (2005): 515–23.

Sheriff, Abdul. "Race and Class in Zanzibar." *Afrika Spectrum* 36, no. 3 (2001): 301–18.

Shivji, Issa G. *The Legal Foundations of the Union in Tanzania's Union and Zanzibar Constitutions*. Dar es Salaam: Dar es Salaam University Press, 1990.

Shivji, Issa G. *Pan-Africanism or Pragmatism? Lessons of Tanganyika–Zanzibar Union*. Dar es Salaam: Mkuki na Nyota/Addis Abeba: OSSREA, 2008.

Smith, William E. *We Must Run While They Walk. A Portrait of Africa's Julius Nyerere*. New York: Random House, 1971.

Speller, Ian. "An African Cuba? Britain and the Zanzibar Revolution, 1964." *Journal of Imperial and Commonwealth History* 35, no. 2 (2007): 1–35.

Stürmer, Martin. *The Media History of Tanzania*. Ndanda: Ndanda Mission Press, 1998.

Werbner, Richard. "Beyond Oblivion: Confronting Memory Crisis." In *Memory and the Postcolony: African Anthropology and the Critique of Power*, ed. Richard Werbner, 1–17. London: Zed Books, 1998.

Wilson, Amrit. *US Foreign Policy and Revolution: The Creation of Tanzania*. London: Pluto Press, 1989.

Medicines of hope? The tough decision for anti-retroviral use for HIV in Zanzibar, Tanzania

Nadine Beckmann

Institute of Social and Cultural Anthropology, University of Oxford, Oxford, UK

The provision of free anti-retroviral treatment for AIDS in Zanzibar since March 2005 is the result of enormous struggles at a global scale and has provided immense relief for sufferers. At the same time, the new "medicines of hope", as they quickly became known, have produced new uncertainties about how best to respond to HIV/AIDS, both for the infected individual and for the society at large. ART programmes make possible a biologised, pharmaceutical life. Drawing on three case studies this paper shows how HIV-positive people struggle to make decisions in an environment characterised by deep uncertainties about the nature and causes of HIV/AIDS in particular, and about the continuity of Zanzibari society in general. It argues that health interventions cannot be orientated to "life itself"; they must be attuned to the contexts in which life takes place. Analysing people's actions and behaviours in the context of their lives-as-lived throws light onto apparently irrational decisions and emphasises the importance of an in-depth understanding of local moral worlds and social contexts.

Introduction

Responding to intense activist mobilisation, the past decade has seen a significant turn in the global response to HIV/AIDS: while in the 1980s and 1990s approaches to HIV/AIDS in low-income countries had strongly focussed on prevention, and anti-retroviral treatment (ART) was regarded as economically and logistically unfeasible, by the early 2000s intense activism had succeeded in redefining treatment access as being a moral imperative and a public health necessity.[1] As a result, in December 2001, UNAIDS for the first time publicly announced its support for anti-retroviral treatment for all in need. Generic drug production had radically lowered the cost of treatment, and new funding instruments were created in a concerted effort to roll out free anti-retroviral treatment of AIDS in the global South.

Over the first decade of the twenty-first century, resources made available for anti-retrovirals (ARVs) have vastly expanded, and funding streams rapidly shifted from prevention towards treatment since the first mass ART programmes were started. By the end of 2011, approximately eight million people were on anti-retroviral treatment,[2] out of an estimated 14.8 million in immediate need. However, the epidemic continues to be outpaced by the rate of new infections, and funding for

AIDS interventions has started to flat-line. As the sustainability of widespread long-term treatment becomes increasingly questionable, new solutions are called for, and recent debates about 'treatment as prevention' have demonstrated growing enthusiasm for finding a pharmaceutical solution for AIDS, both through renewed commitment to finding a cure for AIDS[3] and through intensifying treatment coverage and the more strategic use of ART, including the prophylactic treatment of HIV-negative people classified as being at high risk of becoming infected.[4]

This shift from prevention and clinical care towards an increasing emphasis on access to drugs is indicative of a broader trend towards a pharmaceuticalisation in the realm of public health.[5] But while anti-retrovirals may first have appeared as magic bullets in the fight against AIDS, recent studies on ART[6] and on other mass drug administration programmes[7] have demonstrated manifold problems with access, adherence, and monitoring and evaluation of such programmes. Allen and Parker[8] in their analysis of widely varying rates of treatment uptake for neglected tropical diseases (NTDs) point to the importance of differences in socio-economic contexts and highlight patients' concerns about side effects, the rationale for treatment (particularly in the absence of symptoms), and barriers to drug access due to implementation design. Many of these concerns resemble those encountered in the treatment of AIDS.

At the same time, anti-retroviral treatment poses additional problems, due to its long-term nature and the importance of adherence to a strict treatment regimen. For the first time, large-scale, complex, lifelong treatment for the management of a chronic disease has been implemented in low-income countries, and many of the issues that arise are comparable to those known from the management of chronic conditions elsewhere, including the difficulty of adjusting life to the treatment regimen, treatment fatigue, the ambiguity of people who are sick but fit at the same time, and their constant uncertainty about what they are capable of in the face of the ebbing and surging of symptoms and side effects. Moreover, biomedical management of chronic conditions creates tensions between individuality and sociality:[9] medication and recommendations about healthy lifestyles focus on the individual and tend to overlook the difficulty of making special arrangements for one household member, especially in the presence of poverty and generally high levels of ill health, as experienced by many of my informants. These issues highlight the embeddedness of treatment uptake and outcomes in social processes and the need for strong social support in the management of long-term conditions.

Yet, treatment programmes that focus predominantly on drug access rely heavily on the construction of an individual self who is responsible for their own health and promote a notion of life that is chiefly biological, concerned with physical survival, or "life itself"[10] above all else. This contrasts sharply with my informants' views on the treatment. While obviously concerned about survival, they emphasise their social and moral personae whose actions and experiences are profoundly impacted upon by their social contexts and local moral worlds. Their notion of life is one more akin to what Fassin has called "life as such":

> The course of events which occurs from birth to death, which can be shortened by political or structural violence, which can be prolonged by health and social policies, which give place to cultural interpretations and moral decisions, which may be told or written – life which is lived through a body (not only through cells) and as a society (not only as species).[11]

Such life-as-it-is-lived is a dynamic process, rather than a biological given, operated through discourses, programmes, decisions and actions which invoke and rework a situated form of moral reasoning in order to provide a possible guide to action.[12]

Anti-retroviral treatment

The struggle for access to anti-retroviral treatment in low-income countries has been long and arduous, and is far from over. Debates ranged from economic feasibility to patent issues, generic drug production and quality control, the problems of ensuring treatment adherence and widespread access in areas that lacked infrastructure, qualified personnel, and storage and distribution facilities. Throughout, it was assumed that demand was not going to be a problem. On the contrary, it was feared that demand would be so high that already overburdened health care centres would not be able to cope with the wave of people in need for treatment. And indeed, in many places this is exactly what happened. In the early days of treatment rollout, for example, clinics in Dar es Salaam had to decline new patients, and since 2010 drug shortages were reported in several sub-Saharan African countries.

When free ART was introduced in Zanzibar, a small island archipelago off the Tanzanian coast, in March 2005, it met a population that was largely "treatment-naïve": within weeks, HIV-positive people went from the occasional provision of paracetamol and anti-fungal creams to access to state-of-the-art medication that most had not even known existed. It was a historic point in time that would shape HIV-positive people's lives significantly: the "drugs of hope", as they quickly became known in Zanzibar, would bring back to life those who were almost dead and offer the prospect of a future as "normal", productive and reproductive members of society. And yet the intense excitement that one may have expected was lacking. Overall the treatment programme here has been successful, and members of ZAPHA+, the islands only support group for HIV-positive people, were excited about the prospect of treatment becoming available. However, when talking to my informants individually, I found that many were cautious about coming forward for treatment and were carefully weighing their options.

From the perspective of public health experts and medical doctors, treatment literacy – defined as "the capacity to interpret information about HIV/AIDS prevention, testing and care",[13] which includes the commitment to biomedical "explanatory models"[14] and ideally a process of conversion into responsible, active patient-citizens ready to stick to their side of their "treatment contract"[15] – is the single most important factor in ensuring correct anti-retroviral treatment adherence. Patients must undergo compulsory pre-treatment education sessions and be able to demonstrate sufficient treatment literacy to become eligible for the initiation of treatment. Failure to accept or adhere to anti-retroviral treatment is frequently explained by patients' ignorance and irrationality. However, lack of knowledge is not the main reason for low treatment uptake or adherence. As Niehaus[16] suggests, far from being ignorant about HIV/AIDS, people show a super-abundance of information, provided by multiple diverse discourses, including conventional medical, religious, and lay discourses and rumours. This suggests that other factors are impacting on the efficacy of anti-retroviral treatment programmes. In Zanzibar, these barriers include persistent HIV-related stigma, alternative diagnostic and healing approaches in a context of medical pluralism, widespread poverty and marginalisation, issues of gender, and concerns over individual agency and loss of control.

The complexity of HIV/AIDS epidemics requires us to look beyond statistical measures in evaluations of treatment programmes and provide a contextualisation of the ways in which ARVs are experienced.[17] An understanding of the social-cultural, religious, economic, historical and political context in which treatment programmes are rolled out is crucial to conceptualise people's actions, highlights how structural factors constrain their ability to make choices, and unveils the rationality beyond apparently irrational decisions. Methodologically, such an approach implicates the need for long-term, in-depth ethnographic studies that analyse not only the "facts" (of treatment uptake and adherence, CD4 counts and recovery rates), but also their underlying meanings.

While the new drugs have provided immense relief and transformed the situation of HIV-positive people from one of death and despair into one of hope and the prospect for a future, they have also produced new uncertainties about how best to respond to HIV/AIDS, both for the infected individual and for society at large. Drawing on three case studies I show how HIV-positive people struggle to make decisions in an environment characterised by deep uncertainties about the nature and causes of HIV/AIDS in particular, and about the continuity of Zanzibari society in general. Emphasising the processional nature of disease and the importance of a contextual approach, this paper shows how interpersonal connections, individual experiences and emotions, and moral considerations at the time take precedence over concerns about physical survival, and points to the profound importance of social relationships and a view of life whose value is as much social as it is biological.

The data presented in this paper derive from 15 months of ethnographic fieldwork in Zanzibar in 2004 and 2005 and several follow-up visits in 2007, 2008, 2010 and 2011. Living with a local family and working closely with members of the Zanzibar Association for People Living with HIV/AIDS (ZAPHA +), Zanzibar's only support group for HIV-positive people, I participated in the group's daily activities, visited members' homes, and accompanied them to group events and on their visits to hospitals, relatives, and friends. Material was collected through qualitative methodology, using participant observation – a method resting on the in-depth study of social contexts and critical events particularly appropriate to a setting where shame and danger dominate people's lives.

An "immoral" infection: HIV/AIDS in Zanzibar

The Tanzanian AIDS epidemic is strongly regional, with grossly differing prevalence rates in different geographical areas.[18] Zanzibar is considered a low prevalence region in sub-Saharan Africa; while Tanzania's overall adult prevalence rate reached an estimated 6.2% in 2007,[19] Zanzibar's estimated HIV prevalence was 0.6% in 2003, with women showing infection rates that are four to six times higher than their male counterparts.[20]

Public discussion of HIV/AIDS in Zanzibar takes a strongly moralistic stance, playing on tropes of moral decay, outside influence and an overall increase in immorality.[21] Zanzibaris explain the comparatively low HIV-rates in the islands with their Muslim lifestyle, which many hold to protect its adherents from infection. Indeed, a large governmental AIDS commission sign at one of the major crossroads in Zanzibar Town reads: "Our Zanzibari morals are an important protection against AIDS." The fact that rates have been rising is regarded as an indicator for the breakdown of Zanzibari culture and proof of moral decline, and is frequently mentioned as a sign that "the end is nigh". It is difficult to calculate the influence of Islam on the unfolding of Zanzibar's HIV epidemic. While access to casual sex with multiple partners appears to be more restricted than, for example, in nearby Dar es Salaam, which has a much higher prevalence rate of 8.8%,[22] polygamy is common and non-marital sexual relationships are managed with a high degree of secrecy, which often precludes condom use. Condoms in general are not widely available, especially in rural areas, and difficult to access for unmarried people. Geographical isolation during the first years of the epidemic due to travel restrictions until the early 1990s, as well as the fact that the islands have not yet experienced a high-intensity generalised epidemic and have been offering good coverage of anti-retroviral treatment since 2005, may be important factors that contribute to the relatively low prevalence rates.

Nevertheless, the perceived threat of AIDS in the population is high, and there is a great sense of uncertainty about the nature and the magnitude of the epidemic. This uncertainty has been heightened through HIV awareness campaigns that emphasise that one "cannot tell who is HIV-positive by the looks of a person" (*huwezi kumjua mwenye UKIMWI kwa macho*) especially in times of anti-retroviral treatment. The epidemic has acquired a distinctive position that transcends the sphere of illness and medicine, and for the people of Zanzibar – as in other parts of Tanzania, Africa, and indeed the world – it has a meaning far beyond the individual suffering it causes.

While awareness of the major HIV transmission routes is high, the source of AIDS is located in the divine sphere: the prominent perception among religious leaders and the general population is that AIDS is a divine retribution (*adhabu ya Mungu*) for increasing immorality, embedding the pandemic in a local Muslim discourse on the erosion of Zanzibar's culture. In fact, the framing of AIDS as incurable led many to question whether it was a disease at all, since the Qur'an states that there is a cure for every disease. Therefore, many argued, AIDS had to be a direct punishment from God. The close association made between HIV/AIDS and what is classified as "immoral behaviour" in Zanzibar, with a particular emphasis on illegitimate sexuality, has resulted in severe stigmatisation of HIV-positive people.[23]

It must be pointed out that discourses which connect sexually transmitted diseases to illicit sexual behaviours are not solely informed by Muslim perceptions of sexual impurity and moral loss, but also reflect biomedical notions of disease in sub-Saharan Africa. In colonial Zanzibar, the hospital context, as a racially divided social arena, created opposing human categories along the lines of racial distinctions. As Vaughan argues, colonial medical discourse "operated by locating differences in the body, thereby not only pathologising them but also naturalising them".[24] Consequently, in the creation of the colonial subject in Africa, notions of intelligence, character, and sexuality, and the mental and physical by-products of the human body, like diseases and insanity, followed notions of race.[25] In missionary discourse these diseases of race, associated especially with sexuality, were transformed into "diseases of immorality".[26] Indeed, HIV and other sexually transmitted diseases (STD) were labelled *wagonjwa wa uasherati*, "diseases of sexual promiscuity" in educational posters produced by the Ministry of Health. Henceforth, public education against promiscuity and an emphasis on "zero-grazing" (i.e., faithfulness to one, or a small, geographically close set of sexual partners), has been an important element in HIV prevention campaigns.[27]

Uncertainty about HIV/AIDS in Zanzibar is counteracted by placing the disease in locally meaningful discourses about moral norms and values in a changing world, thereby restoring some sense of security and guidance for action. Knowledge of the biological processes involved in HIV transmission does not preclude this conceptualisation of AIDS in moral terms. Rakelmann, for example, points out that in Botswana the concept of the virus is entirely compatible with the idea of divine punishment: the virus explains *how* an individual is infected, and the sinful way of life explains *why*.[28] Zanzibaris argue, "If God wants to punish somebody, a condom won't stop Him – He'll just let the condom break", thus subordinating knowledge about biomedical concepts of infectious agents travelling from one body to the other to the notion of divine punishment for immoral behaviour.

Such discussions have sparked a strongly conservative response to AIDS in Zanzibar: the return to a life of Muslim values is promoted, and public discourse on sex and condoms is discouraged as fuelling promiscuous behaviour. In this context, many HIV-negative people initially were opposed to the costly treatment for people who, in their eyes, were largely responsible for their fate, fearing that the provision of treatment could lead to an even further relaxation of sexual mores.

"Medicines of hope": Living with anti-retroviral treatment

Within ZAPHA+, the island's only group for HIV-positive people, the promises the new treatment held were eagerly awaited and its success was celebrated: people who had been dying recovered miraculously, voluntary testing numbers shot up, and the trends quickly started to shift from final stage clinical diagnoses of AIDS towards early stage diagnoses of HIV as increasing numbers of people came to test. The introduction of routine testing has reinforced this trend. Yet, while these observations point to the success of the anti-retroviral treatment programme at the population level, individual patients' trajectories suggest that anti-retroviral treatment is often regarded as problematic, and neither treatment uptake nor adherence was guaranteed.

In Zanzibar at the time of treatment rollout, awareness of ART was low, and even within ZAPHA+ few members had heard of the drugs. Only the chairwoman Consolata had been on a regular ART regime financed by her former employer, an international aid agency director, and one other member had used the drugs for some months before having to stop treatment due to the high cost. Only a handful of members had witnessed the drugs' remarkable potential, seeing Consolata's body recover quickly through the treatment. It is perhaps not surprising, therefore, that lobbying for access to treatment had not been a priority within ZAPHA+; the incentive for this came from external volunteers, including myself. Members spoke of their desire to live longer so they could make sure their children would grow up safely, and to regain strength so that they could work again and would not have to be a burden to their families any longer. "*Maisha yangu, kwa kweli, yameshaisha*, to be honest, my life is already finished", a mother of five told me, "if I could only live until my children have finished school, I would be grateful." To achieve this, ZAPHA+ members used various strategies: they tried to eat what they had learned to be a healthy diet, they boosted their immune systems with an array of vitality-enhancing substances and techniques, ranging from vitamin supplements bought at the pharmacy to prayers, they used hospital and traditional medicines to treat opportunistic infections, as well as protective medicines provided by traditional healers, and they constantly strove for creating and maintaining an inner peace which is considered vital for ensuring a healthy body. Anti-retroviral treatment, at first, seemed just one more addition to this array of strategies.

Consequently, ZAPHA+ members asked for comprehensive information about the ways the drugs would work in their bodies. They wanted to know of the advantages and disadvantages of starting the treatment and an expert assessment of their individual health statuses by a doctor, so that each person could make an informed decision about whether to initiate the treatment, or rather to rely on established and trusted ways of handling the infection, including balanced nutrition and care for one's health (*kutumia chakula bora na kulinda afya*), and the use of various traditional medicines. This call for informed decision-making about their course of treatment is not taken for granted in the biomedical setting in Zanzibar: the hospital environment is characterised by a strong hierarchy that prescribes that patients should follow the doctor's advice without questioning, and health personnel often strengthens their authority by avoiding detailed explanation of diagnoses or treatment plans.

There has been much discussion of patients' non-compliance to treatment regimes in less-developed countries, with the biomedical community frequently blaming the patients for their alleged ignorance and obstinacy.[29] Responsibility has become obligatory for the "active biological citizen", Rose and Novas[30] have pointed out: once informed about current illness, susceptibilities, and predispositions he is obliged to take appropriate steps in order to minimise illness and conduct life responsibly in relation to others. The enactment of such responsible behaviour has become routine and expected and built into public health measures; it lies at the heart of the biomedical profession's expectations – and their subsequent disappointment with "non-compliant" patients.

But in developed countries, reports point mainly to patient- and treatment-related factors explaining low adherence, including substance abuse, the complexity of dosing and the "pill burden" as well as side effects. In sub-Saharan Africa, on the other hand, financial constraints have been identified as a major obstacle to treatment adherence, including transport costs, hospital user fees, lack of food, but also long waiting times in the hospitals, fear of stigmatisation, side effects and lack of counselling.[31] Additionally, many of my informants complained that doctors and nurses are often unsympathetic, unfriendly and prejudiced towards HIV-positive people. Finally, there is a general lack of explanation by health workers about what impact specific medicines have on the body and how different pills and injections work. As a result, people (and this includes HIV-negative people) often do not know the differences between medications they are prescribed, their names, the ways the active ingredients have an effect on their bodies, and why they were prescribed this drug and not another. Patients sometimes divide or exchange medications, following colour schemes and pill sizes that are associated with effectiveness for specific complaints, rather than considering the drugs' bio-medically active ingredients. Reporting from a small private research centre in Burkina Faso, on the other hand, Nguyen shows that essential to the success of its AIDS treatment programme has been the physician's ability to foster an institutional culture that enables – in Foucault's terms – disciplined patients. This was achieved by dissolving the hierarchy between patients and physicians through familiarity and friendly treatment and by instilling a culture of explanation.[32] Nguyen's account is not the only one pointing in this direction: Paul Farmer, for example, has long argued against the perceived ability of individuals in poor countries to follow the rational choice model promoted by biomedical physicians, and draws on various cases that show that when barriers against access to effective care were removed the differences between the survival rates among the poor and the wealthy disappeared.[33]

The following case studies shed light on the complexities involved in apparently irrational decisions around anti-retroviral treatment, emphasising how – within the limits of structural constraints – people actively make choices and carefully weigh the potential consequences. They demonstrate the deep social embeddedness of decisions about ART, which are bound up in social, economic, political, and moral contexts.

The risky commitment to life-long treatment: Fatma and Amila

Fatma and her daughter Amila's lives were quite characteristic of the experience of living with HIV/AIDS in Zanzibar. Fatma was 27 years old when I met her the first time at ZAPHA+. She was born in Pemba and married off at the age of 14. She did not really want to get married, but she did not want to appear ungrateful and oppose her parents. After she had one son, her husband divorced her and left her with the child; she was forced to go back to her parents' house where she lived for a few years. But the pressure on her to get married again was mounting, so finally she agreed to become the third wife of an older "Arab" man (as she described him), which is not uncommon for a divorced woman. This man's first two wives had failed to produce any offspring. Fatma noticed early on in the marriage that her husband was constantly suffering from headaches and other ailments and that he was taking Panadol almost every day. Nevertheless, she got pregnant and gave birth to a daughter, Amila. Seven months later, her husband suddenly died. Only then did she find out that he had died of AIDS and had known of his HIV-positive status when he married her. But he was afraid to die without having any children. So when he tested HIV-positive, he married a second wife and four months later a third – Fatma. He left three wives and his only daughter HIV-positive, the little girl being close to death in the summer of 2005. After her husband died, Fatma went back to her father's family, a household of 22 people, all relying on one income. She did not think that she had done anything wrong, but she still felt ashamed about her HIV infection and was afraid of her family's reaction if they found out; surely they would send her away and call her a prostitute, so she had not yet managed to tell her family about her disease.

Evidently, this situation made it difficult to keep up with strict treatment regimens and even to obtain the nutritious food that is vitally important for people living with an immunodeficiency disorder. Although Fatma had not told anybody yet, she thought that some of her family members suspected that she suffered from AIDS, as they refused to eat from the same plate as her and her daughter. Asked about her dreams, about how she envisages her future, she replied:

> *sasa hivi nipo tu*, I am just here now. . . . I can't do business because I get too tired, and I have to take care of the child. And if the people find out that you're HIV-positive they won't buy anything from you anyway. Everybody is afraid of you, they don't even give you any sympathy. When I was a child I dreamt of studying, I wanted to be a teacher or a doctor, but now I'm too old to study. The sun has already set, why should I study anymore?

While her own CD4 was still fine then, her daughter's health status was very poor and the doctor advised Amila should start the treatment. This gave Fatma hope to see her child grow and get better. On the other hand she was also very worried: would the drugs be available in the future? She did not even have the money to buy basic food, let alone expensive Western drugs. And would her daughter have to take pills for the rest of her life? Would it not be better to use vitamin supplements, or take her to the traditional healer to "build up" her body first? After much deliberation, Fatma decided to start the treatment.

Amila was one of the first children in Zanzibar to receive anti-retrovirals, and when she started the treatment she was already very sick; I thought she was going to die. Although she was very good in swallowing all the medications, she often could not keep them inside: she was feverish, could not eat, and constantly vomited. Her mother, being almost illiterate, at first had problems in administering the right dosage (paediatric ARVs come in fluid form and must be mixed and dosed with the help of a syringe) and filling in the monitoring forms. Moreover, Fatma always had to be there and administer the drugs herself, because nobody else in the family knew about her and her daughter's health status, so when there was no food in the house, or Fatma was away, Amila missed her dose. Despite these problems, Amila slowly started to get better, and seeing her again in July 2007, I could hardly believe that this was the same child. The sad-looking tiny girl, who never smiled nor spoke, had grown into a healthy-looking five-year-old who happily played with the other children.

However, by then Fatma's own health status had deteriorated and the doctor advised her to start treatment, too. Yet, although she had seen her daughter regain strength and grow over the past two years, Fatma did not think she would take the drugs herself. She said:

> I've got them at home, but I thought I'd better wait until I have more food to eat. You know how it is at home, I only eat one meal a day, and often not before 2 or 3 pm. These medicines are strong – how can I swallow them without having eaten?

While Fatma could justify spending an extra amount of money on food for Amila, because she was a child and obviously ill, she could not put herself before other members of her family and expect them to provide her with more food than they had, especially her father, the head of household and sole breadwinner. This would have stretched her social support network too much. She was not even visibly very ill – no more than the others, at least, who also suffer from bouts of malaria and other infections. It took her another five months until she finally decided to use the life-prolonging treatment that her body so urgently needed.

Fatma's story elucidates several of the uncertainties brought up by the treatment of AIDS in Zanzibar. Firstly, there is a strong fear of dependency in the context of distrust of the government and the international donors: Fatma had learned from experience that promises made by the government were not necessarily reliable,[34] and the behaviour of international donors was completely out of her control: after the 1995 election riots, for example, most international donors had pulled out of projects in the islands, leading to service delivery projects being starved of funds. Moreover, corruption was thriving in Zanzibar, and hospital staff suspected of starting to charge for the drugs once the funding agency handed the project over to the local authorities. Embarking on a life-long treatment programme therefore meant giving up agency to a large extent and becoming dependent upon authorities that are far beyond "normal" people's control and may have hidden agendas. Whyte, van der Geest and Hardon[35] point to the ambiguity of control inherent in the use of medicines, highlighting the constant field of tension between self-control over the infection versus society's control over the sufferer, which patients have to negotiate. ARVs offer the opportunity to regain some control over one's body and life, providing the patient with the strength and health to resume productive and reproductive activity. At the same time, ART also meant giving up a good deal of control over one's life and handing it over to an unreliable government and to donors who are fickle in their attachment.

Patients were very aware of these uncertainties: the first question always asked in information sessions on anti-retroviral medication was: "Will the drugs be available and still free of charge in two, five, 10 years' time? What happens if the donors pull out?" In their research on the channels ARVs flowed through in Uganda before the introduction of free treatment in June 2004, Whyte et al.[36] point to the necessarily tough prioritising of family funds and the resulting intra-familial moral dilemmas, the terrible decisions of triage, and the growing awareness of inequity that result from the availability of ARVs for payment of a fee in a country where most people cannot afford them. My research participants' concerns were well-founded, as none of them would be able to pay for anti-retrovirals without seriously stretching their social support network and using resources that are greatly needed for other investments – in fact, most of them could not pay for the drugs at all. At the same time, the rollout of free anti-retrovirals in combination with a crumbling public welfare system and an increasing withdrawal of the state from the provision of social services as part of neoliberal reform packages painfully draws to attention the combination of biological inclusion and social exclusion which features in Biehl's[37] critique of contemporary biopolitics of AIDS in Brazil.

Another concern many have with top-down biomedical interventions are the hidden agendas suspected to form their background. Although Fatma had not mentioned this explicitly, other programmes have triggered such discourses. The colonial government's anthrax immunisation project, for example, was widely regarded as an attempt to kill the people's cattle, and led to severe riots in the country that finally resulted in the strengthening of party politics.[38] In 2008, a vaccination campaign sparked violent riots in several hospitals in the country. Family planning messages, likewise, were taken to be motivated by the West trying to limit the reproduction of the African people and to impose their lifestyle upon Africans, with condom promotion in particular being viewed as fuelling the immorality that had already started to spoil Zanzibar society. To what extent these kinds of discourses play a role in the treatment of AIDS still needs to be seen in the future.

Fatma also had concerns about the nature of the medication itself and its effects on the body. Her worries about the side effects need to be considered in the context of constant food insecurity and her experience with Amila and some other HIV-positive friends. Western medicines are perceived as very potent, and therefore potentially dangerous. In the hierarchy of medicines in the area, Western pills rank second to injections only. At the same time, there is not much knowledge about the ways specific drugs work in the body of the patient – pills are often discriminated by their colour and size, rather than the specific illness they are supposed to treat. Rumours about biomedical technologies, such as pills or condoms, causing cancer, impotence, barrenness, or miscarriages are omnipresent and partly supported by medical evidence.

Finally, vitality enhancing medicines, including vitamin supplements sold over the counter at the pharmacy, certain nutritious foods, and a range of traditional medicines that aim specifically at strengthening the body, are popular and often preferred to hospital medicine, especially in cases of paediatric AIDS. Even in the case of "normal" illnesses, parents often ponder for days about subjecting their children's small, vulnerable bodies to the potential toxicity of medicines. Another girl of Amila's age, for example, had developed painful fungal infections in her mouth. She could not eat anymore, lost weight rapidly, and had constant fevers. The doctors advised to start her on AVRs, but her caretaker declined, being too concerned about the dangers of the medication. She decided to boost the girl's general health status by buying expensive vitamin supplements and to wait until the child could eat again. Despite her caretaker's efforts, the girl died a few months later.

Together, these concerns form the context in which Fatma made her decision: despite seeing her daughter improve significantly over the past two years with the help of ARVs, she chose not to start the medication, as the risks of committing to the lifelong treatment for her seemed to outweigh the benefits. However, such decisions are not final, and individuals change their minds, for example when they start feeling ill, or when their life circumstances change. With deteriorating health and constant counselling by ZAPHA+ peers, Fatma finally started treatment in July 2007, but her adherence was patchy, reflecting her strained social relations and economic position. Such intermittent treatment trajectories highlight the processional nature of illness, with individual actors often taking different positions in the course of the illness, both in trying to explain the cause of the suffering, and in the preferred routes of treatment.

Fatma had been confronted with the grim reality of the disease through her daughter's illness – AIDS was omnipresent for her. Her concerns about treatment revolved around issues of availability of food and drugs, around the strong side effects, and the difficulties of adhering to the treatment regime when she could not fall back on the support of her family. In the end, reflecting on the stigmatisation she had experienced, she said: "Why would I want to live longer, if nobody wants me around anymore anyway?" Her only reason to live, she thought at the moment, was to make sure her daughter was taken care of and in the end this swayed her decision towards starting the treatment in 2007. However, she stopped treatment again when she got pregnant three years later for fear of harming the unborn child, and died shortly after the baby's birth.

Measuring life-time left: Tausi

With Tausi, a 30-year-old woman, the situation was different. Tausi was working and her regular income made her economically independent. Therefore, food, and even moderate payment for medication, was not such a problem for her. She largely trusted in biomedicine, and once she had started the treatment, she did not have problems with adhering to the regime. In her case, the decision to start using ARVs was complicated by the fact that the accessibility of the treatment forced her to face her health status again.

She explained: "When I had my initial HIV test and it was positive, I thought my life had stopped. Everybody says: AIDS kills – and I had it." Then she joined ZAPHA+, where she learned about the difference of "living with HIV" and "being sick with AIDS", which is emphasised in HIV/AIDS education sessions. Tausi embraced the international discourse of living with hope, and slowly started to accept her infection. In her quest for normality she did everything she could to redefine her condition in a positive way and to live a "normal" life. This is often perceived as denial by outside onlookers; but Tausi had never denied her diagnosis. She was aware of it every day, but she refused to accept that she was going to die any time soon.

When the drugs became available, however, her carefully built construct was tested and fundamentally shaken. The CD4 count that every HIV-positive person was advised to take to establish disease progression painfully called to her mind that she was not, in fact, leading a normal life, that the infection was still there and might have progressed. But she felt healthy and strong, so she was not too worried. There were others, who were sick all the time and very skinny. They would have to start the medication. On the day before her CD4 test she said: "I feel great, I have gained weight, and even my mother finally starts to believe that I will live and grow old with the infection." And yet, it turned out that her CD4 was well below 200 and she had to start ART immediately. She was devastated. This test was such a shock to her that she later told me: "Receiving this diagnosis was worse than getting the initial HIV-positive result. I thought, now I really am going to die."

Tausi's case is exemplary of the thoughts and fears of many of my informants when treatment finally became available. While being excited about the comforting assurance that now there was something you could do once you fell ill, only few people were eager to start treatment. Rather, the accessibility of medication served as a reassurance, an opportunity for those times far away when the virus would take over the body. For as long as possible, however, a life without the strong drugs was desired. At the same time, the repeated confrontation with the disease was emotionally distressing, especially for those who felt healthy. After all the efforts to build up their new life after the HIV test, carefully constructing a fragile sense of normality in which they are HIV-positive, but not sick with AIDS, now their health status was revised again. The initial HIV test had shattered my informants' lives and drew a boundary, segregating them from the world of the living, the "normal", HIV-negative members of society. Through the CD4 count again boundaries are drawn – this time within the community of PLHA, once more segregating members who had tried to build up new networks of solidarity. Becoming eligible for treatment initiated the person into the group of "proper" AIDS patients. It meant that the end was near, that the person's life-time was running out.

But it was not merely the confrontation with the infection that was distressing to my informants. The nature of the test itself, its biomedical claim to authority and absolute truth, was considered problematic. While diagnoses by traditional healers are usually produced in collaboration with the patient and other members of the social network, and are always open for reinterpretation and adjustment, the CD4 count pushes the individual into a passive position. This process of measuring a person's health status, and thereby their remaining life-time, transforms persons into patients and takes away their agency, subjecting them to "objective" tests that often do not reflect how healthy a person feels. Again, an anonymous lab test would decide about their lives – after spending so much energy on getting their lives under control after the initial test. The diagnosis was thus sometimes questioned and trust in the authority of the health personnel and quality of counselling once more played a crucial role in deciding on the best course of action.

Competing authorities: Aziza

The story of Aziza, a young woman who died in June 2005, brings up a completely different set of issues that influence a person's decision about whether to use anti-retroviral treatment. Aziza had been diagnosed with final stage AIDS and was in hospital. She had had an HIV test before, which was positive, but she did not believe in the diagnosis. Instead, she trusted in the expertise of a traditional healer who had diagnosed her with a witchcraft affliction (*kurogwa*) and administered anti-witchcraft medicine, purgatory agents that made her vomit and caused diarrhoea in order to expel the witchcraft agent from her body. By the time she was admitted to the hospital she was severely dehydrated and weak. But even in the hospital, and despite repeated counselling, she carried on with the anti-witchcraft medicine. She finally died all by herself, because her family never visited her in the hospital – they only came to pick up her corpse when they were informed that she was dead.

Aziza's story reminds us of the fact that there are experts other than biomedical doctors, who are consulted and trusted by the majority of the population. And there are theories of disease causation that differ from the biomedical model of infectious agents invading the body. Lab-based diagnostics and anti-retroviral treatment have to compete with these models, and if we consider the local context, the witchcraft idiom becomes quite appealing. In an environment where AIDS equals adultery and immorality, and the victims face stigmatisation even by those closest to them, the witchcraft explanation requires an analysis of the whole network of social relations and thus deflects blame away from the individual, placing responsibility on the larger group.

Moreover, an explanation using the witchcraft idiom (or the notion of divine retribution) opens up possibilities and routes for action: healers are consulted and different treatments are tried out – each offering the prospect of a cure. And while my informants praised the introduction of anti-retroviral treatment, a cure (*kupona kabisa*) is what they were really hoping for. Consequently, the majority had already tried out one or several traditional treatments that promised to eradicate the virus completely, and frequently news about some new medicine against AIDS arrived. People went home to their villages to seek out their own healers, and bought medicines from all over the country, from places as far away as Kagera (where the Tanzanian epidemic had started and thus people were assumed to have a lot of experience with treating it), Dubai or Saudi Arabia. In 2011, six years after treatment rollout, thousands flocked to rural Loliondo to drink a "miracle brew" conceived in a local pastor's dream, and many died en route. Herbal concoctions (*dawa za miti shamba*), the composition of which would come to the healer in a dream or through the help of spirits, and fumigations (*fukizo,* "incense burning"), often in combination with Qur'anic supplication (*dua*), were administered and supported through prayer and abstinence, following the way of the scriptures.

Traditional doctors seemed to be making a good business out of this,[39] to the extent that in 2004 all advertisements that claimed to offer a cure for AIDS were made illegal. This is, however, not to say that their attempts were all purely focussed on making a profit. Some healers seemed to be genuinely concerned about finding a cure and I came across several cases where treatment was offered for free. Stories about successful cases came up again and again and kept kindling hopes, despite the fact that most of my informants were repeatedly disappointed. After all, who knew what the real cause of the treatment failure was? According to Parkin, religious and spiritual beliefs survive empirical challenges because faith may always be invoked to provide answers that biomedicine or traditional herbalism do not: along the lines of the principle of secondary elaboration as enunciated by Evans-Pritchard in his study of Azande divination and cure, the apparent failure of divine or spiritual treatment can always be ascribed to the improper performance of the ritual and procedure; Muslim prayers said before a biomedical treatment, for example, must be said sincerely and properly, if they are to work. This is consistent with the view in Zanzibar today that the Qur'an is the ultimate medicine and source of scientific knowledge,[40] and is supported by the belief that God can cure any disease.

ARVs, the doctors clearly emphasise, cannot offer such a cure. Yet, the definition of illness as having an infectious agent hide somewhere in the body, waiting for its chance to strike, for many was hard to understand: "If you are not ill (*kama huumwi*), if you don't feel pain, or lie in bed, but go out to do your work as usual, then how can you be sick?" a young man explained. "What does being sick mean, then? I might have a virus in my body, so what? I'm not sick." In Zanzibar, as elsewhere in the region, illness is associated with incapacitation. Health, here, is the absence of illness, of pain, weakness, and the inability to work. If ARVs can restore the body to a state in which it functions as good as normal, then for many this meant that the person is healthy again. Indeed, when I revisited the island over the following years, some of my informants had stopped taking the drugs, considering themselves cured when they started to feel better.

However, these were a minority; most ARV receivers had remained on treatment, especially those who had been with ZAPHA+ since before treatment was available. They had experienced the treacherous nature of AIDS, with periods of succumbing to illness, temporarily getting better after the treatment of opportunistic infections and worse again only a short time after. They had found ways to explain the work of the virus and of the drugs in people's bodies, and continuously argued against stopping the treatment. "The ARVs put the virus to sleep (*virusi vimelala*)," they explained, "it hides and rests somewhere in your body....But when you stop the treatment the virus comes back stronger than ever and kills you very quickly." The view of the virus as a "bug" (*dudu*) which can be put to sleep was combined with local views on appropriate behaviour and the effects of sex on the body in explanations that emphasise the need to refrain from excessive sexual activity: "When you have sex the blood becomes hot and flows faster; this wakes up the virus and it begins to circulate through your body", a ZAPHA+ member explained.

Never promising more than a longer life span, in official medical education sessions ART was presented as *dawa za kurefisha maisha*, "medicines to prolong life". But despite all the new kinds of uncertainties the new treatment has provoked, in ZAPHA+ discourse they soon became *dawa za matumaini*, "medicines of hope". Anti-retrovirals build up the body, it was argued, so that it endures until finally a real cure will be found. In this sense, ARVs may be classed as yet another, albeit powerful, vitality enhancing medicine. This is supported by the heavy emphasis laid on techniques to guard one's health (*kulinda afya*) through quality nutrition, appropriate amounts of rest and exercise, and a morally sound lifestyle. Much trust is invested in the prospect that a cure will be found one day, either through biomedicine or "traditional" healers. Thus, the diagnosis of HIV in the end is not as final as it may have seemed – some scope for hope, and for action, always remains.

Hoping for a good death

At the same time, most of my informants had accepted the thought that they would most likely die from AIDS one day. But how would this death come about, under the new anti-retroviral treatment? The anti-retrovirals prolong patients' lives – but would they in the end still die as terribly as their fellow sufferers before? This was one of the most pressing questions always posed in conversations about ART. Dying from AIDS was clearly a "bad death": One day, Rahma, an HIV-positive woman in her 50s and long-term member of ZAPHA+, brought photographs of her late sister for me to look at. The first picture showed a big, laughing young woman in a bright, colourful dress. "This is before her infection," Rahma explained. The next one showed the same woman, weighing a little less maybe, but smiling, with beautifully smooth and clear skin. "This is in April, after she had just received the diagnosis." The last picture features Rahma, sitting on a bed next to her sister on the day before she died. Amina and Khamis, two other members who are watching together with me, are as shocked as I am at the sight of this wasted body – we cannot recognise the woman from before; she is mere skin and bones, covered in rash, looking ancient. "This is a bad disease," Amina said quietly, and I could read her thoughts: Will I die like this? The prospect of escaping from this fate, of growing old and dying in dignity, is what the "medicines of hope" symbolised for my informants. Whether it will be fulfilled is hard to say; from a biological point of view, if the treatment fails the virus is no longer suppressed and the disease progresses to AIDS.

Many of those ZAPHA+ members who had witnessed the introduction of ART are still alive today because of the drugs, and actively promote treatment uptake and adherence as peer counsellors and home-based carers. Newly diagnosed patients therefore encounter a better organised network of peer support and information within ZAPHA+ and the HIV clinic. Nevertheless, there are signs that drop-out rates are increasing, for a number of reasons. Fear of stigmatisation still makes it difficult to take the drugs when in the company of others, e.g., at work or within the family, and social and economic support and home-based care programmes have been reduced significantly due to funding cuts. Moreover, widespread treatment provision and routine testing policies have brought AIDS into public discourse and result in many now being tested in early stages of infection not yet having suffered from serious opportunistic infections, thus lacking the powerful experience of the drugs' work in restoring their health. Without the experience of severe symptoms it has become increasingly difficult to convince people to stick to lifelong treatment regimes. These are issues which will need consideration with maturing treatment programmes across the region.

In Zanzibar, specifically, religious and moral concerns pose additional hurdles. Fasting during Ramadhan, for example, is an important religious requirement and a highly respected social activity, but interferes with the strictly time-bound treatment regimes. While the sick are exempted from fasting in Islamic doctrine, HIV-positive people on treatment face competing messages about their status: clinic staff emphasise the "chronically sick" identity of PLHA, whose lives depend on following the strict treatment regimes. At the same time, according to the language of international HIV/AIDS programmes, successful treatment restores patients' health and affords them a "normal life, just like any other person". Many are eager to take part in the collective experience of Ramadhan, others are worried about having to explain why they do not fast. An elderly widowed woman in the rural east, whose health was poor, explained: "I'm not sick, I'm just disabled (*siumwi, ni mlemavu tu*). Even if you bring that Islamic scholar again to lecture me, I won't stop fasting!" As a result, clinic staff report falling CD4 counts and rising opportunistic infections during and after Ramadhan in the islands.

Yet, most people in Zanzibar were treatment-naïve and by 2011, ART resistance was still low. Death was not a pressing worry anymore. Concern was focused once more on the topic which preoccupied most people's lives: impoverishment and the difficulty of making a living in what was perceived as an increasingly tough life, *maisha magumu*.

Conclusion

The vignettes in this paper show how patients make sense of and respond to the uncertainties of illness and treatment through social relations. They demonstrate that the social, economic, moral, and political contexts in which mass treatment programmes are rolled out are profoundly important for treatment uptake and adherence. In their decision-making, people fall back on previous experience of the healthcare system and with promises made by the government and international donors, they consider their network of social relations, moral concerns and individual emotional factors. Treatment literacy played a relatively minor role in predicting the success or failure of anti-retroviral treatment in Zanzibar; rather, concerns revolved around questions of control and agency, limiting structural factors, and alternative aetiologies in the context of medical pluralism.

These findings confirm Allen and Parker's[41] claim that a pharmaceutical approach is not sufficient to tackle complex epidemics like HIV/AIDS. Health interventions cannot be orientated to "life itself"; they must be attuned to the contexts in which life takes place: the family, the community, the structural inequalities that make some treatment decisions and practices of self-care easier and others more difficult. ART programmes make possible a biologised, pharmaceutical life. But life-as-lived must be shared with others. Therefore, shifting funding streams to drug provision without a comprehensive prevention and clinical care approach, and expecting patients to make the "right" choices in the face of structural constraints and competing messages, ignores the fact that patients are persons, social beings who relate with and depend on others to survive and live a good life.

Analysing people's actions and behaviours in the context of their lives-as-lived throws light onto apparently irrational decisions and emphasises the importance of an in-depth understanding of local moral worlds and social contexts. Life with a chronic illness is a messy, emotional and uneasy process that involves uncertainty, anxiety and self-doubt, a need for sharing with others in a similar situation, and for support and kindness from service providers. In the global North, AIDS today is largely addressed as a chronic illness, with support systems going far beyond the dispensing of drugs. In the global South, however, AIDS continues to be treated in emergency mode, as an acute infection which first and foremost requires pharmaceutical treatment, while social support programmes such as home-based care, peer support, and livelihood provision are increasingly cut in order to get more patients on the treatment registers. What these case studies clearly show is that the management of a life-long chronic condition cannot be tackled on a biological basis alone. Treatment has to be made meaningful and embedded in people's social lives in order to work and achieve patients' commitment to adherence.

Notes

1. For a detailed account of the global AIDS Treatment Access Movement, albeit presented largely from a US point of view, see Smith and Siplon 2006.
2. UNAIDS, *Together We Will End AIDS*, 9.
3. UNAIDS Press Release, "Inaugural Global Scientific Strategy."
4. WHO News Release, "'Strategic Use' of HIV Medicines."
5. Biehl, *Will to Live*.
6. Biehl, *Will to Live*; Nguyen, *The Republic of Therapy*.
7. Cf. Parker et al., "Border Parasites"; Allen and Parker, "The Other Diseases of the Millennium Development Goals" and "Will Increased Funding . . . Make Poverty History?"
8. Allen and Parker, "Will Increased Funding . . . Make Poverty History?"
9. Whyte, "Chronicity and Control."
10. Rose, *The Politics of Life Itself*.
11. Fassin, 2009: 48.
12. Ibid.
13. Schenker, *HIV/AIDS Literacy*, 3.
14. Kleinman, "Concepts and a Model".
15. Beckmann, "Responding to Medical Crises" (forthcoming).
16. Niehaus, "Part I: Bushbuckridge", 18.
17. McNeill and Niehaus, "Conclusion", 119.
18. Cf. Leshabari et al., "Youth Mobility and Unprotected Sex."
19. UNAIDS, *Report on the Global AIDS Epidemic 2008*, 215.
20. ZAC, *Report on Situation and Response Analysis of HIV/AIDS in Zanzibar*, 1.
21. Beckmann, "AIDS and the Power of God."
22. TACAIDS/ZAC/NBS/OCGS/Macro International Inc. 2007.
23. Beckmann, "AIDS and the Power of God."
24. Vaughan, *Curing Their Ills*, 13.
25. Nisula, *Everyday Spirits and Medical Intervention*, 244. Some observations on patterns of condom use in casual sexual encounters on the tourist beaches in Zanzibar suggest that these racial notions still live on today: several backpackers said they often used condoms with African lovers, less frequently with other white travellers.
26. Vaughan, *Curing Their Ills*, 66–67. Note, for example, reports from the Zanzibar Medical Officer in which the prevalence of venereal diseases was attributed to the natives – particularly the women – being ignorant, immoral and engaging in casual prostitution (Nisula, *Everyday Spirits and Medical Intervention*, 243).
27. Iliffe, *East African Doctors*, 223.
28. Rakelmann, "Local Interpretations of AIDS in Botswana", 45–6.
29. Cf. Farmer on tuberculosis and antiretroviral treatment (*Infections and Inequalities*, 191–9, 208, 268–71).
30. Rose and Novas, "Biological Citizenship."
31. WHO, *From Access to Adherence*, 1, 7
32. Nguyen, "Antiretroviral globalism, biopolitics, and therapeutic citizenship", 139.
33. Farmer, *Infections and Inequalities*, 266–71.
34. One may only think of the allegedly free provision of education and health care, which in fact both had to be paid for.
35. Whyte, et al., *The Social Lives of Medicine*.
36. Whyte et al., "Treating AIDS."
37. Biehl, *Will to Live*.
38. Babu, "The 1964 Revolution."
39. Payments usually ranged between TSH 150000 and TSH 500000 – expensive, but not unaffordable. Many of my informants had mobilised their social networks to raise it.
40. Parkin, "In Touch Without Touching."

41. Allen and Parker, "Will Increased Funding...Make Poverty History?"

References

Allen, T., and M. Parker. "The Other Diseases of the Millennium Development Goals: Rhetoric and Reality of Free Drug Distribution to Cure Poor's Parasites." *Third World Quarterly* 32 (2011): 85–115.

Allen, T., and M. Parker. "Will Increased Funding for Neglected Tropical Diseases Really Make Poverty History?" *The Lancet* 379, no. 9821 (2012): 1097–8.

Babu, A.M. "The 1964 Revolution: Lumpen or Vanguard?" In *Zanzibar Under Colonial Rule*, eds. A. Sheriff, and E. Ferguson, 220–48. London: James Currey, 1991.

Beckmann, N. "AIDS and the Power of God: Narratives of Decline and Coping Strategies in Zanzibar." In *AIDS and Religious Practice in Africa*, eds. F. Becker, and P.W. Geissler, 119–54. Leiden: Brill Publishers, 2009.

Beckmann, N. "Responding to Medical Crises: AIDS Treatment, Responsibilisation and the Logic of Choice." In special issue "Therapeutic Knowledge, Health, Crises and Processes of Diversification and Mainstreaming", eds. G. Alex, K. Krause and D. Parkin. *Anthropology and Medicine* 20 (Forthcoming).

Biehl, J. *Will to Live: AIDS Therapies and the Politics of Survival.* Princeton: Princeton University Press, 2007.

Farmer, P. *Infections and Inequalities: The Modern Plagues.* Berkeley: University of California Press, 2001.

Fassin, D. "Another politics of life is possible." *Theory, Culture and Society* 26, no. 5 (2009): 44–60.

Iliffe, J. *East African Doctors: A History of the Modern Profession.* Cambridge: Cambridge University Press, 1998.

Kleinman, A. "Concepts and a Model for the Comparison of Medical Systems as Cultural Systems." *Social Science and Medicine* 12, no. 1 (1978): 85–93.

Leshabari, M.T., S.F. Kaaya, J.Z. Killewo, and J.K. Mbwambo. "Youth Mobility and Unprotected Sex as Key Factors in the Spread of the AIDS Virus in Tanzania." In *Social Change and Health in Tanzania*, eds. K.H. Heggenhougen, and J.L.P. Lugalla, 31–46. Dar es Salaam: Dar es Salaam University Press, 2005.

McNeill, F., and I. Niehaus. "Conclusion." In *Magic: AIDS Review 2009*, eds. F. McNeill, and I. Niehaus, 115–9. University of Pretoria, Centre for the Study of AIDS, 2009.

Nguyen, V.-K. "Antiretroviral Globalism, Biopolitics, and Therapeutic Citizenship." In *Global Assemblages: Technology, Politics, and Ethics as Anthropological Problems*, eds. A. Ong, and S.J. Collier, 124–44. Oxford, Blackwell Publishing, 2005.

Nguyen, V.-K. *The Republic of Therapy. Triage and Sovereignty in West Africa's Time of AIDS.* Durham: Duke University Press, 2010.

Niehaus, I. "Part 1: Bushbuckridge: Beyond Treatment Literacy." In *Magic: AIDS Review 2009*, eds. F. McNeill, and I. Niehaus, 17–59. University of Pretoria, Centre for the Study of AIDS, 2009.

Nisula, T. *Everyday Spirits and Medical Intervention: Ethnographic and Historical Notes on Therapeutic Conventions in Zanzibar Town.* The Finnish Anthropological Society. Saarijarvi: Gummerus Kirjapainooy, 1999.

Parker, M., T. Allen, G. Pearson, N. Peach, R. Flynn, and N. Rees. "Border Parasites: Schistosomiasis Control Among Uganda's Fisherfolk." *Journal of Eastern African Studies* 6, no. 1 (2012): 98–123.

Parkin, D. "In Touch Without Touching: Islam and Healing." In *On Knowing and Not Knowing in the Anthropology of Medicine*, ed. R. Littlewood, 194–219. Walnut Creek: Left Coast Press, 2007.

Rakelmann, G.A. "'We sat there half the day asking questions, but they were unable to tell where AIDS comes from....' Local Interpretations of AIDS in Botswana." *Africa-Spektrum* 36, no. 1 (2001): 35–52.

Rose, N., and C. Novas. "Biological Citizenship." In *Global Assemblages: Technology, Politics, and Ethics as Anthropological Problems*, eds. A. Ong, and S.J. Collier, 439–63. Oxford, Blackwell Publishing, 2005.

Rose, N. *The Politics of Life Itself. Biomedicine, Power, and Subjectivity in the Twenty-First Century.* Princeton: Princeton University Press, 2007.

Schenker, I. *HIV/AIDS Literacy: An Essential Component in Education for All. EFA Global Monitoring Report.* Paris: UNESCO, 2006. Background paper.

Smith, R.A., and P.D. Siplon. *Drugs into Bodies: Global AIDS Treatment Activism.* Westport, CT: Praeger, 2006.

Tanzania Commission for AIDS (TACAIDS), Zanzibar AIDS Commission (ZAC), National Bureau of Statistics (NBS), Office of the Chief Government Statistician (OCGS), and Macro International Inc. 2008. *Tanzania HIV/AIDS and Malaria Indicator Survey 2007–08.* Dar es Salaam, Tanzania: TACAIDS, ZAC, NBS, OCGS, and Macro International Inc.

UNAIDS. *Report on the Global AIDS Epidemic 2008.* Geneva: UNAIDS, 2008.

UNAIDS. *Together We Will End AIDS.* Geneva: UNAIDS, 2012.

UNAIDS Press Release. Inaugural Global Scientific Strategy Towards an HIV Cure Launched Ahead of the XIX International AIDS Conference in Washington DC, 19 July 2012. http://www.unaids.org/en/resources/presscentre/pressreleaseandstatementarchive/2012/july/20120719prhivcure/ (accessed August 22, 2012).

Vaughan, M. *Curing Their Ills: Colonial Power and African Illness.* Stanford: Stanford University Press, 1991.

WHO. *From Access to Adherence: The Challenges of Antiretroviral Treatment. Studies from Botswana, Tanzania and Uganda.* WHO, 2006.

WHO News Release, 12.7.2012. "'Strategic Use' of HIV Medicines Could Help End Transmission of Virus". http://www.who.int/mediacentre/news/releases/2012/hiv_medication_20120718/en/index.html (accessed August 22, 2012).

Whyte, S.R., M.R. Whyte, L. Meinert, and B. Kyaddondo. "Treating AIDS: Dilemmas of Equal Access in Uganda." *Journal of Social Aspects of HIV/AIDS Research Alliance* 1, no. 1 (2004): 14–26.

Whyte, S.R., S. Van der Geest, and A. Hardon. *The Social Lives of Medicine.* Cambridge: Cambridge University Press, 2002.

Whyte, S.R. "Chronicity and Control: Framing 'Non-communicable Diseases' in Africa." *Anthropology and Medicine* 19, no. 1 (2012): 63–74.

ZAC. *Report on Situation and Response Analysis of HIV/AIDS in Zanzibar.* Zanzibar AIDS Commission, 2003.

Chasing imaginary leopards: science, witchcraft and the politics of conservation in Zanzibar

Martin Walsh[a] and Helle Goldman[b]

[a]*Wolfson College, University of Cambridge, UK;* [b]*Norwegian Polar Institute, Tromsø, Norway*

The Zanzibar leopard (*Panthera pardus adersi*) is (was) a little-known subspecies endemic to Unguja island. Rapid population growth and the expansion of farming in the twentieth century destroyed leopard habitat and decimated their natural prey, bringing them into increasing conflict with people. Villagers explained the growing number of attacks on their children and livestock by supposing that the leopards responsible for them were owned by witches and sent by them to do harm. Following the Zanzibar Revolution in 1964, localised efforts to act on this theory culminated in an island-wide leopard eradication and witch-finding campaign, supported by the government. By the 1990s state-subsidised hunting had brought the leopard to the brink of extinction, and most zoologists now presume it to be extinct. However, many islanders believe that leopard keepers are still active in rural Unguja and sightings of leopards continue to be reported. Beguiled by such narratives, visiting researchers and local conserva-tionists have continued to pursue these elusive felids. In this paper we describe and analyse a series of unsuccessful "kept leopard chases", including abortive calls by government officials for the capture and display of domesticated leopards. These quixotic efforts show no signs of abating, and the underlying conflicts of knowledge and practice remain unresolved, posing a challenge to the theory and practice of conservation not only in Zanzibar but also further afield.

Introduction

This paper describes conflicting ideas and proposals about the Zanzibar leopard (*Panthera pardus adersi*), a much-feared predator which is (or was) endemic to Unguja island. Conservation biologists will recognise this as an example of "human-wildlife conflict" that has parallels with other cases of human-carnivore and especially human-felid conflict,[1] a field of study and practice that has its own literature and guidelines for intervention.[2] Anthropologists have long pointed out that the human dimensions of "people-wildlife conflicts" are often ignored or misunderstood.[3] Attempts to redress the balance through the implementation of community-based conservation initiatives have had only limited success,[4] though some applied anthropologists and ethno-biologists remain optimistic about the prospects for conservation and development based on indigenous knowledge and practice.[5] The case of the Zanzibar leopard, however, provides few grounds for optimism. Despite the emergence of hybrid discourses about this elusive creature, the gulf between scientific and local understandings is arguably greater than ever.[6] This apparent incommensurability has seen foreign conservationists and NGOs on Zanzibar turn away from leopard conservation and focus their attentions elsewhere.

The sections below outline the development of these different discourses about the Zanzibar leopard: scientific, local ("indigenous"), and hybrid. The latter are broadly categorised in turn into the hybrid discourses of outside observers, including conservationists, and the hybrid discourses of Zanzibaris, among them government staff responsible for the development and implementation of the nation's conservation policies and programmes. We have paid particular attention to these because not only do they demonstrate the persuasiveness of local narratives about leopards, but because they bring to the fore an epistemological and practical dilemma that remains unresolved: how can conflicting knowledge about the leopard and proposed practices pertaining to it be reconciled? It will become clear that we are not disinterested parties, but have played a role in the events we describe, with the aim of improving scientific understanding and actions in relation to both the Zanzibar leopard and the different narratives and proposals about it. At the same time we believe that this case has wider implications for conservation policy and practice, and seek to bring these out in the concluding section of the paper.

Science: the Zanzibar leopard in the wild and museums

A number of nineteenth century visitors to Zanzibar noted the presence of leopards on Unguja,[7] but they did not become subjects of close scientific attention until the second decade of the 20th century. The first collected skin and skull, which came from the vicinity of Chwaka on the east coast of Unguja, was sent to the British Museum in 1919 by Dr. William Mansfield Aders, the Zanzibar Protectorate's Economic Biologist.[8] Aders also wrote a short paragraph on the leopard for a book chapter about the natural history of Zanzibar.[9] Another administrative officer, John Henry Vaughan, sent a second skin to London in 1929.[10] The mammal specialist there, Reginald Pocock, told Vaughan that he had named the two specimens from Zanzibar as a "local race" of leopard.[11] Pocock's formal description of the Zanzibar leopard was later published in a major review of the taxonomy of African leopards.[12] It was identified as a distinct subspecies of leopard and named *Panthera pardus adersi* in honour of Aders and his collection of what was now designated as the type. In his letter to Vaughan, Pocock asked for additional specimens. A mounted leopard was presented to the Zanzibar Museum around this time, and two skins and skulls were sent to the Harvard Museum of Comparative Zoology in 1939 and 1940, but another one was not presented to the British Museum until 1984.[13] All of these were collected by British officials in Zanzibar.

Otherwise the colonial authorities' interest in the Zanzibar leopard was primarily instrumental, linked to its economic value and relation to the maintenance of social order. For many years local trappers were paid by government for killing leopards, which were vilified for preying on livestock in particular.[14] During and immediately after the Second World War, when agricultural production was intensified on Unguja, reports of leopard predation on livestock increased, and a number of attacks on people and especially children were also brought to the government's attention.[15] However, some British officials argued that leopards were in fact benefiting farmers and so helping economic development. This position was most clearly articulated by

R.H.W. Pakenham before and after he rose to become Senior Commissioner in the Zanzibar Provincial Administration. Pakenham insisted that leopards should not be treated as "vermin", because they preyed on animals which caused direct damage to crops. In 1950 therefore the leopard was added to the schedule of protected wild animals, while an order was drawn up that allowed the killing of leopards on permit whenever they became a local nuisance.[16] Needless to say, rural Zanzibaris continued to take matters into their own hands, trapping and hunting leopards regardless of the legal protection afforded to them and outside of the provisions of the new legislation.

After the Zanzibar Revolution in 1964 local practice became national policy. The wildlife protection decree and its amendments were ignored and leopards were hunted down as vermin. It was left to a handful of external scholars to renew and maintain scientific interest in the Zanzibar leopard. Based on a review of museum material and photographs, Dobroruka questioned its classification as an island endemic, suggesting instead that it should be assimilated to a mainland subspecies.[17] Kingdon re-examined the specimens in the British Museum, confirmed the distinctiveness of the Zanzibar leopard, and discussed the possible reasons for this.[18] Pakenham, who had continued to research and write about the fauna of Zanzibar in his retirement, updated earlier work and reviewed existing knowledge of the leopard in his meticulous study of *The Mammals of Zanzibar and Pemba*. Apart from incidental references and a brief report of leopard hunting and the preparation of skins, little information came from Unguja itself until the early 1980s, when Tanzanian wildlife researchers were working on the island. Issai Swai provided an up-to-date description of the status and distribution of the Zanzibar leopard in his thesis about wildlife on the island.[19] He also described the only reported sightings (even now) of the leopard by researchers: "Within the period of the study I succeeded to see one wild leopard at Mapopwe study area [. . .] and Fatina Omari in 1981 (pers. comm.) sighted a leopard at Jozani study area."[20] Unfortunately no one followed up with further fieldwork on the leopard, and nothing more was written about this elusive mammal until the 1990s, by which time some external authorities had begun to assume that it was extinct.[21]

Interest in the Zanzibar leopard was revived when foreign donors and NGOs promoting a conservation agenda began working closely with the Government of Zanzibar. Tony Archer, a Kenyan wildlife consultant, played an important role in bringing the Zanzibar leopard to everyone's attention. He began asking about it on a visit to Jozani Forest in 1991,[22] and continued to gather information during subsequent work, in particular when undertaking antelope surveys for the FINNIDA-funded Zanzibar Forestry Development Project.[23] Archer encouraged and advised many of the researchers who followed, including ourselves. In 1994–95 three students wrote papers about the Zanzibar leopard.[24] Their studies provided useful new information about the leopard and local beliefs about it, discussed in more detail below. In 1995 the Jozani-Chwaka Bay Conservation Project (JCBCP) was started as a collaboration between CARE Tanzania and the Commission for Natural Resources in the (then) Ministry for Agriculture, Livestock and Natural Resources. This was Zanzibar's first integrated conservation and development project, led by a British Project Manager working with the Head of Conservation in the Sub-Commission for Forestry. The Zanzibar leopard was very much on the project's early agenda, reflecting in part Archer's influence. This led directly to the proposal for a survey of practices and beliefs threatening the Zanzibar leopard, which we undertook ourselves.[25]

The work of Archer and others had given credence to local claims that some leopards were bred and kept in captivity by rural Zanzibaris for nefarious purposes, and indeed further investigation of these claims was one of the main objectives of our 1996 survey. It did not take us long to realise that the detailed leopard-keeping narratives that we recorded were not grounded in any real practice of leopard domestication, but are part of a complex of witchcraft beliefs that could be analysed in standard anthropological terms (summarised in the next section). In addition to investigating indigenous knowledge and belief about the Zanzibar leopard, we elicited detailed histories of leopard hunting and analysed available statistical records of leopard kills from the 1980s through to the year preceding our study. We also gathered numerous reports from villagers and forest station staff of recent leopard sightings, leopard attacks on livestock, and sightings of pugmarks. On the basis of all of the evidence that we had examined, we concluded that a small population of leopards remained on Unguja, though it was probably on the brink of extinction. We argued that further research and a conservation programme were urgently required to stave off the imminent extinction of the Zanzibar leopard, and suggested a number of ways in which this might be approached.[26] Following our study, Goldman began to draft a leopard conservation programme for JCBCP, and South African wildlife researchers Chris and Tilde Stuart were recruited to determine the leopard's current status and distribution. Assisted by Goldman, the Stuarts made field observations, undertook camera-trapping and conducted interviews in select areas that were thought to be prime leopard habitat. However, the results of this search were disappointing, and having failed to find any conclusive evidence of leopards, the Stuarts concluded that the Zanzibar leopard was either extinct or as good as.[27] Discouraged by this result, and the implication that further action would not be worthwhile, JCBCP shelved the draft leopard conservation programme and turned its attention to other conservation and development initiatives that were proving rather more promising and were well-supported by the international conservation community.

The Zanzibar leopard continues to be reported as extinct, though the evidence for this remains equivocal[28] and some sources have assumed its continuing existence.[29] The WWF *Strategic Framework for Conservation 2005–2025* for the Eastern Africa Coastal Forests Ecoregion lists "Population status of the Zanzibar leopard is known" as an indicator to be achieved by 2015.[30] In common with the Stuarts' survey in 1997, camera-trapping exercises undertaken in different parts of the island in 2003 and since the end of 2008 have failed to produce any photographs of leopards.[31]

Local understandings: domesticated and kept leopards

If the Zanzibar leopard has been an object of favourable interest among British colonial authorities, zoologists, other researchers and conservationists, most islanders take an entirely negative view of the leopard. Their intense fear and loathing for leopards stems in part from the status of the species as the island's largest and most dangerous predator and is also rooted in the animal's strong association with witchcraft. Central to these beliefs is the notion that malevolent individuals deploy "domesticated" leopards to perform evil deeds for them, chiefly terrorising people for whom they bear ill-will, including family members and fellow villagers. Beliefs about this form of witchcraft include details about how such leopards are secretly bred, trained and moved about among the members of the leopard-sharing associations that own them.[32] Such witches are fearfully respected and gossiped about; under normal circumstances, though, they are not openly accused.

According to these beliefs there are "wild" leopards as well as "kept" ones, distinguished by their behaviour. Domesticated leopards are those encountered near settlements and cultivated fields, which frighten or attack livestock and people, or which do not immediately flee upon being seen. Leopards spotted deep in the bush, promptly evading human contact in the manner characteristic of most wild animals, are likelier to lack owners. Sudden unusual illness, such as vomiting "leopard hairs" or death subsequent to a leopard encounter, is considered proof of its domesticated status, as are the bearing and suggestive statements of a suspected leopard keeper in the area.

These beliefs are grounded in a broader complex of Zanzibari ideas about sorcery and witchcraft,[33] and show interesting parallels with patterns of belief regarding large carnivores and other predatory wild animals elsewhere in Sub-Saharan Africa and further afield.[34] Beliefs about leopards, like witchcraft beliefs in general, readily explain particular occurrences of misfortune and attribute them, ultimately, to human failings and interpersonal conflict. Within local discourse, the logic of these beliefs is virtually impervious to assault, although adherence to these ideas is not quite universal among Zanzibaris.

Their association with witchcraft can be seen to have provided leopards with a measure of protection since the dread of the witch's retribution that would follow from harming a domesticated leopard is very great. Ordinarily, killing a leopard is to be avoided at all costs and a hunter who inadvertently shoots one (mistaking it, at night, for other wildlife) takes pains to conceal all evidence of the event in case it was a "kept" leopard. However, rural Zanzibaris have periodically overcome this fear and attempted to reduce the perceived threat posed by "kept" leopards and their "keepers" through collective action at various scales through the colonial era. Older, localised initiatives in which public oathing ceremonies were directed against leopard keepers, or leopards were openly trapped and killed, were superseded after the 1964 Revolution by a national drive to exterminate leopards and neutralise witches known as the Kitanzi Campaign.[35]

The precise timing of the Kitanzi Campaign and the details of how it unfolded have not been documented and the accounts that informants gave us are incomplete and inconsistent. What is not disputed is that the campaign was spearheaded by a man called Kitanzi Mtaji Kitanzi, who had once played a leading role in public oathing in Makunduchi, in southern Unguja. In 1967 or 1968, President Karume, a "moderniser" alarmed by the perceived effects of witchcraft on the nation's development, supported Kitanzi in a national campaign.[36] The campaign was carried out by organised units of officials who were authorised to arrest suspected witches.[37] While suspected witches, including leopard keepers, were being taken into custody and detained for varying lengths of time, another arm of the campaign focused on exterminating leopards. Led by Kitanzi's brother's son Abdallah Banga, this effort involved as many as 25 or so hunters, issued with guns by the government and protected and strengthened through various forms of magic. For the first time, leopard meat was consumed – in secret by campaign participants and on some accounts also more openly, by children as well as adults.[38] It is not known how many leopards were killed in this campaign by the time it ended some time after the assassination of Karume in 1972.

The conclusion of the Kitanzi Campaign did not stop the killing of leopards, however. Leopards continued to be shot by the National Hunters, a loose organisation of mostly urban-based men whose contribution to vermin control on Unguja was subsidised by the state. Local hunting groups based in rural areas also killed leopards from time to time. Although the colonial laws protecting leopards had never been repealed, they were completely ignored. Exterminating vermin – including leopards – was official policy and was linked with the goal of self-sufficiency in food production.[39] According to the National Hunters' records, roughly 100 leopards were killed in the decade from 1985. In the mid-1990s – at around the same time as leopard conservation became topical as a result of revived interest among researchers in the Zanzibar leopard's fate – the reported figure suddenly fell to zero, and the leopard was listed as a protected species in 1996 wildlife protection legislation.[40] As noted already, camera-trapping efforts have failed to produce any photographs of leopards, and to our knowledge no other indisputable evidence of the survival of a leopard population has turned up, in spite of continuing rumours of leopard sightings and leopard attacks on livestock.

Hybrid discourses about the Zanzibar leopard

As the work of Agrawal and others might lead us to expect, the contrast that we have drawn so far between scientific and indigenous discourses is not always so sharp.[41] In this section we will describe two kinds of hybrid discourse about the Zanzibar leopard, and the actions and proposals stemming from these. The first set of cases sees visiting researchers and others incorporating Zanzibari beliefs into their knowledge and practice. The second set shows Zanzibaris themselves grafting conservation proposals onto local ideas about leopard-keeping.

Kept leopard chases

The first published references to leopard-keeping were made by British colonial officials and missionaries. All of them were careful to refer to this as something that local people believed, implying that they themselves did not.[42] However, there is also evidence to suggest that some of the British in Zanzibar were prepared to accept local statements about leopard-keeping at face value. One of these was Geoffrey Wilkinson, an agricultural officer who spent three years based in Chwaka and Hanyegwamchana in the east of Unguja at the height of the panic about leopard predation. In 1949 he saw an old male leopard that had been trapped near Chwaka, and was told that it was believed to be a leopard which had taken a baby from the Mudir's house.[43] Recalling this event more than half a century later, he wrote: "I, together with all the villagers of Chwaka were convinced that the leopard must have been taken by its owner (an Mchawi [witch]) to the house with the definite intent of taking the babe."[44] There is none of the caution here that Pakenham and others displayed in print. It is unlikely that Wilkinson was the only expatriate in Zanzibar during the colonial period to be persuaded by leopard-keeping narratives, and indeed Pakenham himself seemed prepared to believe that leopards were being tamed when he first wrote about this practice in his field notebooks.[45]

We have relatively little documentary evidence for the decades following the Zanzibar Revolution, before the impacts of political and economic liberalisation began to be felt in the archipelago. Tanzanian researcher Issai Swai's 1983 MSc thesis was one of the first to be written about wildlife and conservation in the islands. He devoted a whole section of his study to the Zanzibar leopard, and reported matter-of-factly that "leopards were tamed and used by witch-craft practitioners", naming a Zanzibari forest guard as his source for this information.[46] Swai evidently tried to follow up on this, but to no avail: "Attempts to be shown a domesticated leopard failed because they are domesticated in secrecy."[47] In later life he remained in no doubt that leopards were indeed domesticated on Unguja.[48] His dissertation was supervised by Alan Rodgers, then a lecturer in the Department of Zoology in the University of Dar es Salaam and one of Tanzania's leading conservationists. It is interesting that Swai's reference to leopard-keeping was allowed to stand, though subsequent leopard chases make it less surprising.

The opening up of Zanzibar to mass tourism in the 1990s brought increasing numbers of outside visitors into contact with rural Zanzibaris. One of these was the Budapest-born Lajos Josza, better known now as the Swiss adventurer and environmentalist Louis Palmer. Josza visited Jozani Forest in September 1994 while on a cycling tour of Africa.[49] After seeing a reference to the Zanzibar leopard at the reserve entrance, he cycled to a nearby village where he was shown and took photos of leopard claws. His hosts offered to take him to see and photograph a leopard in a cave if he paid them 100 US dollars. When they reached the cave they only found leopard scratch marks and faeces, the identification of which was later confirmed from photos. Josza settled with his guides for 50 dollars. The next day he viewed the stuffed leopard in the Zanzibar Museum and then went to the office of the Sub-Commission for Forestry in Maruhubi, where he learned more about the Zanzibar leopard and was entertained with leopard-keeping narratives:

> The belief in these leopards is unshakeable – it belongs to Zanzibar like its palm trees and beaches. "Could I see a captured leopard?" I ask, but the Director gives a sign of refusal: "No! Nobody would ever admit to know who could have such a cat. He could himself be cursed and become a leopard. And this would be worse than any disease in the world."[50]

Enthused by his experience, and told by forestry officials that they had been unable to raise funds for leopard conservation, Josza determined to help. On his return to Switzerland, he reported his findings to the WWF and was later put in contact with Peter Jackson, the Chairman of the IUCN/SSC Cat Specialist Group; the result of this was that modest funds were secured to search for hard evidence of the leopard's continued existence on the island, paying for the Stuarts' survey in 1997.

Before this happened, a new generation of wildlife researchers had already begun to actively engage with leopard-keeping narratives. Although he did not indicate this in his written reports, the Kenyan wildlife consultant Tony Archer was intrigued by the possibility that leopards were indeed being kept by rural Zanzibaris. His principal informant on leopards and leopard-keeping seems to have been the same as Swai's, a Jozani Forest officer who also assisted subsequent leopard researchers and was one of our own interviewees in 1996. Walsh had a number of discussions with Archer about the Zanzibar leopard in 1995 and 1996. During one conversation that included the JCBCP Project Manager and a researcher attached to the project, Archer talked at length about leopard-keeping and what he understood about it. There were, he had been told, at least five kept leopards on the island, and he knew of an offer to be shown one in return for a payment of 50,000 Tanzanian shillings (approximately 100 US dollars). The closest parallel he knew to leopard-keeping on Zanzibar was hyena-rearing in western Tanzania, and he told the story of how a colonial game ranger at Itigi had once come across a trapped hyena that was dressed in a shirt and trousers.[51]

The first of the studies inspired by Archer was a paper on "The Status of the Zanzibar Leopard." The author, Scott Marshall, was an American studying with the School for International Training (SIT), which organises attachments for students throughout Tanzania. Using an interpreter, Marshall interviewed hunters in villages around Jozani in late 1994, and also joined Tony Archer in trying to bait leopards in the forest. One of these attempts, using a chicken, produced fresh leopard spoor, but no live sighting. Marshall collected some basic information about leopard-keeping and recorded that:

> I received several offers from people to show me a domesticated leopard for large quantities of money. I could not afford to pay the required price for many of these offers, so I was not able to capitalise on a lot of potential information. In almost every case, I was not able to see any physical evidence of a leopard without paying a price. I was able to see the claws of a "Konge" leopard [one of a number of locally recognised varieties] killed by a hunter three years ago. Many other people promised to show me faeces, spoor prints, and even an actual leopard, but none followed through on their promises.[52]

Marshall's is the first report of a researcher or other visitor being asked for money to be shown a kept leopard. Whether or not this was a new initiative in response to his and Archer's requests, it certainly became a common phenomenon in the years that followed, replacing the earlier practice of offering leopard skins for sale.[53]

Marshall's work was followed up in April/May 1995 by another young SIT student, Benjamin Selkow. Whereas Marshall had been attached to the Zanzibar Forestry Development Project, Selkow worked directly with the Sub-Commission for Forestry in the Commission for Natural Resources. His paper, "A Survey of Villager Perceptions of the Zanzibar Leopard", was based on interviews with hunters in 15 villages, and covered much the same ground as his fellow American's study. Whereas Marshall was in general noncommittal, Selkow seemed to have no doubts about the reality of leopard-keeping, but discussed it as though it was an important practice to be investigated.[54] He also made of point of asking whether leopards might be publicly exhibited in a zoo or holding pen, a subject we discuss at greater length in the next section. Like Marshall, he was offered the possibility of being shown kept leopards, but could not afford the high prices that people asked:

> I had offers to see trained leopards, but the price for me was too much. But, for a funded research project, the sum (two-hundred US dollars) is very easily managed.[55]

This statement exhibits a degree of naivety, and not just about the budgets of research projects. Researchers like Selkow had evidently become "fair game" for enterprising villagers claiming to have access to kept leopards – never their own, but usually those of absent friends or kin.

This included Tanzanian and even Zanzibari researchers. Khamis A. Khamis was a student in the College of African Wildlife Management at Mweka. Although his fieldwork spanned a much longer period, his "Report on the Status of Zanzibar Leopards from 15th Dec. 1994 to June, 1995 in Different Times at Zanzibar" was much shorter than the papers written by his American predecessors. Again, he worked through the Sub-Commission for Forestry and his research focused on the area around Jozani. Khamis was more cautious than Selkow, and although he listed "Facts of Tamed Leopards", he took care to note "But I failed to get the evidence of the truth of these points."[56] He did, however, pay 10,000 shillings for permission to photograph the skin and claws of a leopard said to have been killed in September 1993.[57] He is the only researcher to admit actually paying like this, and this may have encouraged would-be leopard "entrepreneurs" to continue asking, as they certainly did.

As we have seen the CARE-funded JCBCP began in 1995. The Project Manager, Rob Wild, was influenced by Tony Archer at an early stage and was clearly intrigued by elements of the leopard-keeping narratives that he heard and also read about in existing reports. In addition to employing Goldman and then funding the anthropological survey led by Walsh, he also approved a number of attempts to secure photographic and other evidence for leopard-keeping. In 1996 he told us that one project informant had promised to show a kept leopard for 20,000 shillings, but then claimed that he had to get permission to do so from his mother and that she had said that it would take a week to prepare the necessary protective medicine. This came to nothing.

Thabit Kombo, who was the Head of Conservation and Wild's counterpart, later recalled a number of similarly unsuccessful kept leopard chases.[58] In 1996 or thereabouts a camera purchased with GEF (Global Environment Fund) money was given by the project to the *Sheha* (local government administrator) at Cheju, who promised to get a picture of a leopard. But the camera ended up broken and they got no pictures at all. The project was ready to pay 150,000 shillings for pictures, but the *Sheha* had to return the money that was advanced to him when he failed to get any after a period of months. On another occasion the JCBCP Project Manager camped at Charawe hoping to see a leopard but came away with nothing. Thabit himself was also drawn into these activities, and in 1998 or so a former classmate told him that one of his close relatives was a leopard keeper. It was arranged that they could view the leopard in a cave at Bambi, and agreed that they would pay 200,000 shillings for this. However, when they turned up at Bambi on the appointed day they were told that the leopard owner had gone to Zanzibar Town. They did not pursue the offer again after this disappointment. In 1999 he was told by a Jozani Forest guard that three (presumably kept) leopards had been born in a cave at Ukongoroni. The guard promised to take him to see the cubs, but did not, and there was no further follow-up of this report.

Another JCBCP staff member, Derek Finnie, also later recalled a number of incidents.[59] Around November 1999 two people came separately to the project office claiming to be able to show them leopards. About two weeks separated these two incidents. Finnie had only recently started work at Maruhubi and was not fully aware of what was happening. He went himself with the first claimant out to a village (he had no idea where this was) and was taken to a place on the edge of the settlement where there were two or three houses. However, there was no sign of a leopard, and being new to Zanzibar, he was unable to understand the Swahili explanation of what had happened and why their trip had been fruitless. The second person claiming to be able to show staff a leopard did not come back a second time to the office and no more was heard of that. Finnie also remembered a subsequent occasion when there was a leopard skin in the office for several days. The project had offered money for it and he thought that this may have been paid, but was not sure at the time. However, the skin was measured and it was decided that it must be from a continental African leopard (*Panthera pardus pardus*) because it was too big to be a Zanzibar leopard. This implies that the project had been duped, and perhaps even persuaded to part with money for what might have been an illegally obtained and traded skin from the Tanzanian mainland.[60]

The next incident that we were personally involved in was the Wangwani case. This was not a kept leopard chase as such, but illustrates the fruitless pursuit of leopard material whose outcome was allegedly influenced by the fear of leopard-keeping. In April 2002 Walsh was told by a JCBCP officer, Ali Ali Mwinyi,[61] that the previous August he and others had come across leopard tracks at Wangwani in north-west Jozani, and followed these to an apparent kill, the remains of a male suni antelope. Ali had collected one of its horns and also leopard faeces from the site of the kill, which he had brought back to Maruhubi, where they were kept in bottles. Walsh asked to see them, but after a quick search neither Ali nor Thabit Kombo could find anything, and were told that these precious relics had probably been thrown away by the cleaners or other staff. It was suggested that this was not just an accident, but because of the fear which leopard-linked objects can induce: any normal person with these beliefs would want to get rid of them. Ali then gave Walsh the name of a Jozani Forest Guard who had been at Wangwani with him and might be able to provide more details of the original find.[62] This guide subsequently provided a detailed account that differed in a number of ways from Ali's. He agreed, however, that they had collected leopard faeces, adding that the men in the patrol (eight in all) were quite apprehensive about this, afraid that it was a kept leopard and knowing that keeping such objects was a dangerous thing to do.[63] Ali later said that he had kept this material on his desk for some time, but that it had indeed been thrown out by the office cleaners, a fate that had also befallen leopard scat collected by Goldman some years earlier.[64] Goldman herself followed up on the Wangwani case in January 2003. Two of the other men who had been in the original patrol took her to the site of the antelope kill and provided accounts that were at variance with both those given to Walsh. They could not cast any light on the loss of the material collected by Ali, but like others in the party were clearly steeped in leopard-keeping lore and not entirely happy with the collection of leopard faeces.[65] Subsequent efforts by Goldman to find out more produced more discrepancies, but did at least result in the finding of the original data record of the patrol.[66]

In January 2003 Department of Commercial Crops, Fruits and Forestry (DCCFF) staff also told Goldman about an ongoing kept leopard chase in Marumbi. This was said to have begun three months earlier with reports of leopard predation on livestock and the sighting of a leopard entering and then exiting a local man's house. DCCFF employees were sent to follow up on these reports, and one of them saw the house of the supposed leopard keeper together with a structure at the back that would allow a leopard to come and go. The visitors met with the deputy *Sheha* to talk about events, but were spooked into silence when they realised that the alleged leopard keeper was lurking nearby. A DCCFF team returned again in January 2003, and their leader asked the deputy *Sheha* to collaborate in an attempt to get a photo of the kept leopard. The deputy was very reluctant to agree to this and clearly afraid, but was told that as a government employee he had no option but to cooperate: after all, foreign researchers had come all the way from Europe to do this work. Eventually the deputy *Sheha* yielded, but it was agreed that when the researchers returned with a camera they would have to pretend that they were doing something else, like surveying monkeys or birds. Back in Zanzibar town, the team leader approached Goldman, who was then photo-trapping in Jozani Forest, hoping that she would carry out the plan, for which transport and money for accommodation and a payment to the *Sheha* were all required.[67] But with limited time and resources at her disposal, and bothered by significant discrepancies in the story as related by different key people, Goldman did not pursue it. She left Zanzibar shortly after this, and if there were further efforts to track down the Marumbi leopard they were not brought to our attention.

During fieldwork in rural Zanzibar leopard keepers were often pointed out to us and/or named. We were presented with a number of opportunities to engage in our own kept leopard chases, but did not follow up on these other than by investigating caves and other sites where leopards and leopard signs were said to be found (Goldman in particular, when working for JCBCP). The Marumbi case is worth highlighting though because it is an example of Zanzibari conservation staff themselves being drawn into a kept leopard chase, and then seeking the collaboration of external researchers.

Displaying kept leopards

Whereas foreign researchers have sometimes been beguiled into believing that leopard-keeping is really practised on Unguja, some Zanzibari researchers and others have sought to reconcile their own witchcraft beliefs with conservation science in a quite different way, by proposing that kept leopards be displayed to the public and tourists in particular. Zanzibar had a zoo (of sorts) in the period after the Revolution, and exotic animals have been displayed from time to time. In the mid-1990s a small private zoo, Zala Park, that houses mainly reptiles and amphibians, was established in Muungoni village near to Jozani Forest. But it seems most likely that the modern idea of displaying leopards arose in response to the research that was being undertaken at that time. One of the questions that SIT student Benjamin Selkow asked his interviewees in 1995 was: "Hypothetically, how would you feel if a zoo or holding pen with a Zanzibar leopard was built somewhere in Zanzibar?"[68] He reports:

> I received a mixed response to the proposal of a Zanzibar leopard holding pen. The majority supported the hypothetical plan and thought it was a good idea for a variety of reasons. Some said the present generation (those under forty years of age) has only heard about and had never seen a leopard and probably would not unless there was a zoo. Others said it was a good way to educate people about its history without them feeling threatened because it would be in a cage (and there would be some gratification in seeing "the pest" caged). Many supported the idea because it would attract more tourists which would help the local businesses as well as being a source of government revenue.

> Several interviewees were against this proposal or would support it with some reservations. One man suggested breeding leopards to increase the population, and then distribute them to zoos at hotels around the island for educational and revenue

purposes. A hunter from Upenja was quite adamant against breeding them, saying that only two to four should be kept. He wanted all offspring to be killed because he believed that they should only be for exhibition and not re-introduced into the wild. Another man said it would be a good idea for future generations, but not for the present because there is still too much "aggressive fear". A hunter from Paje supported this and said that exhibiting a Zanzibar leopard would [be] touching too sensitive an area with locals. He proposed exhibiting a mainland sub-species as a first step. Finally, several interviewees thought it would be a bad idea because the zoo would shame hunters, exhibit a creature that had too many superstitious and magical issues associated with it, and make owners vengeful because the respect by fear status that owners enjoy would be downgraded.[69]

Did Selkow help to plant the idea of a leopard pen or zoo? We may never know, but certainly by the time that we began joint fieldwork in July 1996 it was not a new idea. Walsh's field assistant, who was an experienced hunter and former Secretary of the government-subsidised *Wasasi wa Kitaifa* (National Hunters' organisation), enthusiastically asked a number of our interviewees whether it would be feasible to persuade leopard keepers to display their leopards to the public and fee-paying tourists. The same idea also came up in the discussion that followed our end-of-fieldwork presentation to JCBCP and other government staff.

In October 1996 Goldman and a colleague in the Commission for Natural Resources, Wahira J. Othman, were assigned to investigate a proposition that had been made to the Commission. They drove down to Kizimkazi to meet with four men who were proposing to capture and display leopards. At that time Kizimkazi was just beginning to become known for its dolphin tourism. The men claimed to have seen a leopard in the area in recent months, and were firm believers in leopard-keeping, expressing the possibility that all leopards might be kept leopards. But they were not worried by being associated with witchcraft, because they planned to keep leopards in the open, in a zoo along the lines of Zala Park. They opined that it would cost around 300,000 shillings to purchase or capture a single leopard. Once they had a leopard in captivity, they would display it in an enclosure among bushes near the shore. This would be some 30×20 metres in size, and quite high. They also planned to build a reception area and small restaurant, at a cost of some 700,000 shillings. At this point in the conversation it seemed that they might be angling for support from the Commission, but they did not ask for this explicitly. Leopard keepers would show them how to train leopards. They wanted to start with two: a male and a female. One in a group of men suggested that they might kill surplus leopards and sell the skins, but one of his colleagues countered that they would set them free in the bush. Before taking leave, Wahira let them know that the Commission would consider their idea, but that if it was approved, it would only be on a trial basis. On their way back to Zanzibar Town Goldman expressed her doubts about the proposal to Wahira, and did not hear about it again.

In January 2003, an employee at the Department of Regional Administration informed Goldman, in confidence, that he knew someone who had obtained two leopards in Jambiani for the purpose of displaying them to tourists. The animals were purportedly being secretly kept in captivity in Chwaka until the man had made the necessary preparations to exhibit them.[70] Goldman expressed interest in seeing the leopards as the government employee proposed, but he subsequently failed to contact her. So, like other captive leopards rumoured to exist, this pair remained elusive.

The leopard display idea clearly did not wither and die following the dissemination of our final report, in which we made it clear that we thought leopard-keeping to be wholly imaginary.[71] Indeed it surfaced in a quite unexpected place, in a debate in the Zanzibar House of Representatives in April 2003, when the Deputy Minister for Agriculture, Natural Resources, Environment and Co-operatives declared that his ministry would be happy to buy leopards to display them to tourists. At least this is how it was reported in the press:

Government is ready to buy Leopards

THE MINISTRY for Agriculture, Natural Resources, Environment and Co-operatives in Zanzibar has said that it is ready to buy Leopards if people come forward to sell them, reports MWANTANGA AME.

This announcement was made the day before yesterday in the hall of the House of Representatives in Zanzibar town. It was made by the Deputy Minister and Representative for Uzini constituency, Tafana Kassim Mzee, when he was contributing to the debate about starting a special fund.

He declared that his Ministry was ready to buy Leopards so that they could be displayed in tourist areas.

The Representative pointed out that some tourists already came to Zanzibar to see snakes. If Zanzibar had enough Leopards for the purpose then revenues could be raised accordingly.

Tafana said that if the country had these animals they would increase government income, and he asked for citizens to sell them to the state.

He let it be known that the long-held fear that anyone caught with a Leopard would be punished was a thing of the past, and that the government had no plans to do that again.

"There's a fear that if anyone appears with a Leopard, then he'll feel the noose around his neck. Get rid of that fear: my Ministry is ready to buy Leopards; I declare that we will buy those Leopards", he said.

Another Representative who contributed to this debate, Brigadier-General (Rtd.) Adam Mwakanjuki, said that in the past Zanzibar had a lot of Leopards, but that now they had disappeared.

He said that it was good that the Ministry was thinking of obtaining these animals so that they could be put in a special reserve and the government make money.

He said that it was sad that Zanzibar now only had one specimen of that animal in the museum at Mnazi Mmoja in Zanzibar town.[72]

To anyone who has studied the history of Zanzibar leopard-killing since the Revolution, this statement represents an ironic turnaround. Adam Mwakanjuki was one of the original revolutionaries, and for many years the Minister of Agriculture responsible for a policy that classed leopards as vermin and contradicted the legal protection that the law was supposed to offer to them.

Perhaps not surprisingly, rumours about the availability of leopards for purchase have continued to circulate. In July 2011 we received emails from an unknown correspondent, purporting to be a man born in Makunduchi, offering to procure a pair of Zanzibar leopards for us in return for the princely sum of 10 million US dollars. The same email was also sent to two Canadian film directors and their associates who had earlier (in 2009) posted a proposal for a film about the Zanzibar leopard on the web.[73] Not wishing to encourage scams of this kind, none of us replied. Visiting the (renamed) Department of Forestry and Non-Renewable Natural Resources later in the same month, Walsh was told a rumour about the presence of a pair of kept leopards at Mtende, to the south of Makunduchi village.[74] In January 2012 Walsh's research assistant in Uroa told him that he had been contacted by phone and offered one million shillings if he could obtain a young leopard. The would-be buyers were said to be foreigners who already possessed a pair of leopards and were operating through intermediaries in Jozani to procure more.[75] Later in the year he reported that a group of sellers had been found, but that one of the leopard's owners had pulled out of the deal at the last minute.[76] Meanwhile, back in Forestry headquarters, Ali Ali Mwinyi was telephoned by people claiming to have a pair of young leopards for sale in Paje. However, when he attempted to negotiate a visit by Walsh to authenticate the leopards prior to purchase, his contacts reneged on a previous agreement to allow this. When asked who might want to buy these leopards, he named a senior official in his Ministry who was, he emphasised, acting in a private capacity. This well-educated man, who is familiar with our research on the Zanzibar leopard, was said to be eager to obtain leopards for display and the income this could generate.[77]

Conclusion: hybridity and incommensurability

Our own view, as we have already made clear, is that these kept leopard chases and proposals for their purchase and display are quixotic enterprises, pursuits of the imaginary. While some Zanzibaris have clearly had their eyes on making a fast buck, both foreign and local researchers have all too often fallen for or been unwilling to reject narratives of leopard-keeping. This is perhaps not entirely surprising. The persistence of witchcraft beliefs in contemporary Tanzania and other parts of Africa is now the subject of a large literature,[78] and it is not unusual for Westerners to take some of these beliefs on board. Indeed it is not unknown for anthropologists to suspend disbelief and get caught up in the occult.[79] The same presumably also happens to natural scientists, though there might be less opportunity for its expression in their professional work.

In the case of the Zanzibar leopard, the reality is that there is a continuum of falsifiable knowledge and unfalsifiable belief (and so "hybrid discourses") along which different people's views at different times might be placed. Some researchers have never been persuaded by leopard-keeping narratives. Long residence in East Africa and a working knowledge of Swahili has not insulated others, but in some cases it seems to have increased their gullibility, as well as their thirst for more knowledge. And so, for example, Tony Archer's interest in the Zanzibar leopard and leopard-keeping ultimately led to our own research and the rapid realisation that it had the same ontological status as many other African witchcraft beliefs, at least as these are understood in the mainstream.[80]

In some respects this case invites interpretation in the terms discussed by Agrawal and indeed this is how we have structured the paper. Here is a more recent summary of his well-known argument:

> Initial studies of indigenous knowledge (and its analogues such as local, practical, or traditional) sought to underline its difference from scientific knowledge (and its analogues such as western, rational, or modern) along a variety of methodological and contextual criteria. But most scholars have now come to accept that there are no simple or universal criteria that can be deployed to separate indigenous from western or scientific knowledge. Attempts to draw a strict line between scientific and indigenous

knowledge on the basis of method, epistemology, context-dependence, or content, it is easy to show, are ultimately untenable.[81]

There is more to the Zanzibar leopard's fate, though, than different constructions of knowledge. It is about the practice that both stems from and informs knowledge, and the reality that underlies both. However hybrid the discourses have become, there is still a fundamental disagreement at the heart of different proposals for the conservation (or not, as the case may be) of the Zanzibar leopard. This disagreement concerns the very existence and nature of the animal that zoologists have called *Panthera pardus adersi* and that most Zanzibaris know simply as *ch'ui*, "the leopard". As recent decades have shown, there is no easy way to bridge the gulf between conflicting understandings of the leopard and the different practices that they comprise and entail. The simplest way out for conservationists has been to believe that the Zanzibar leopard is extinct, or so close to extinction that it is not worth saving. Instead they have focused attention on more visible and charismatic species (dolphins and the endemic Zanzibar red colobus) and on the conservation of the seascapes and landscapes that sustain the island's greatest biodiversity. These are perfectly reasonable things to do, but by turning away from the issues that this case raises, they have left the Zanzibar leopard suspended between science and belief.

Conservation scientists have not been particularly troubled by either the demise of the Zanzibar leopard – leopards are not threatened globally – or the persistence of anecdotal reports of its survival, interesting though these might be from an ethnographic and an epistemological point of view. We would argue, however, that the case of the Zanzibar leopard raises awkward questions for the policy and practice of conservation not only in Zanzibar, but also more generally. Over the past two decades, participatory engagement and the incorporation of local knowledge in conservation initiatives have become standard recommendations. As we know from existing critiques of participatory development and community-based conservation, their implementation is frequently far from perfect, the blame for this being variously laid on failures of agency (e.g., poor planning and execution), the obduracy of structure (e.g., of hegemonic power) or combinations of both.[82] Naïve optimism about the value and assimilability of local knowledge often survives these critiques, and simple conceptions of this knowledge and its possession are rarely subjected to the same kind of detailed examination. Our study of the Zanzibar leopard illustrates what can happen when local knowledge and its transformations are exposed to critical scrutiny. In this case it reveals a deep and in some respects widening divide between scientific knowledge and the hybrid discourses of many Zanzibaris, including local conservationists trained in conservation science. The gulf in interpretation is arguably unbridgeable, and has led to sharply conflicting proposals for action (or inaction as the case may be). The challenge this poses to conservation is how to act when such incommensurabilities emerge. It helps, of course, to recognise them in the first place, and we hypothesise that many more cases of this kind are waiting to be described.

Acknowledgements

We are indebted to everyone who has helped us in our research, including all of our sources in Zanzibar, named and unnamed in the text. A version of this paper was presented at the VIII European Swahili Workshop (*Contemporary Issues in Swahili Ethnography*), University of Oxford, 19–21 September 2010. We are grateful to Iain Walker for providing us with this opportunity, to other participants in the workshop for their perceptive comments, and to our two anonymous *JEAS* reviewers for helping us to improve the paper. The usual disclaimer applies.

Notes

1. Woodroffe, Simon, and Rabinowitz, *People and Wildlife.*
2. For example Nowell and Jackson, *Wild Cats*; Inskip and Zimmermann, "Human-Felid Conflict."
3. Knight, "Introduction."
4. Berkes, "Community-based Conservation."
5. For example, Sillitoe, "Ethnobiology and Applied Anthropology."
6. Compare Agrawal, "Indigenous Knowledge."
7. For example Burton, *Zanzibar*, 198.
8. Walsh and Goldman, "Updating the Inventory," 4.
9. Mansfield-Aders, "Natural History of Zanzibar and Pemba," 329.
10. Walsh and Goldman "Updating the Inventory," 4.
11. Natural History Museum Archives, London, Pocock to Vaughan, 11 December 1929.
12. Pocock, "Leopards of Africa," 563.
13. Walsh and Goldman, "Updating the Inventory," 4–5.
14. Zanzibar National Archives, file AB4/434, "Destruction of Leopards", 1922–48, and correspondence therein.
15. For details see Walsh and Goldman, "Killing the King."
16. Zanzibar Protectorate, *Wild Animals Protection (Amendment of Schedule) Order, 1950*, Government Notice No. 29, 11 March 1950; *Wild Animals Protection (Exception) Order, 1950*, Government Notice No. 30, 11 March 1950.
17. Dobroruka, "Zur Verbreitung des 'Sansibar-Leoparden'."
18. Kingdon, *East African Mammals*, 351; also *Island Africa*, 45.
19. Swai, "Wildlife Conservation Status," 19–20, 48, 52–53.
20. Ibid., "Wildlife Conservation Status," 53.
21. For example, Nowell and Jackson, *Wild Cats*, 27, Fig. 6.
22. Archer, Collins, and Brampton, "Report on a Visit," 65.
23. Archer, *Survey of Hunting Techniques*, 2, 17.
24. Marshall, "Status of the Zanzibar Leopard"; Selkow, "Survey of Villager Perceptions"; Khamis, "Report on the Status."
25. Goldman and Walsh, *Leopard in Jeopardy.*
26. Ibid., iii–iv.
27. Stuart and Stuart, *Preliminary Faunal Survey.*
28. Goldman and Walsh, "Is the Zanzibar Leopard Extinct?"
29. Nahonyo et al., *Biodiversity Inventory.*
30. Mugo, *Eastern Africa Coastal Forests*, 16.
31. Goldman and Winther-Hansen, "First Photographs"; Siex, *Protected Area Spatial Planning*, 28.
32. This account is based on Goldman and Walsh, *Leopard in Jeopardy*, 5–15.
33. Ingrams, *Zanzibar*, 465–477; Goldman, "Comparative Study," 349–357, 371–378; Arnold, "Wazee Wakijua Mambo."
34. Evans-Pritchard, *Witchcraft*; Middleton and Winter, *Witchcraft and Sorcery*; Marwick, *Witchcraft and Sorcery*; Moore and Sanders, *Magical Interpretations*; Stewart and Strathern, *Witchcraft.*
35. Walsh and Goldman, "Killing the King."
36. "Makamo avilaani vitendo vya uchawi," *Kweupe*, 12 August 1967; see also Swai, "Wildlife Conservation Status," 20; Archer, *Survey of Hunting Techniques*, 17.
37. Walsh and Goldman, "Killing the King."
38. Shabani Imani Ali, interviewed by Helle Goldman, Pete, Zanzibar, 19 January 2003, and Ameir Mohammed, interviewed by Helle Goldman, Oslo, Norway, 29 May 2008.
39. Khamis, "Report on the Status," 6.
40. Zanzibar Revolutionary Government, *The Forest Resources Management and Conservation Act no. 10 of 1996.* The approximately 90 vertebrate and 13 invertebrate species in

Appendix 1 "are to be totally protected year round and . . . are to be accorded the highest conservation action and work priority."

41. Agrawal, "Dismantling the Divide."
42. Abdy, "Witchcraft", 237–238; Ingrams, *Zanzibar*, 471; Pakenham, *Mammals*, 49.
43. The Mudir was an administrative officer who presided over a number of *Shehas* and their territories.
44. Letter from Geoffrey D. Wilkinson to Martin Walsh, 4 August 2004.
45. Natural History Museum, Tring, Manuscript Collection of Richard Hercules Wingfield Pakenham (1906–1993), natural history notebook X, entry dated 25 July 1948.
46. Swai, "Wildlife Conservation Status," 20.
47. Ibid., 52.
48. Conversation with Martin Walsh, Iringa, 23 May 2001.
49. The following is based primarily on Josza's published account of these events (Palmer, *Verrückt Nach Dieser Welt*, 35–38) and a telephone conversation and email exchange with Helle Goldman on 6 and 8 March 2005 respectively.
50. Palmer, *Verrückt Nach Dieser Welt*, 38. This English translation from the German text was kindly drafted by Winfried Dallmann in Tromsø, and has only been slightly amended. The allusion to metamorphosis may be based on a misunderstanding, and Josza admitted to Helle Goldman that he had difficulty in interpreting what was said. It is more likely that he was told about the leopard-like behaviour (including growling and barking) that is said to be exhibited by people who have come into contact with leopards and/or angered their keepers.
51. Conversation with Martin Walsh and others, Zanzibar, 15 June 1995. Walsh has heard similar stories in south-west and south-central Tanzania.
52. Marshall, "Status of the Zanzibar Leopard," 11–12.
53. See Goldman and Walsh, *Leopard in Jeopardy*.
54. Selkow, "Survey of Villager Perceptions," 6, 12.
55. Ibid., 26.
56. Khamis, "Report on the Status," 4.
57. Ibid., 6–7.
58. Thabit Kombo, interviewed by Martin Walsh, Maruhubi, Zanzibar, 5 April 2002.
59. Derek Finnie, interviewed by Martin Walsh, Ngome Kongwe, Zanzibar, 6 April 2002.
60. Another JCBCP staff member who had been involved in this case later told Walsh that local "experts" had viewed the skin and rejected a Zanzibar provenance. It was also known to have been brought to Maruhubi by businessmen in need of cash. Ali Ali Mwinyi, interviewed by Martin Walsh, Maruhubi, Zanzibar, 8 April 2002.
61. Ali Ali Mwinyi, who features more than once in this paper, worked as a research assistant on our 1996 study.
62. Ali Ali Mwinyi, interviewed by Martin Walsh, Maruhubi, Zanzibar, 5 April 2002.
63. Ramadhani Khamis Suleiman ("Mcheju"), interviewed by Martin Walsh, Jozani Visitors' Centre, Zanzibar, 7 April 2002.
64. Ali Ali Mwinyi, interviewed by Martin Walsh, Maruhubi, Zanzibar, 8 April 2002. Our interest in locating this leopard material derived in part from the possibility of using it for genetic analysis.
65. Jarahani Mcha Mkanga and Khatibu Zuberi Khatibu, interviewed by Helle Goldman on a visit to Wangwani, Jozani Forest, Zanzibar, 11 January 2003.
66. Field Data Collection Form, "Wangwani mangroves", dated 19 August 2001.
67. Sheha Idrissa Hamdan, meeting with Helle Goldman, Zanzibar Town, 23 January 2003.
68. Selkow, "Survey of Villager Perceptions," 12. This is the English version of a question that was translated into Swahili by his interpreter.
69. Ibid., p. 20.
70. This conversation took place at Vuga, Zanzibar, 23 January 2003.
71. Goldman and Walsh, *Leopard in Jeopardy*.
72. Mwantanga Ame, "Serikali Iko Tayari Kununua Chui," *Zanzibar Leo*, April 13, 2003. Our translation from the Swahili original.
73. Emails from Mohammed D. Babu to Martin Walsh, Helle Goldman, Adam Gray, Andrew Gray and others, dated 8 July 2011. The film proposal, entitled "The Ghost Leopard of

Zanzibar", named Walsh as a participant. The film was not made and the proposal has since been removed from the web.
74. Ali Ali Mwinyi, in discussion with Martin Walsh, Maruhubi, Zanzibar, 20 July 2011.
75. Msellem Abdalla Abdalla, in conversation with Martin Walsh, Pongwe, Zanzibar, 19 January 2012.
76. Msellem Abdalla Abdalla, in conversation with Martin Walsh, Pongwe, Zanzibar, 4 August 2012.
77. Ali Ali Mwinyi, in discussion with Martin Walsh, Maruhubi, Zanzibar, 30 July 2012.
78. For example Abrahams, *Witchcraft*; Moore and Sanders, *Magical Interpretations*.
79. For example, Turner, "Reality of Spirits"; Willis, *Some Spirits Heal*.
80. Compare Evans-Pritchard, *Witchcraft*.
81. Agrawal, "Dismantling the Divide," 293.
82. See, for example, Berkes, "Community-based Conservation"; Cooke and Kothari, *Participation*; Escobar, "After Nature."

References

Abdy, Dora M. "Witchcraft amongst the Wahadimu." *Journal of the African Society* 16 (1917): 234–41.

Abrahams, R.G., ed. *Witchcraft in Contemporary Tanzania*. Cambridge: African Studies Centre, 1994.

Agrawal, Arun. "Dismantling the Divide between Indigenous and Scientific Knowledge." *Development and Change* 26 (1995): 413–39.

Agrawal, Arun. "Indigenous Knowledge and the Politics of Classification." *International Social Science Journal* 54 (2002): 287–97.

Archer, A.L. *A Survey of Hunting Techniques and the Results thereof on Two Species of Duiker and the Suni Antelopes in Zanzibar*. Report to FINNIDA/Forestry Sector, Commission for Natural Resources, Zanzibar, 1994.

Archer, A.L., S. Collins, and I. Brampton. "Report on a Visit to Jozani Forest, Zanzibar." *East Africa Natural History Society Bulletin* 21 (1991): 59–66.

Arnold, Natalie. "Wazee Wakijua Mambo/Elders Used to Know Things!: Occult Powers and Revolutionary History in Pemba, Zanzibar." PhD diss., Indiana University, 2003.

Berkes, F. "Community-based Conservation in a Globalised World." *Proceedings of the National Academy of Sciences of the United States of America* 104 (2007): 15188–93.

Burton, Richard F. *Zanzibar; City, Island, and Coast* (Volume I). London: Tinsley Brothers, 1872.

Cooke, Bill, and Uma Kothari, eds. *Participation: The New Tyranny?* London and New York: Zed Books, 2001.

Dobroruka, L.J. "Zur Verbreitung des 'Sansibar-Leoparden', *Panthera pardus adersi* Pocock." *Zeitschrift für Säugetierkunde* 30, no. 1964 (1932): 144–6.

Escobar, Arturo. "After Nature: Steps to an Antiessentialist Political Ecology." *Current Anthropology* 40 (1999): 1–30.

Evans-Pritchard, E.E. *Witchcraft, Oracles and Magic among the Azande*. Oxford: Clarendon Press, 1937.

Goldman, Helle. 1996. "A Comparative Study of Swahili in Two Rural Communities in Pemba, Zanzibar, Tanzania." PhD diss., New York University, 1996.

Goldman, Helle, and Martin Walsh. *A Leopard in Jeopardy: An Anthropological Survey of Practices and Beliefs which Threaten the Survival of the Zanzibar Leopard* (Panthera pardus adersi). Report to Jozani–Chwaka Bay Conservation Project, Commission for Natural Resources: Zanzibar, 1997.

Goldman, Helle, and Martin Walsh. "Is the Zanzibar Leopard (*Panthera pardus adersi*) Extinct?" *Journal of East African Natural History* 91 (2002): 15–25.

Goldman, Helle, and Jon Winther-Hansen. "First Photographs of the Zanzibar Servaline Genet *Genetta servalina archeri* and Other Endemic Subspecies on the Island of Unguja, Tanzania." *Small Carnivore Conservation* 29 (2003): 1–4.

Ingrams, W.H. *Zanzibar: Its History and its People*. London: Frank Cass, 1931.

Inskip, C., and A. Zimmermann. "Human-Felid Conflict: A Review of Patterns and Priorities Worldwide." *Oryx* 43 (2009): 18–34.

Khamis, Khamis A. "Report on the Status of Zanzibar Leopards from 15th Dec. 1994 to June 1995 in Different Times at Zanzibar." Certificate student paper, College of African Wildlife Management, Mweka, 1995.

Kingdon, Jonathan. *East African Mammals: An Atlas of Evolution in Africa. Vol. IIIA, Carnivores.* Chicago: University of Chicago Press, 1977.

Kingdon, Jonathan. *Island Africa: The Evolution of Africa's Rare Animals and Plants.* Princeton: Princeton University Press, 1989.

Knight, John. "Introduction." In *Natural Enemies: People-Wildlife Conflicts in Anthropological Perspective*, ed. John Knight, 1–35. London and New York: Routledge, 2000.

Mansfield-Aders, William. 1920. "The Natural History of Zanzibar and Pemba." In *Zanzibar: The Island Metropolis of Eastern Africa*, ed. F.B. Pearce, 326–39. London: T. Fisher Unwin, 1920.

Marshall, Scott. "The Status of the Zanzibar Leopard." Student paper, SIT Study Abroad, Zanzibar, 1994.

Middleton, John, and E.H. Winter, eds. *Witchcraft and Sorcery in East Africa.* London: Routledge and Kegan Paul, 1963.

Marwick, Max, ed. *Witchcraft and Sorcery: Selected Readings.* Harmondsworth: Penguin, 1970.

Moore, Henrietta, and Todd Sanders, eds. *Magical Interpretations, Material Realities: Modernity, Witchcraft and the Occult in Postcolonial Africa.* London: Routledge, 2001.

Mugo, K., ed. *Eastern Africa Coastal Forests Ecoregion: Strategic Framework for Conservation 2005–2025.* Nairobi: WWF Eastern Africa Regional Programme Office, 2006.

Nahonyo, C.L., L.B. Mwasumbi, S. Eliapenda, C. Msuya, C. Mwansasu, T.M. Suya, B.O. Mponda, and P. Kihaule. *Biodiversity Inventory of Jozani–Chwaka Proposed National Park, Zanzibar.* Technical report for CARE Tanzania/Department of Commercial Crops, Fruits and Forestry, Zanzibar, 2002.

Nowell, Kristin, and Peter Jackson, eds. *Wild Cats: Status Survey and Conservation Action Plan.* Gland, Switzerland: IUCN, 1996.

Pakenham, R.H.W. *The Mammals of Zanzibar and Pemba Islands.* Harpenden: Privately printed, 1984.

Palmer, Louis. *Verrückt Nach Dieser Welt: Abenteur zwischen Himmel und Erde.* Bielefeld: Delius Klasing Verlag, 2005.

Pocock, Reginald I. "The Leopards of Africa." *Proceedings of the Zoological Society of London* II (1932): 543–91.

Selkow, Benjamin. "A Survey of Villager Perceptions of the Zanzibar Leopard." Student paper, SIT Study Abroad, Zanzibar, 1995.

Siex, Kirstin S. *Protected Area Spatial Planning for Unguja and Pemba Islands, Zanzibar.* Report to the World Wide Fund for Nature (WWF), Wildlife Conservation Society, New York, 2011.

Sillitoe, Paul. "Ethnobiology and Applied Anthropology: Rapprochement of the Academic with the Practical." *Journal of the Royal Anthropological Institute* 12 (2006): S119–42.

Stewart, Pamela J., and Andrew Strathern. *Witchcraft, Sorcery, Rumors, and Gossip.* Cambridge: Cambridge University Press, 2004.

Stuart, Chris, and Tilde Stuart. *A Preliminary Faunal Survey of South-eastern Unguja (Zanzibar) with Special Emphasis on the Leopard* Panthera pardus adersi. Unpublished report, African–Arabian Wildlife Research Centre, Loxton, South Africa, 1997.

Swai, Issai S. "Wildlife Conservation Status in Zanzibar." MSc diss., University of Dar es Salaam, 1983.

Turner, Edith. "The Reality of Spirits: A Tabooed or Permitted Field of Study?" *The Anthropology of Consciousness* 3 (1992): 9–12.

Walsh, Martin, and Helle Goldman. "Killing the King: The Demonization and Extermination of the Zanzibar Leopard/Tuer le Roi: La Diabolisation et l'Extermination du Leopard de Zanzibar." In *Le Symbolisme des Animaux: L'Animal Clef-de-Voûte dans la Tradition Orale et les Interactions Homme–Nature/Animal Symbolism: The 'Keystone' Animal in Oral Tradition and Interactions between Humans and Nature*, ed. E. Dounias, E. Motte-Florac and M. Dunham, 1133–82. Paris: IRD, 2007.

Walsh, Martin, and Helle Goldman. "Updating the Inventory of Zanzibar Leopard Specimens." *CAT News* (Newsletter of the IUCN/SSC Cat Specialist Group), 49 (2008): 4–6.

Willis, Roy. *Some Spirits Heal, Others Only Dance: A Journey into Human Selfhood in an African Village.* Oxford: Berg Publishers, 1999.

Woodroffe, R., T. Simon, and A. Rabinowitz, ed. *People and Wildlife: Conflict or Co-existence?* Cambridge: Cambridge University Press, 2005.

Constructing translocal socioscapes: consumerism, aesthetics, and visuality in Zanzibar Town

Paola Ivanov

Ethnological Museum–National Museums in Berlin–Prussian Cultural Heritage Foundation

In examining the burgeoning practices of conspicuous consumption of imported commodities in contemporary Zanzibar Town, this contribution seeks to go beyond simplifying interpretations of non-Western consumerism by focusing on the significance of aesthetics and beauty in Zanzibar's social life. Following Alfred Gell, aesthetics is seen as a "technology of enchantment". It deploys its effectiveness in an agonistic as well as unifying sense in the course of ceremonial exchanges of the gift of beauty, which in turn serves as a veiled disclosure of socioeconomic and moral values in a Muslim world characterised by the habitus of "covering". It is argued that the topic of aesthetics, which is mostly neglected by anthropology, provides a clue to a deeper understanding of key processes of constructing difference and value, as well as of community building in Swahili societies. Such a perspective reveals specific, culturally shaped patterns not only of consumerism, but also of relating to the social and material world which cannot be subsumed under Western models.

Theory and practice of research: anthropology, consumerism, and aesthetics

The focus of this contribution is on aesthetics, a topic that is unorthodox from the perspective of social anthropology, and, in connection with this, on visuality – a slightly less unusual topic. The reasons for the negative attitude held by anthropology towards aesthetics will be addressed later. However, it should be stressed that my exploration of this issue did not arise from theoretical considerations prior to fieldwork, but inevitably emerged from research experience in Zanzibar – it is one of those topics that are suggested for analysis by the subject of study itself.

Originally, my research in Zanzibar focused on consumption, a topic that has gained new relevance in the context of the debate on globalisation. Using the capital Zanzibar Town as an example, my study aimed at examining how identity and personhood are constituted by means of goods in Zanzibar's postcolonial society, and what role is played in that process by the consumption of things coming from "outside", including contemporary global goods.[1] The theoretical background of that question is the long history of translocal interconnectedness of the Swahili-speaking Muslim polities of the East African coast. Having emerged since the late first millennium CE within the commercial and religious networks interlinking the littoral regions of the Indian Ocean as middlemen communities in the trade between the maritime regions and the East African hinterland and interior, Swahili towns were (and are) characterised by the continuous integration of people, ideas, and things that have their origin in the aforementioned places. Imports from the Indian Ocean region, such as glazed earthenware and Chinese porcelain, many different kinds of textiles, glass, jewellery, and cosmetics had paramount cultural relevance in the coastal towns. Following integration into the world market in the nineteenth century, commodities from Europe and North America began to flow in as well.[2]

Within the current debate on globalisation and on processes of appropriation, the overriding question that imposes itself from this long history of interconnectivity at the Swahili coast is: to what extent can locally specific patterns of constituting the person and identity by means of goods and consumption be found in Zanzibar, and how do these patterns interact with historical transformations?[3] In that context, consumption is not viewed from the older, semiotic perspective, but from that of practice theory, and thus defined as a practice that is socially shaped while at the same time shaping society: practices of consumption do not merely reflect pre-existing structures and meanings, but contribute to the latter's creation by objectifying, reproducing, and modifying them. This approach also implies a focus on the relationship between subject, object, and society, on which the modes of consumption are based, as well as on the role played by materiality and embodiment in that context. According to the view now generally held in research, the subject is created in relation to its social and material environment. This, however, is interpreted in very diverse ways by various scholars.[4] Furthermore, the question arises as to how far the spread and appropriation of today's global goods entail the adoption of some "modern" consumer culture, or consumerism, of Western imprint and of the corresponding patterns of subject formation and social integration – that is, according to prevalent interpretations: individualisation, a striving for distinction, the formation of lifestyles, and the emergence of milieus defined by the latter.[5] Or is there, on the contrary, a historically founded local practice of consumption that only outwardly, by using the same things, resembles its Western-modern counterpart?[6]

In the Swahili coastal towns in general, but particularly in Zanzibar Town due to the rapid increase in commodity flows following economic liberalisation in the 1980s, there is today a pronounced competition by means of imported goods and fashions which are locally chiefly conceptualised as "European" or "Arab".[7] The female sphere is at the very centre of this competitive consumption, which is most obvious at opulent wedding ceremonies as well as at other family festivities such as the newly introduced children's birthday parties. It also strongly manifests itself in women's clothing and adornment. However, emic appraisal does not focus on the opulence *per se*, but on "beauty", *uzuri*: the beauty of furnishings or decoration, of a ceremony, or a person. Women engage in a virtual cult of beauty into which they invest much effort and money (Figure 1). Moreover, there is a general emphasis on the beauty of Zanzibari women which forms a basis of communal identity: in 2006, a debate arose about whether the newfangled beauty contests that had become increasingly popular in mainland Tanzania should be held in Zanzibar as well. Muslim tradition seemed to forbid this, yet the slogan "all Zanzibari women are beautiful, and thus we do not need any beauty contests" offered a solution accepted by most.

But let us return to the topic of consumption. With regard to such extreme forms of consumption, in particular of global ("Western") goods, by "Southern" societies, scholarship offers a repertory of simplifying formulas. On the one hand, these betray a

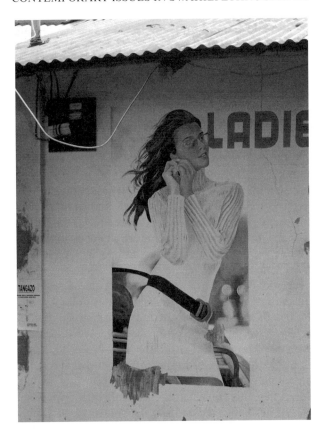

Figure 1.   Wall painting advertising a beauty salon. Zanzibar Town, Mlandege (Photo Klaus Raab, 2006; © Paola Ivanov).

puritan, at times denunciatory, attitude towards something that appears to be an exaggerated obsession with outward appearance. On the other, there is an uneasiness and a feeling of estrangement on the part of scholars with a Western education in the face of the use of "our" goods in unexpected ways, by unexpected people, and in unexpected environments; at the bottom line, this is perceived as ridiculous by Western or Western-influenced sensibilities, even though this perception is never made explicit. For that reason, the postcolonial interpretations, which imply that the unfamiliar appropriations are expressions of "ironies" undermining the "hegemonic" symbolic orders that are being replicated,[8] have an air of exoticism. The subversion occurs only in the eyes of the postcolonial beholder who takes "Western" meanings as a benchmark.

While such impressionistic interpretations of processes of appropriation have largely given way to a serious, actor-focused analysis of the creative adaptation of global cultural forms to the respective local social and cultural environment,[9] the reasons for the appropriation in the context of consumption remain unclear in the final analysis. It is apparently assumed that the brave new world of goods exerts some kind of "fatal attraction"[10] which unfolds automatically: neo-liberalism is thus affirmed. So-called economies of desire are commonly thought to develop on the basis of consumption serving as a key to "modern" lifestyles. The appropriation of global goods is thus interpreted as a way of taking possession of things as symbols of (Western) modernity, or is viewed exclusively as a localisation of Western "consumer culture".[11]

The lavishness of consumption can be reduced to a simple formula as well: to the concept of "conspicuous consumption" which emphasises the wealth of the actors and thus creates prestige and status – a formula that was coined by economist Thorstein Veblen at the turn of the nineteenth/twentieth centuries. Alternatively, recourse is taken to the concept of demonstration, or communication, of status by means of (exaggerated) consumption, according to the interpretation of fashion given by sociologist Georg Simmel, or the structuralist point of view later advanced by Mary Douglas and Baron Isherwood.[12] While all these analyses interpret consumption as a practice, they essentially view it as a means used for representation or communication: of wealth or of status.

All these models do not allow for the possibility that consumption may be about something different as well, even about "beauty" and aesthetics, as is the case in Zanzibar. In anthropology, aesthetics has an even worse reputation than consumption. This is due to the misconception that whenever social and cultural phenomena in non-Western societies do not correspond to modern Western definitions, this implies that they are non-existent. While this is tantamount to asserting, for example, that acephalous societies do not have any political system – an idea that has already been discarded in the founding period of social anthropology – this misconception has long persisted with regard to aesthetics.[13] The study of aesthetic forms of expression remained reserved to the anthropology of art; dealing with allegedly "traditional" aesthetic phenomena that fit into the Eurocentric category of fine arts, it has lived a shadowy existence within the discipline to this day.

Apart from a peculiar reluctance to study the beautiful within the context of respectable social science, this constellation is mainly due to an absolutisation of the Western definition of aesthetics which basically goes back to Immanuel Kant. The term "aesthetics" (derived from Greek *aisthesis*, "sensory perception") was introduced into philosophy in the mid-eighteenth century by Baumgarten as the "science of perception" and, more specifically, as the "science of sensible cognition".[14] In the writings of Kant, the term has two meanings: on the one hand (and often neglected), it continues to refer to the "science" of perception or, more precisely, of the "sensuous faculty" or "sensibility" as the foundation of cognition. This is what Kant calls "transcendental aesthetic".[15] On the other hand, his understanding of this term corresponds to today's general definition of aesthetics as the judgement about what is beautiful: in his terminology, the "pure aesthetic judgement" or "judgement of taste".[16] According to Kant, this is defined by the disinterested, free feeling of pleasure which becomes awakened and excludes the wish to enjoy, possess, and also to understand the beautiful object. However, the judgement of taste is not arbitrary, but rather determined by the harmonious union – a "free play" – of the faculties of imagination and understanding: the subject feels itself.[17]

The bourgeois understanding of "art" (limited to literature, music, the visual and performing arts) developed from this second definition, including the ideological connotation of "artistic beauty", the cult of the genius, the invention of the "connoisseur", and other almost religiously charged attributions and attitudes. The "lower" senses – touch, taste, smell – are excluded from that understanding, and the same is true for mundane, material and bodily beauty; after all, such beauty serves specific purposes, evokes desire, arouses interest in pleasure, and does not seem to allow for a harmonious interplay with reason and an association with morality.[18] This classical concept of aesthetics as detached from the sphere of everyday life is the reason for the negative attitude towards it on the part of the social sciences.

Does this imply that, in accordance with the interpretations offered by the social sciences, we are thus merely dealing with demonstration and maybe with distinction in Zanzibar, based on the last universal: the undifferentiated human desire for material things, and particularly for things of "Western" modernity? And does it imply that this desire is possibly coupled – and this would mean that we are dealing with still more universals – with a passion for finery and/or a readiness for submission to sexualised male fantasies that is innate in women's very nature?

In order to clarify these questions, let us return to the ethnographic context. While I will use the definition of aesthetics in the comprehensive meaning of sensory perception, the quality of experience, that is, "beauty", is definitely important as well, at least when it comes to analysing aesthetics in Zanzibar.

Reciprocal exchange, beauty, and respect: the paradox of veiled disclosure

To begin with, it is remarkable that the so-called ostentatious display by means of consumption is found in a cultural context shaped by Muslim religion, where the contrast between showing and not-showing and between seeing and not-seeing plays a focal role. Indeed, if one examines the everyday practices that serve to create the subject as well as spatial and temporal order in Zanzibar, "covering" (Kiswahili: -sitiri, noun: sitara), that is, the material and immaterial "shielding" of the person and of social spaces, can be identified as the basic principle of experiencing and shaping the world.[19] This "shielding" is constantly negotiated and implemented anew in practice, both at the material and the immaterial levels: first, by covering the bodies not only of women, but also of men, who have to observe Muslim clothing rules as well (their covering has to reach beneath their knees and shoulders). It is also realised in people's behaviour, which is very self-restrained and polite in terms of speech and demeanour on the part of the women *and*, again, also of the men. This reserved behaviour aims at protecting everything that is conceived as "intimate", ranging from people's bodies and feelings to all family matters, and thus might cause embarrassment to someone if exposed. People take great pains to make sure that no personal or family matters do become public. These are for the most part not matters that might be called "improper" or even "immoral" – actually, the Western concept of shame is too narrow to grasp these practices.

Sitara is the material and immaterial protection that safeguards the purity of intimacy and the family. Hence, it is put into practice by separating and shielding spaces (again, both materially and immaterially) according to an "intimacy gradient"[20] (Figure 2). The sharp dichotomisation between public = masculine and private = feminine space, which is considered a characteristic feature of Muslim societies,[21] is not found in Zanzibar. Rather, we are dealing with gradients of social closeness and the purity or impurity associated with them. There are subtle nuances, ranging from the "pure", protected house, which is associated with the lady of the house and requires the lowest degree of veiling, to the neighbourhood, more or less busy streets, and finally to the place associated with maximum impurity and thus requiring the highest degree of protection – the market place, that is, the site of anonymous commodity exchange. Insofar as women go there at all, many of them will wear the face veil *niqab* (usually nicknamed *ninja* in allusion to the Japanese warriors coming from popular culture).

Yet "covering" or "shielding" is not to be viewed as an abstract norm, but can most aptly be characterised as a habitus as defined by Bourdieu: that is, as a disposition

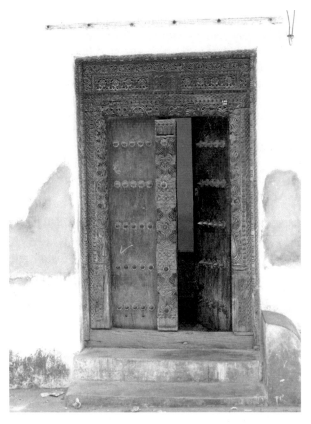

Figure 2. Zanzibar door, Stone Town: aesthetic design of items separating spaces (Photo Klaus Raab, 2006; © Paola Ivanov).

created by practice and in turn creating practice, which is entrenched in the body itself as a "matrix of perceptions, appreciations, and actions".[22] Rather than being merely discursive and communicative, *sitiri* is primarily performative, sensuous, and existential. The entire (relational) person with his or her material and immaterial "covers" is undergoing changes in relation to his or her social environment.[23]

Abidance by this material and immaterial "covering/veiling" creates the basic social value of *heshima*, which can be broadly translated as respect, reputation, and honour. Contrary to the prevalent interpretation of honour in Muslim societies as being a purely male attribute, which is frequently also applied to the Swahili, in Zanzibar *heshima* is considered a female quality as well.[24] However, the most important feature of *heshima* is that it, too, is not an abstract behavioural norm or value. It is only within the practice of interaction that it is negotiated and produced, not exclusively in material terms, yet including the latter. As has already been observed by Middleton, *heshima* is generated in the ongoing interactions through reciprocal exchange between persons or groups, that is, in the form of a gift exchange as defined by Mauss.[25] By means of polite, reserved demeanour, by language and bodily expression including clothing, one pays respect both to oneself and one's *vis-à-vis*. The latter, in turn, by displaying appropriate demeanour and dignified appearance, also shows respect both to himself/herself and to the person with whom he/she is interacting. Whoever violates the *sitiri*, however – that is, whoever is too "open" (*wazi*) in his/her behaviour, body posture, language, or dress – brings *aibu* (shame) not only upon himself/herself, but also upon the addressee. A person's material attributes, such as "modest dress", and his/her appearance in general, which is shaped by the habitus of *sitiri*, thus do not serve the purpose of representing *heshima*, but aim at creating the latter, which for that reason is also embodied in the person as a whole.

Within the system just outlined, any overt and public display of wealth does not only offend against self-restraint and respect and is explicitly negatively sanctioned by Muslim religion, which forbids any arrogance based on possessions because the rich and the poor are equal before God. Any overt demonstration of wealth is, moreover, a dangerous exposure that may make other people envious of a person's qualities or material wealth, and thus attract the evil eye. To "see" something has an aggressive quality in Zanzibar, and to be "seen" means to make oneself vulnerable. Due to a mixture of all these feelings, people carefully avoid displaying possessions and boasting about their resources and capabilities in everyday life. However, the ceremonial and performative events are definitely about displaying.[26] Beauty offers a way out of the dilemma; it is like a protecting veil, mediating between display and non-display. This becomes particularly manifest at the wedding festivities, *harusi*. From a Western perspective, this is the complex of ceremonies where the element of display is most pronounced; from the emic perspective, these festivities are all about beauty.

Before further elaborating on this point, it is necessary to comment briefly on the understanding of beauty, *uzuri*, in Zanzibar (Figure 3). The local conception does not make a distinction between outer and inner beauty: *uzuri* implies material, physical, and moral beauty, that is, it includes behaviour, piety, and purity. Like almost everywhere except in modern Western societies, beauty – including beauty in a material sense – is inseparably associated with purity and sacredness. Purity (*usafi*) is also a condition that is both spiritual and physical and can be experienced sensuously. This becomes apparent, for example, in the "purifying" effect of fragrances, most notably *udi* incense,[27] which are used for beautification and, at the same time, expel all impurities, ranging from bad smells to spirits – an effect frequently attributed to fragrances in Muslim societies. Still, this concept of beauty does not imply that no distinction is made in Zanzibar between the "interior" and "exterior" of a person. Quite on the contrary: as will be shown below, the discrimination between these two aspects is of crucial importance. However, as has already been observed by Marilyn Strathern, there are cultural differences in the articulation between the inner and the outer self.[28] For the time being, it can be stated that beauty is not an outer mask in Zanzibar; instead, it can give expression to inner qualities.

The key episodes of the wedding festivities which focus on beauty (and in Western eyes, on conspicuous consumption) are those where the bride is "presented". Depending on the family's financial means, legal marriage is followed by a series of episodes that are chiefly reserved to the female guests and are celebrated very lavishly. These episodes are generally either referred to by the English word *celebration* or by the Swahili term *sherehe*, which has a much stronger emotional connotation of joy and exultation. The most important of these episodes are a *maulidi* ceremony celebrating the Prophet's birthday, which is usually Arab-inspired in style (Figure 4), and an event with music and dance called by the English word of *reception*, which shows European influence in its style (Figure 5). While *receptions* may be attended by both sexes, this is only rarely practised in Zanzibar as compared to mainland

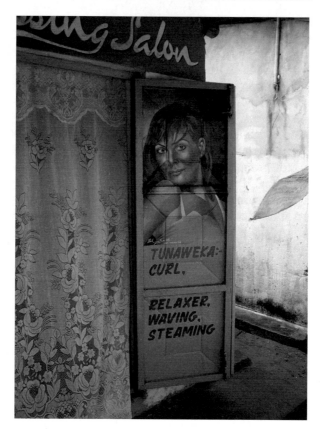

Figure 3.   Door painting advertising a hairdresser's shop. Zanzibar Town, Magomeni (Photo Klaus Raab, 2006; © Paola Ivanov).

Tanzania. Depending on the hosts' religiosity or taste, one of these two ceremonies is performed. More affluent people will usually host both.

In the context of marriage as a rite of passage, these episodes of the *harusi* constitute the phase of reincorporation. They have been preceded by a liminal phase of physical preparation and transformation, which is undergone separately by the bride and groom and is of particular importance for the bride because her beauty is "brought out" in the course of this phase. Then, in the reincorporation phase, she is "presented" (*ku-onesha*), nowadays often together with the groom, on an elaborately decorated stage to the female guests who act as representatives of the community. The audience "sees" the bride and thereby acknowledges her; in that process, the judgement (and thus all conversation) focuses on her beauty. In this way, the bride becomes reintegrated into society in her new role as an adult young woman.[29] At the same time, marriage implies a change in status for the two families as well. Conceived as two "sides" (*supande*), they have now become united and are also reincorporated into society in this new status. For that reason, every detail of the "presentation" ceremony (decoration of the premises, music, food) is evaluated, too – and this word is to be taken literally, because everyone with a practised eye can tell from every single item how expensive the wedding has been. The hostess, that is, the mother of either the bride or the groom, is "praised" for her accomplishment by being presented with (usually small) banknotes (*ku-tunza*).

126

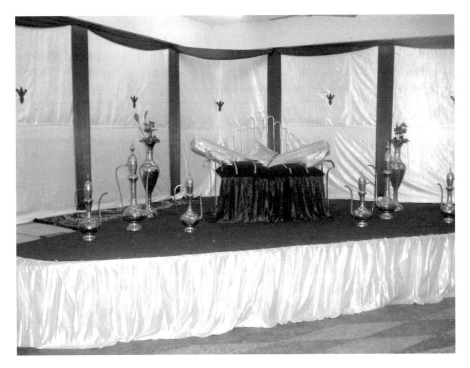

Figure 4.   Stage for a wedding *maulidi* celebration made by Hussein Hamid Mansab (Photo and © Hussein Hamid Mansab, 2006).

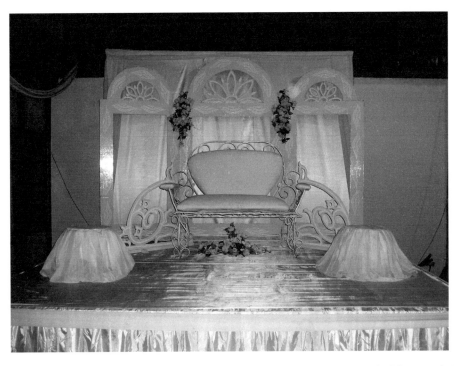

Figure 5.   Stage for a wedding *reception* made by Hussein Hamid Mansab (Photo and © Paola Ivanov, 2006).

The entire ceremony can be interpreted as reciprocal exchange aiming at the creation of *heshima*, respect. The hostess honours the participants by bestowing the gift of beauty upon them, and by giving them the feeling that they are cherished guests. This is effected by the exquisitely designed invitation cards (sometimes imported from Dubai or North America), the selected decoration of the ceremonial room, the distribution of food, beverages, and scents – perfume oil, rose water, *udi* incense, and a special rosette of flowers and aromatic leaves, the *kikuba* – as well as (optionally) by presenting the guests with additional gifts, usually cloths or objects of decoration. This aesthetic presentation is the return for a series of weddings previously attended by the hostess herself; the interactions of the past are thus found at each wedding in a condensed form. The guests, in turn, honour the hostess by participating in the event and by giving recognition to both the bride and the hostess. In addition, they "give" her respect by means of their own aesthetic performance, that is, their adornment, perfume and the new, exquisite clothing they have donned (it is considered shameful to show up at a wedding in clothes that are not newly bought or tailored), as well as by means of their contribution to the enhancement of the aesthetic and emotional intensity of the ceremony by dancing and uttering cries of joy (Figure 6). At the same time, this reciprocal exchange provides the community's moral sanctioning of the marriage, that is, recognition of the moral value of both the bride and groom and the marriage as a whole, as a union of the two families – only a wedding between socially equal families is considered a "beautiful" wedding.

In this process of exchange, too, material goods and aesthetic elements do not represent respect, but generate respect. Beauty serves as sensuous sublimation of the economic capacity and social ties of a family, which in Swahili are summarised by the key term *uwezo* (economic and social ability) and are the prerequisite for hosting an expensive, or "beautiful", wedding; beauty also sensuously sublimates the *uwezo* of the participants, which makes their aesthetic accomplishment possible, as well as the shared common moral values.[30] The material and spiritual beauty/purity of women, ceremonies, and houses, which is generated by means of decommodification[31] and is invested into the reciprocal exchange of *heshima*, is the condensed, veiled disclosure

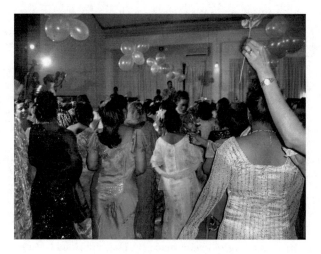

Figure 6.   Women dancing at a wedding *reception* (Photo and © Paola Ivanov, 2006).

of economic, social, and moral values in the form of aesthetic elaboration and civilisedness – the only possible form in the world of "not overtly showing". It is this very paradox of covering/veiling, and not simple demonstration, that generates prestige and status, particularly for the family hosting the event, but also for the guests.

Aesthetics and epistemology of presentation

However, Zanzibari patterns of consumption diverge even more from the concept of conspicuous consumption for purposes of demonstration, or communication, of wealth or status, as well as from the above-mentioned conceptualisations of "Western" consumerism that are projected onto non-Western societies.

First of all, this applies to the epistemic realm. Within the context of a different aesthetic genre (poetry in Yemen), Caton interprets the composition of poems as a "glorious deed" that generates honour. In this context, he refers to a "dialectic of history": not only do the glorious deeds of the past cast their splendour onto the present lives of actors; the latter's glorious deeds in the present can also glorify their past.[32] The same is true of the "big wedding" in Zanzibar,[33] which "big families" are obliged to host because otherwise the honour of their past would become diminished as well. Conversely, such weddings can also help individuals who aspire to higher social status to construct a respectable past. Moreover, a similar spatial and temporal amplification also exists in the immediate context of a particular wedding as a "glorious deed". Rumours about the glory of the wedding are already spread in its run-up phase. These rumours relate to remarkable details, for example, that the bride will wear a particularly expensive dress from the United States, that the stage for the presentation of the bride will boast a completely new design, or that a very large number of guests will attend the wedding, including persons of high standing. After the wedding, the guests take the aesthetic gifts with them and thus continue to spread the fame of the "great deed", even non-verbally:[34] by means of the perfume that still sticks to the participants when the ceremony is over, the flower rosette that is being kept and treasured, the cloths and objects of decoration that were presented as gifts, the additional, packaged food that is taken home, and even the carrying bags that held this food and are subsequently used when people go shopping in town (which means that one can always tell who has been at which wedding). The new media of photography and – in particular – video are also used to present the great deed over and over again; I deliberately do not use the word "represent" in this context. Showing the photo album or the video of the wedding, for example on the occasion of receiving visitors, makes the glorious deed present again, and thus newly generates respect.

This spatial and temporal amplification has an epistemological consequence: from an epistemological point of view, we are not dealing with a regime of representation, in the sense of (re)presenting something that is distant in terms of time and space. Since honour is created anew with every act of display of the aesthetic elements, we are dealing with a contemporaneous event, that is, with a *presentation* by means of aesthetics: the repeated and yet ever new display of something perceived as ever present – namely, the honour of actors.

This epistemic background explains one of those principles of Zanzibari aesthetics that seem most peculiar from an external point of view, a principle that in turn disproves the presupposition that "consumerism" is invariably associated with individualistic distinction and with milieus defined by lifestyle hedonism; thus, a further divergence of Zanzibari patterns of consumption from conceptualisations of "Western" consumerism becomes manifest. On the one hand, it is true that from the local perspective it is important to offer "new", extraordinary things at a ceremony, and thus to be the talk of the town (for example, hot dogs as a new, exceptional dish: Figure 7). Yet aesthetics as a whole, both in ceremonies and in general, neither meets the criteria of some "creative individualism", nor is it patterned after some versatile "postmodern hedonism", both of which are decisive factors in Euro-American consumerism. Quite to the contrary, aesthetics complies with largely homogenous, collectively shared patterns which, while putting an emphasis on always presenting something "new", basically generate similitude – or, to use Foucault's term, "resemblance":[35] between the different ceremonies, the different home furnishings and decorations, or the different clothing styles.

Part of this similarity results from the very fact that material goods, as well as their sources of supply and models for manufacture, are scarce resources. Yet this is not the main point. A comparison with the European Middle Ages may be elucidating here, that is, with the time prior to the epistemic rupture which – as has been outlined, for example, by Bruno Latour and Michel Foucault – caused a change from a regime of presentation (or of "resemblance") in the Middle Ages to a regime of representation in the modern age.[36] According to Latour, in medieval painting religious images were the medium used to make the sacred events of the past present again; the main criteria for their veridicity were their uniqueness (a scene was shown to the beholder for the first time), and at the same time their conformity with all other images of the same kind.[37] Zanzibari aesthetics is very similar to this: on the one hand, it is claimed that each presentation is unique; on the other, the consistency of expression constitutes an aesthetic ideal that confers veridicity upon each presentation and enables respect to be generated. However, this ideal does also allow for minor variations. The qualities that produce an increase in respect are objectified by exactly these subtle differences: a person's preferences (that is, her/his personality), his/her competences (*akili*, that is, his/her good taste), and his/her

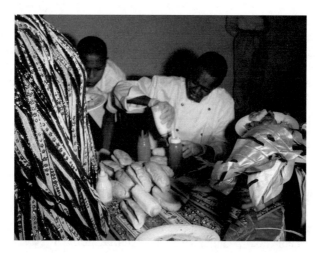

Figure 7.   Serving hot dogs during a wedding *reception* (Photo and © Paola Ivanov, 2006).

uwezo, the economic and social ability to provide oneself with the appropriate things. The "craving" for the latest goods and fashions is thus not due to some universal desire to set oneself off from the rest of society, as has been postulated by Georg Simmel with regard to fashion in Europe – an interpretation that has been applied to non-Western societies in a generalising manner as well.[38] It is due to the increase in *heshima* gained by being "the first" – individual, family, or group – to present a style that is new and at the same time in accordance with all other presentations. The goal is not individualism and differentiation, but concordance and, at the same time, elevation.

Civilised beauty: aesthetics of translocality, exclusion, and competition

Based on the above, it is possible to further enlarge upon the social context of beauty in Zanzibar. From a social perspective, aesthetics and taste do not only generate distinction in Bourdieu's sense,[39] but also exclusion. With regard to the wedding ceremonies, Appadurai's concept of the "tournaments of value" can be applied,[40] in which not merely status is negotiated but "the disposition of the central tokens of value in the society in question".[41] The transformation of socioeconomic values into beauty and respect leads to the emergence of a collective awareness of urban "civilisedness", which is the key criterion for membership in the community. In that process, the actors are socially positioned in a field of tension between hierarchical poles defined in terms of aesthetics, which separate those who are "civilised" and possess honour from those who are not (or less) "civilised" and possess no (or less) honour.[42]

In this context it also becomes apparent why imported, and not local, goods are invested in the competitive consumption. In coastal society, which was based on mercantile exchange, the highest socioeconomic values were, and still are, of a translocal nature. Historically, imports objectified the relationships of an individual or family within the translocally extended commercial networks of kinship, clientele, and alliance.[43] Yet even today, both trade and access to goods do not only depend on the financial means of actors, but in particular on the networks of relationships maintained by Zanzibari families, which today extend to Europe and North America due to migration. This social component finds expression in the very key term *uwezo*, which combines the meanings of economic and social "power". Within the context of the reciprocal exchange of respect, it is precisely this translocal socioscape that is objectified and aesthetically embodied by the consumption of things than come from "outside": we are dealing with a form of mimesis, or mimetic appropriation, of the aesthetics of the "outside" partner(s), with the purpose of constituting and elevating the person.[44] This, and not some automatism innate in human nature, is the reason for the striking "desire" for all global things coming from outside, and accounts for the importance of these goods in the creation of the highest value of civilisation within reciprocal exchange.

It is known that the coastal communities' former ideal of civilisation, which was linked to "free" or "gentle" birth (*uungwana*) as opposed to descent from slaves, came to be associated with the new Omani rulers in the nineteenth century and transformed into the quality of *ustaarabu*, "becoming an Arab". Today the most important aesthetic-hierarchical poles between which status is constituted in Zanzibar (Figure 8) are "Arab" (high-status, civilised, beautiful, endowed with honour) versus "African" (low-status, uncivilised, not beautiful, lacking honour),

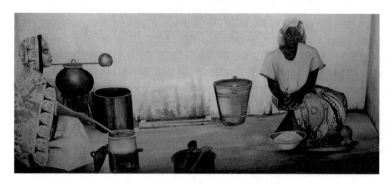

Figure 8.   Painting in the House of Wonders Museum, Zanzibar Town: reconstruction of a nineteenth-century kitchen scene with an "Arab" mistress and an "African" slave (Photo and © Paola Ivanov, 2006).

and "urban" (high-status, sophisticated) versus "rural" (low-status, rough). This reveals the trait of exclusiveness inherent in the ideal of civilisation: whoever does not have honour, that is, whoever is a "barbarian" (*mshenzi*) from the mainland, an "outlaw" (*mhuni*), or in some cases even a "rustic person" from the countryside (*mshamba*), is excluded from the community based on the values of "civilisation" and "respect" – a fact that has all too often been politically exploited.[45]

Two points are notable with regard to these essentialising dichotomies. First, they are conceptual distinctions that do not reflect historical reality. With regard to similar pairs of opposites, such as "Hellenes" and "barbarians", the German historian Reinhart Koselleck has coined the term "asymmetrical antonyms".[46] He emphasises that the political impact and "inherent suggestive power" of such "strict dualisms" "[must] not mislead us into inferring that the mutual relations referred to, and often engendered, by them [dualisms] can also be historically interpreted, and pinned down, as dualisms". Particularly in the face of the devastating political instrumentalisation of the "Arab"–"African" dichotomy in Zanzibar, which has surfaced again and again since political mobilisation in the 1950s and the 1964 revolution, it is crucial to heed Koselleck's warning that "neither social nor political history . . . [is] ever identical with its conceptual self-articulation".[47] Second, the analysis of the practice of *heshima* exchange shows that "Arabness" is primarily one pole in a hierarchy founded on aesthetics; it is hardly ever based on actual descent but is rather a result of the mimetic embodiment of the privileged relations maintained by the inhabitants of the Swahili coast with the Arabian peninsula. These ties have become further consolidated in recent times due to politically or economically motivated migration, as well as to the economic growth of the Gulf States – particularly Dubai, which has become the primary hub for the flows of goods in the entire Indian Ocean region. Claims to high status continue to go along with an aesthetic preference for everything "Arab", which since the late nineteenth century has been, to varying degrees, accompanied by an appropriation of things defined as "European" or "Western", that is, of the attributes of the newly arrived powerful partners.

Let us now turn to the high degree of competition also involved in the reciprocal exchange of respect. This aspect has been most aptly analysed by Bourdieu in his discussion of honour among the Kabyles. In this context, he refers to a "*dialectique du défi et de la riposte*" (dialectics of challenge and counter-challenge) which can theoretically be continued *ad infinitum* because the virtual dishonouring inherent in the challenge or gift always calls for a counter-challenge or a counter-gift.[48] In this sense, too, consumption in Zanzibar is "competitive" or "agonistic" rather than being merely of a demonstrative nature.[49] People try to outdo each other in terms of beauty. However, what is the role of aesthetics in all this? In one passage of the enlarged English edition of the *Theory of Practice*, Bourdieu pointedly stresses how, in the context of relations of honour, aesthetic forms "disclaim" the former's political and economic essence in an "exemplary" way and "thus offer the connoisseurs of beautiful form the enchanting spectacle of an art of living raised to the level of an art for art's sake".[50] Yet, in his works dedicated specifically to the topic he contents himself with the demystification of art and taste as sources of social distinction without enquiring into the specificity of the beautiful and the reasons for the latter's importance and efficacy.[51]

Enchantment and the efficacy of beauty

With regard to this last question, the ideas on art elaborated by British anthropologist Alfred Gell are elucidating. Gell interprets art as a "technology" – that is, an effective action – "of enchantment" for "securing the acquiescence of individuals in the network of intentionalities in which they are enmeshed".[52] According to his reasoning, aesthetic objects are secondary actors. They are a Peircean index, that is, a result or instrument of the agency of social actors, perpetuating the latter's intentionalities. This secondary agency is based on the objects' artistic virtuosity which, according to Gell, accounts for their ability to induce "captivation" and engenders a kind of "cognitive indecipherability" that has a demoralising effect on the beholder, as the latter is faced with the superhuman skill and achievement of the object's creator.[53] The example used by Gell comes from just the paradigmatic situation of competitive, or agonistic, exchange in Melanesia: according to him, the sinuously carved, painted prow boards that used to adorn the boats on the Trobriand Islands were employed as a kind of "psychological weapons". Their aesthetic power had a dazzling effect on the Trobrianders' exchange partners, causing them to give in more readily in the bargaining about the kula shells.[54]

A similar occurrence is found in one of the most pronounced forms of aesthetic competition in Zanzibar, the so-called *rusha roho*, which translates as "to cause someone's spirit to fly" and can best be rendered as "to dispirit (a rival)". In this game of honour, two women wooing a man's favour – for example, two co-wives – engage in a dance contest. Each presents her beauty and female skills (including those of an erotic nature, which are suggested in the *ku-kata kiuno*, a dance with rotating hip movements), as well as her moral value. The latter is based on a successful, harmonious marriage (again including sexuality) that does not disrupt the union of the two families and, in a broader sense, the community. This moral value is objectified in the dance contest by the material benefits bestowed on her by the man, such as jewellery, clothing, or a mobile phone, the latter being not only a gift from the man, but also a means of intimate communication. In the ideal case, one of the rivalling women is supposed to eventually become disheartened and to capitulate (in reality, however, the quarrel will usually escalate).

While this is an extreme manifestation, the efficacy of aesthetic accomplishment within exchange can also be observed in other instances, in fact not only causing demoralisation, but also inducing "positive" enchantment. This actual effect of the aesthetic presentation – the victory won in a contest, generally the achievement of respect or fame – and the further transactions initiated on its basis and thus corroborating its social reality, can be seen as the factors that essentially confirm the efficacy of aesthetics as a technology of enchantment.

In order to understand the positive components of enchantment, we need to look into the most important values of Zanzibari aesthetics. The captivation by beauty cannot be apprehended without considering its sensuous allure on the whole person of the beholder. In Zanzibar, beauty emerges primarily through the interplay of visual, haptic, olfactory, and kinetic elements; most importantly, the qualities that are cherished entail the potential for evoking cross-sensory or synaesthetic associations. The haptic equivalents of lustre as primary and at the same time intermodal sensory quality and, in the visual sphere, of the bright and saturated colourfulness, are the softness and smoothness of surfaces. With regard to olfactory sensation, "coolness", "sweetness" (pleasantness), and "purity" are the counterparts of the visual and haptic qualities. The fragrant, lustrous, and soft quality of the bride's skin, which is effected in the course of her beautification during the wedding ritual by treating her with a special scrub, is paradigmatic in this respect. This sensory interplay is complemented by the swaying, yet self-contained expansion of the body (including the clothing that covers it) in space by means of movement, which in turn is reflected by the fabrics that are draped to decorate and divide spaces. In assembling these correspondences, aesthetics is guided by an overall principle of skilled, harmonious combination of the individual elements. Beauty is "composed" (*ku-tunga*), just like a necklace, or like a poem, which is also perceived as an ornament,[55] and the rules of symmetry and harmony find expression in the prime principle of "*ku-match*" (from English "match"; the corresponding Kiswahili verb *ku-fanana* is considered less refined). This principle refers primarily to colour, but the individual elements are supposed to also harmonise with each other in their "*style*" (*mtindo*), e.g., "Arab", "European", or "traditional". The result is precious, pure, and beguiling. Beauty – to quote Alfred Gell – is suggestive of a "miraculous creation" and thus establishes contact with the supernatural.[56]

These elements, and in particular the enchantment created by the sophisticated composition which leads over to the supernatural, are vividly illustrated by the lyrics of a classic *taarab* song: in "veiled" language (*mafumbo*), a masterly assembled "cluster of flowers" is praised for its beauty and metaphorically identified with the beloved woman; but the description harbours a second metaphorical veil, as it reveals that this specific "cluster" is the flower rosette *kikuba* (Figure 9), which has been mentioned above in the context of wedding ceremonies, and which in turn is a main component of erotic intimacy.

My Cluster of Flowers (*Shada Langu la Maua*)
Beautiful is my cluster of flowers, I'm dying for its colours
It is elegantly arranged, the like of it, I cannot find
To be inserted with jasmines, that is what it deserves
This flower has been, the flower of paradise for her people

Sweet basil and roses, these are its beads
Then flowers of a screw pine are tied to secure them
Its cool scent, is among the qualities of this cluster
How beautiful this cluster is, skilful is its maker

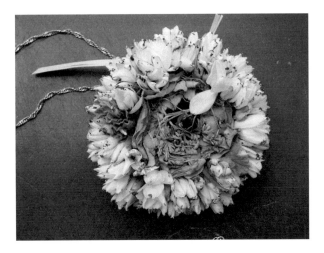

Figure 9. *Kikuba* (Photo and © Paola Ivanov, 2006).

Pachori and pompia[57] you would think an emerald
The way it smell [sic] makes it even more beautiful
It excels in beauty and scent, and its qualities are emphatic
I have but to reward it with all these praises

When placed on the neck, it appears extremely gorgeous
It rests in gentleness, like a food plate and its cover
It attracts the Satan and genies with wings
The angels and spirits, they're all beguiled by it
And they finally all recognise it.[58]

What is also noticeable in this concept of beauty is the parallelism between the aesthetic criterion of harmonious composition on the one hand and the principles that account for social and moral "beauty" on the other. Thus, the following elements are decisive with regard to the wedding ceremonies: first, social symmetry, that is most notably the union of equal partners in marriage (in accordance with the principle of *ku-match*); yet the relative equality of the participants in the ceremony is also of importance. The second principle is social harmony, that is, the social sanctioning of the marriage by society as well as by the parents – a point that nowadays is a critical issue: theoretically, any working young woman can arrange her wedding from her own resources, and even without her family's consent; yet, such a wedding will not be "beautiful". Despite all this, however, the question as to whether this parallelism does allow for further inferences cannot be answered without further analysis. The search for one-to-one correspondences between aesthetic and social forms harbours the risk of over-simplification.

The above discussion shows that the positive efficacy of aesthetics as a technology of enchantment entails a high emotional quality and an intense affective involvement of the person. This positive efficacy may be seen as one reason why in Zanzibar and generally in Muslim societies beauty provides access to the sacred and to the epitome of beauty – God – and why perfumes and incense in particular have a "purifying" effect. Yet in the social context, too, beauty does not only give rise to demoralisation.

Just like any other form of exchange, the ceremonial exchange of aesthetic gifts does not only have an agonistic aspect, but also a unifying one: thanks to the agency of aesthetics, the joint commitment to the production of a ceremony's beauty is emotionally enhanced. This is true for all ceremonies, not just for those reserved for women. At the big *maulidi* ceremonies held in the month of the Prophet's birthday, for example, which are mainly celebrated by the men, a high intensity of aesthetic expression is achieved that contributes to "sanctifying" the whole festivity, to unifying the festive community, and to establishing the spiritual connection with God. Aesthetics in Zanzibar is far from being in accordance with Kant's definition. To best describe the state of pure joy effected by beauty in Zanzibar, the somewhat old-fashioned word "bliss" may be most suitable: enchanted participation instead of distanced contemplation.

Conclusion: ambiguity and visuality in the world of *sitiri*

The preceding analysis allows some conclusions to be drawn about the relationship between the "interior" and "exterior", and the specificity of visuality in Zanzibar. The production of respect and status by means of the practice of veiled disclosure – including the "veil" of (female) beauty – gives free play to ambiguities. Non-visibility through veiling does not imply invisibility, but is equivalent to ambiguous accentuation. Whatever is being veiled is at the same time being emphasised. Yet there is a large measure of uncertainty, because no one can ever tell whether what is behind the veil is indeed what is expected. This ambiguity is inherent in the very nature of veiled disclosure: the "exterior" should correspond to the "interior", aesthetic coherence should be in accordance with moral and social coherence. Yet, it is impossible to ever gain complete certainty. Beauty and veiling can be deceitful, as they may "conceal" a lack of values, or even immorality. There are many stories about women who use their complete veiling to go to bars, or even visit their lovers, without being recognised.[59] On the occasion of any wedding ceremony, there may be much discussion among the participants: has the wedding really been beautiful, or has it rather been too pretentious, too cheap, a failure in terms of aesthetics? Have the guests been treated respectfully enough, or have they rather been dishonoured, for example, by poor catering? Do the male and female "sides" really match each other? And the bride – wasn't her dress too "open", her entire makeup too cheap (even though her family is well-to-do), and: Is she really a virgin?

On the one hand, the ambiguity unfolding in each act of aesthetic exchange engenders a potential for the transformation of cultural forms: whatever creates respect can be subject to change, which becomes apparent, for example, if one takes a diachronic look at the very diverse fashions in female garb and veiling.[60] On the other hand, it gives rise to a large potential for negotiation with regard to the construction of the person: the identities thus created always remain ambiguous to a certain degree. In the end, it is not even possible to rely on what is "seen" in the context of the reciprocal *heshima* exchange. As is frequently stressed in proverbs and conversations, it is ultimately impossible to see into a person, or into a house.[61] This ambiguity, in combination with the fact that the processes of negotiation are about crucial, existential values rooted in the "whole" person emotionally and sensuously, and, based on these values, about social inclusion or exclusion, can be viewed as an important factor that intensifies the social conflicts virulent in Zanzibar.

Above all, however, this ambiguity means that *sitiri*, "covering/veiling", as a habitus and "veiled disclosure" as a means of producing respect imply a specific type of visuality: unlike – at least theoretically – in the West, seeing and representation (including speech) are not the privileged ways of knowing, conceptualised as leading to the cognition of an "outer" world that exists separately from the subject. On the contrary: in the social world of *sitiri*, which is fraught with ambiguity and compartmented into multiple spaces – spaces that always encompass the relational subject in his/her engagement in reciprocal exchange – seeing and representation are charged with aggressiveness and immorality, as they can potentially break up the very principle that is the foundation of the world. People will stress that human vision is not subject to any "screens" or "boundaries": the eye can perceive things that are meant to be concealed from its gaze and, as an envious, non-reciprocal evil eye, even attack what is exposed. Knowledge of the whole truth is reserved to God. The social world, on the other hand, which is subject to constant change in the course of history, is a world of ambiguity and imperfection where people constantly need to secure their respective categories and judgements anew: a struggle that is fought by the very means of aesthetics – the reflection of divine light.

In conclusion, the analysis presented here shows the necessity of keeping to anthropology's principle relating to the historically determined (of course always changeable) specificity of interactive processes taking place within concrete social formations, and to the specificity of the resulting cultural practices. This non-essentialist concept of culture should also apply to studies of seemingly familiar phenomena, such as "consumerism" in Swahili communities, conducted in the context of research on contemporary globalisation processes. In Zanzibar, we encounter a consumerism in its own right. Historically, this consumerism developed in the context of "modern" processes of interconnection spanning spatial distances, just as did its Euro-American counterpart(s): the Swahili coast was no less involved in these processes than were Europe or America. Yet, Zanzibari consumerism can neither be subsumed under "Western" models, nor is it oriented towards "Western modernity". The focus on beauty and aesthetics, which is a research topic considered irrelevant and neglected by social analysis, enables us to gain a deeper understanding of crucial, historically and culturally shaped processes in Zanzibari society: processes of constituting the person in relation to his or her social and material environment on the one hand, and of creating value and community, as well as distinction and exclusion, on the other. This also helps to understand the tensions inherent in the construction of the Swahili communities. Moreover, the focus on aesthetics reveals patterns of perception as well as both epistemological and ontological principles that differ from those of Western modernity. And last but not least, the study of aesthetics enables us to grasp all-encompassing human existential experience, and human capability for deep emotion and transcendence.

If we consider these specificities of Swahili Muslim cultural experience, which is shaped by the habitus of "covering/veiling", and if we bring them into relation with Western concepts of personhood, their relevance in terms of self-awareness becomes apparent as well. Foucault states that the visibility of the isolated individual is the basis of both the constitution of the modern self and modern exercise of power, according to the model of the panopticon, the prison envisioned by the English philosopher Bentham at the end of the eighteenth century, where every prisoner is constantly exposed to the (unseen) guard's gaze, and thus internalises the latter.[62] If Foucault is right, this may also help to explain the visceral, almost irrational Western aversion towards the veil. "Veiling" does not only mean that both the person and intimate, yet definitely communal spaces of action are hidden from the controlling eye (which thus looses the privilege of being unseen); in essence, "veiling" is the very antinomy of the Western subject's self-conception.

Notes

1. My fieldwork in Zanzibar was conducted in 2006 in the context of a research project based at the Chair of Anthropology, University of Bayreuth. I wish to express my thanks to the German Research Society for funding the project, and to Sabine Lang for the translation.
2. Cf. particularly Horton and Middleton, *Swahili*; Pouwels, *Horn and Crescent*; Prestholdt, *Domesticating the World*.
3. Laura Fair has already dedicated some important studies to consumption and popular culture in colonial Zanzibar. Cf. Fair, *Pastimes and Politics*; Fair, "It's Just No Fun."
4. Theoretical approaches range all the way from phenomenological ones (e.g., Ingold, *Perception of the Environment*) to Daniel Miller's dialectical approach (Miller, *Materiality*), the concept of a "dividual" or "distributed person" (e.g., Gell, *Art and Agency*; Strathern, *Gender of the Gift*), and to Latour's revision of the Cartesian ontology itself in *We Have Never Been Modern*, according to which there are no subjects and objects, but only "hybrids".
5. Cf., among others, Campbell, *Romantic Ethic*; Featherstone, *Consumer Culture and Postmodernism*; Slater, *Consumer Culture and Modernity*.
6. See also Prestholdt, *Domesticating the World*, 88–116; Parkin, "Nemi."
7. In reality, most imported things locally conceived as "Arab" or "European" nowadays come from Southeast and East Asia, often via Dubai.
8. Cf., for example, the concept of "colonial mimicry" developed by Homi Bhabha, *Location of Culture*, 121–31. For an anthropological perspective, see Appadurai, *Modernity at Large*.
9. Cf. with regard to consumption Colloredo-Mansfeld, "Consumption"; Hahn, *Consumption in Africa*.
10. Hahn, "Appropriation", 71.
11. For African examples see, among others, Fardon et al., *Modernity on a Shoestring*; Hahn, *Consumption in Africa*; Newell, "Migratory Modernity." With regard to Zanzibar Town, see Burgess, "Cinema, Bell Bottoms." Recent historical research shows that even in the "West" consumerism is only one of various modes of consumption; see Trentmann, "Modern Genealogy."
12. Cf. Veblen, *Theory of the Leisure Class*; Simmel, "Philosophie der Mode"; Simmel, *Philosophie des Geldes*; Douglas and Isherwood, *World of Goods*.
13. Cf., for example, Ingold, *Key Debates*, 249–93.
14. Baumgarten, *Meditationes*, § CXVI; Baumgarten, *Aesthetica*, § 1.
15. Kant, *Critique of Pure Reason*, §§ 1–8. However, Kant is not concerned with immediate sensible perception, but with the latter's "pure" principles – time and space – which pre-structure experience and which in his view are existing *a priori* in the mind.
16. Kant, *Critique of Judgement*, §§ 1–22.
17. Ibid., § 9.
18. Cf. with regard to morality ibid., § 59.
19. Cf. also Parkin, "Blank Banners."
20. Ghaidan, *Lamu*, 75–6.
21. Cf., for example, Bourdieu's classic example of the Kabyle house in *Esquisse*, chap. 2; for the Swahili, Donley-Reid, "Structuring Structure." However, Myers already describes a much more differentiated and flexible use of social space in Zanzibar Town (*Reconstructing Ng'ambo*, 154–62).
22. Bourdieu, *Outline*, 83.
23. Cf. also Ivanov, "Verschleierung als Praxis." "Veiled" language and communication in the coastal societies have already been discussed by various authors, including Bacuez, *De Zanzibar à Kilwa*; Hirsch, *Pronouncing & Persevering*; Swartz, *Way the World is*. The interpretation of "covering" as habitus, however, goes beyond pure communication or discourse.

24. Cf. for the different positions with regard to whether women are attributed honour at the Swahili coast: Hirsch, *Pronouncing & Persevering*, 48–9, 296 n. 32; Bacuez, *De Zanzibar à Kilwa*, 208–30; Swartz, *Way the World is*, 157–75; Middleton, *World of the Swahili*, 192–4.
25. Middleton, *World of the Swahili*, 194; Mauss, "Essai sur le don."
26. In the final analysis, the same is true for everyday life; this, however, cannot be elaborated here.
27. *Udi* is made of agarwood with an admixture of perfume oils.
28. Strathern, "The Self in Self-Decoration."
29. Cf. also Middleton, *World of the Swahili*, 141–56. Of course, the groom is reincorporated into society as an adult as well, but this is less stressed in ritual.
30. Cf. also Fair, *Pastimes and Politics*, 74–109.
31. Cf. Appadurai, "Introduction", 18–27.
32. Cf. Caton, *"Peaks of Yemen"*, 27–8, 35.
33. Cf. already Meneley, *Tournaments of Value*, with regard to Yemen.
34. Cf. Kanafani, *Aesthetics and Ritual*, 100–1.
35. Foucault, *Order of Things*.
36. Latour, "Opening one Eye"; Foucault, *Order of Things*.
37. Latour, "Opening one Eye", 22–3.
38. Cf. Simmel, "Philosophie der Mode"; Simmel, *Philosophie des Geldes*.
39. Bourdieu, *Distinction*.
40. As has already been done by Meneley, *Tournaments of Value*, with regard to Yemen.
41. Appadurai, "Introduction", 21.
42. Cf. also Ivanov, "Cosmopolitanism or Exclusion?"
43. Cf. also Horton and Middleton, *Swahili*, 196–7.
44. The socioscape that is embodied can also be partially imaginative: cf. Ivanov, "Cosmopolitism or Exclusion?"
45. Cf. especially Glassman, "Slower Than a Massacre"; Glassman, *War of Words*.
46. Koselleck, *Vergangene Zukunft*, 211–59.
47. For both quotations: ibid., 214; translation by Sabine Lang.
48. Cf. Bourdieu, *Esquisse d'une théorie*, chap. 1; quotation ibid., 24.
49. Cf. also Beidelmann, "Agonistic Exchange." The agonistic character of gift exchange has been already stressed by Mauss, "Essai sur le don."
50. Bourdieu, *Outline*, 194–5.
51. Bourdieu, *Distinction*; Bourdieu and Darbel, *Love of Art*.
52. Gell, "Enchantment of Technology", 43.
53. Gell, *Art and Agency*, 68–72, 95.
54. Ibid., 69–72; Gell, "Enchantment of Technology", 44–6.
55. Cf. Fuglesang, *Veils and Videos*, 127; Werner and Hichens, *Advice*, stanzas 8–9; Biersteker, "Language, Poetry, and Power", 71–2.
56. Gell, *Art and Agency*, 68.
57. Two kinds of fragrant leaves.
58. Khamis, "Images of Love", 37–8; his translation.
59. For purposes of complete veiling, women will nowadays wear a black, floor-length *buibui* coat, a headscarf (*mtandio* or *hijab*), and a face veil. The former style of complete veiling (*kizorro*, a term derived from the Zorro movies) could be created situationally by manipulating the manner of wearing the older type of *buibui* cloak.
60. Fair, *Pastimes and Politics*, 64–109; Ivanov, "Verschleierung als Praxis", 142.
61. Cf., for example, the proverb *Nyumba husitiri mambo*, "The house conceals matters."
62. Cf. Foucault, *Discipline & Punish*, chap. 3.

References

Appadurai, Arjun. "Introduction: Commodities and the Politics of Value." In *The Social Life of Things: Commodities in Cultural Perspective*, ed. Arjun Appadurai, 3–63. Cambridge: Cambridge University Press, 1986.

Appadurai, Arjun. *Modernity at Large: Cultural Dimensions of Globalization*. Minneapolis: University of Minnesota Press, 1996.

Bacuez, Pascal. *De Zanzibar à Kilwa: Relations conflictuelles en pays Swahili*. Louvain: Peeters, 2001.

Baumgarten, Alexander Gottlieb. *Meditationes philosophicae de nunnullis ad poema pertinentibus*. Hamburg: Felix Meiner, 1983 [1735].

Baumgarten, Alexander Gottlieb. *Theoretische Ästhetik. Die grundlegenden Abschnitte aus der "Aesthetica" (1750/58)*. Hamburg: Felix Meiner, 1988.

Beidelman, T.O. "Agonistic Exchange: Homeric Reciprocity and the Heritage of Simmel and Mauss." *Cultural Anthropology* 4, no. 3 (1989): 227–59.

Bhabha, Homi K. *The Location of Culture*, revised edn. London: Routledge, 2004.

Biersteker, Ann. "Language, Poetry, and Power: A Reconsideration of 'Utendi wa Mwana Kupona'." In *Faces of Islam in African Literature*, ed. Kenneth W. Harrow, 59–77. Portsmouth: Heinemann, 1991.

Bourdieu, Pierre. *Outline of a Theory of Practice*. Cambridge: Cambridge University Press, 1977.

Bourdieu, Pierre. *Distinction: A Social Critique of the Judgement of Taste*. Cambridge, MA: Harvard University Press, 1984.

Bourdieu, Pierre. *Esquisse d'une théorie de la pratique, précédé de trois études d'ethnologie kabyle*. Paris: Éditions du Seuil, 2000 [1972].

Bourdieu, Pierre, and Alan Darbel. *The Love of Art: European Art Museums and their Public*. Cambridge: Polity Press, 1991.

Burgess, Thomas. "Cinema, Bell Bottoms, and Miniskirts: Struggles over Youth and Citizenship in Revolutionary Zanzibar." *International Journal of African Historical Studies* 35, nos. 2/3 (2002): 287–313.

Campbell, Colin. *The Romantic Ethic and the Spirit of Modern Consumerism*. Oxford: Blackwell, 1987.

Caton, Steven C. *"Peaks of Yemen I Summon": Poetry as Cultural Practice in a North Yemeni Tribe*. Berkeley: University of California Press, 1990.

Colloredo-Mansfeld, Rudi. "Consumption." In *A Handbook of Economic Anthropology*, ed. James G. Carrier, 210–25. Cheltenham: Elgar, 2005.

Donley-Reid, Linda W. "A Structuring Structure: The Swahili House." In *Domestic Architecture and the Use of Space*, ed. Susan Kent, 114–26. Cambridge: Cambridge University Press, 1990.

Douglas, Mary, and Baron Isherwood. *The World of Goods*. New York: Basic Books, 1979.

Fair, Laura. *Pastimes and Politics: Culture, Community, and Identity in Post-Abolition Urban Zanzibar, 1890–1945*. Athens: Ohio University Press, 2001.

Fair, Laura "It's Just no Fun Anymore: Women's Experiences of Taarab Before and After the 1964 Zanzibar Revolution." *International Journal of African Historical Studies* 35, no. 1 (2002): 61–81.

Fardon, Richard, Wim van Binsbergen, and Rijk v. Dijk, eds. *Modernity on a Shoestring: Dimensions of Globalization, Consumption and Development in Africa and Beyond*. Leiden: EIDOS, 1999.

Featherstone, Mike. *Consumer Culture and Postmodernism*. London: Sage, 1991.

Foucault, Michel. *The Order of Things: An Archaeology of the Human Sciences*. London: Tavistock Publications, 1970.

Foucault, Michel. *Discipline & Punish: The Birth of the Prison*. New York: Vintage Books, 1995.

Fuglesang, Minou. *Veils and Videos: Female Youth Culture on the Kenyan Coast*. Stockholm: Department of Social Anthropology, Stockholm University, 1994.

Gell, Alfred. "The Enchantment of Technology and the Technology of Enchantment." In *Anthropology, Art, and Aesthetics*, ed. Jeremy Coote, and Anthony Shelton, 40–63. Oxford: Clarendon Press, 1992.

Gell, Alfred. *Art and Agency: An Anthropological Theory*. Oxford: Clarendon Press, 1998.

Ghaidan, Usam. *Lamu: A Study of the Swahili Town*. Nairobi: East African Literature Bureau, 1975.

Glassman, Jonathon. "Slower Than a Massacre: The Multiple Sources of Racial Thought in Colonial Africa." *The American Historical Review* 109, no. 3 (2004): 720–54.

Glassman, Jonathon. *War of Words, War of Stones: Racial Thought and Violence in Colonial Zanzibar*. Bloomington: Indiana University Press, 2011.

Hahn, Hans P. "Appropriation, Alienation and Syncretization: Lessons from the Field." In *Unpacking the New: Critical Perspectives on Cultural Syncretization in Africa and Beyond*, ed. Afe Adogame, Magnus Echtler, and Ulf Vierke, 71–92. Münster: Lit, 2008.

Hahn, Hans P., ed., *Consumption in Africa: Anthropological Approaches*. Münster: Lit, 2008.

Hirsch, Susan F. *Pronouncing and Persevering: Gender and the Discourses of Disputing in an African Islamic Court*. Chicago: University of Chicago Press, 1998.

Horton, Mark, and John Middleton. *The Swahili: The Social Landscape of a Mercantile Society*. Oxford: Blackwell Publishers, 2000.

Ingold, Tim. *The Perception of the Environment: Essays on Livelihood, Dwelling and Skill*. London: Routledge, 2002.

Ingold, Tim, ed. *Key Debates in Anthropology*. London: Routledge, 1996.

Ivanov, Paola. "Verschleierung als Praxis: Gedanken zur Beziehung zwischen Person, Gesellschaft und materieller Welt in Sansibar." In *Die Sprache der Dinge*, ed. Elisabeth Tietmeyer, et al., 135–48. Münster: Waxmann, 2010.

Ivanov, Paola. "Cosmopolitanism or Exclusion? Negotiating Identity in the Expressive Culture of Contemporary Zanzibar." In *The Indian Ocean: Oceanic Connections and Creation of New Societies*, ed. Abdul Sheriff, and Engseng Ho. London: Hurst, forthcoming.

Kanafani, Aida S. *Aesthetics and Ritual in the United Arab Emirates: The Anthropology of Food and Personal Adornment among Arabian Women*. Beirut: American University, 1983.

Kant, Immanuel. *Critique of Judgment*, trans. Werner Pluhar, Indianapolis: Hackett, 1987 [1790].

Kant, Immanuel. *Critique of Pure Reason*, trans. and ed. P. Guyer and A. Wood. Cambridge: Cambridge University Press, 1997 [1781, 1787].

Khamis, Said A.M. "Images of Love in the Swahili Taarab Lyric: Local Aspects and Global Influence." *Nordic Journal of African Studies* 13, no. 1 (2004): 30–64.

Koselleck, Reinhart. *Vergangene Zukunft: Zur Semantik geschichtlicher Zeiten*. Frankfurt am Main: Suhrkamp, 1979.

Latour, Bruno. "Opening One Eye while Closing the Other…a Note on Some Religious Paintings." In *Picturing Power: Visual Depiction and Social Relations*, ed. Gordon Fyfe, and John Law, 15–38. London: Routledge, 1988.

Latour, Bruno. *We Have Never Been Modern*. Cambridge, MA: Harvard University Press, 1993.

Mauss, Marcel. "Essai sur le don; forme archaïque de l'échange." *L'Année Sociologique N.S.* 1 (1923/24): 30–186.

Meneley, Anne. *Tournaments of Value: Sociability and Hierarchy in a Yemeni Town*. Toronto: University of Toronto Press, 1996.

Middleton, John. *The World of the Swahili: An African Mercantile Civilization*. New Haven, CT: Yale University Press, 1992.

Miller, Daniel, ed. *Materiality*. Durham: Duke University Press, 2005.

Myers, Garth A. *Reconstructing Ng'ambo: Town Planning and Development on the Other Side of Zanzibar*. Ann Arbor, MI: University Microfilms, 1996.

Newell, Sasha. "Migratory Modernity and the Cosmology of Consumption in Côte d'Ivoire." In *Migration and Economy: Global and Local Dynamics*, ed. Lillian Trager, 163–90. Walnut Creek, CA: Altamira Press, 2005.

Parkin, David. "Nemi in the Modern World: Return to the Exotic?" *Man* 28 (1993): 79–99.

Parkin, David. "Blank Banners and Islamic Consciousness in Zanzibar." In *Questions of Consciousness*, ed. Anthony P. Cohen, and Nigel Rapport, 198–216. London: Routledge, 1995.

Pouwels, Randall L. *Horn and Crescent: Cultural Change and Traditional Islam on the East African Coast, 800–1900*. Cambridge: Cambridge University Press, 1987.

Prestholdt, Jeremy. *Domesticating the World: African Consumerism and the Genealogies of Globalization*. Berkeley: University of California Press, 2008.

Simmel, Georg. "Philosophie der Mode." In Vol. 10 of *Gesamtausgabe*, 7–37. Frankfurt am Main: Suhrkamp, 1965 [1905].

Simmel, Georg. *Philosophie des Geldes*. Frankfurt am Main: Suhrkamp, 1989 [1907].

Slater, Don. *Consumer Culture and Modernity*. Cambridge: Polity Press, 1997.

Strathern, Marilyn. "The Self in Self-Decoration." *Oceania* 49 (1979): 241–57.

Strathern, Marilyn. *The Gender of the Gift: Problems with Women and Problems with Society in Melanesia*. Berkeley: University of California Press, 1988.

Swartz, Marc J. *The Way the World is: Cultural Processes and Social Relations among the Mombasa Swahili*. Berkeley: University of California Press, 1991.

Trentmann, Frank. "The Modern Genealogy of the Consumer: Meanings, Identities and Political Synapses." In *Consuming Cultures*, ed. John Brewer, and Frank Trentmann, 19–69. Oxford: Berg, 2006.

Veblen, Thorstein. *The Theory of the Leisure Class: An Economic Study of Institutions*. New York: New American Library, 1963 [1899].

Werner, Alice, and William Hichens, eds. *The Advice of Mwana Kupona upon the Wifely Duty (Utendi wa Mwana Kupona)*. Medstead: The Azania Press, 1934.

Integration and identity of Swahili speakers in Britain: case studies of Zanzibari women

Ida Hadjivayanis

Department of Languages and Culture, School of Oriental and African Studies, University of London, London, UK

An interesting feature of a growing number of the recently arrived Swahili-speaking communities in Britain is their parallel integration into the British society alongside their current integration into the newly emerging spread of 'correct Islamic rituals' as opposed to the old traditional 'African Islamic' ways from the Swahili coast. The new rituals with strong authorities offer social, emotional as well as economic support in relation to life-changing factors such as birth, death and marriage, and hence, in a way, adopt the role of the traditional Swahili extended family; although at the same time, they also act as alienating factors. This paper is an initial attempt at examining the extent to which the current integration has changed the cultural values and identities of the Swahili living in Britain. It aims at describing the socio-spatial dynamics and identity formation that has transcended the 'original' Swahili boundaries and how these are intricately linked to religion. To this end, three case studies of Zanzibari women in the recently arrived Swahili-speaking communities of London, Milton Keynes and Northampton will be presented.

Culturally, one of the most important feminine practices among all the Swahili is that of *kujifukiza*, immersing one's body and clothing into fumes of burning incense and heavy Middle Eastern perfumed oils of *udi*. Ideally, the infused *udi* scents, a defining female characteristic, would remain on a woman's clothing for a while. From a young age, girls start to learn about this artistic process which culminates around their wedding day. Interestingly, many Swahili women in Britain recount that these distinguished perfumed scents are seen as 'pungent' and are actually met with disgust and revulsion by those outside the Swahili community. And so we find that, as these women face embarrassment for 'smelling', they are forced to go through a process of calculating the do's and don'ts of integrating into the mainstream British society.

Initially, as a heavily perfumed Swahili woman realizes that she has become an irritation, but nevertheless, does not need to relinquish that integral feminine trait, but can now only practice it in certain spaces and among certain people; as she learns to calculate the spatial and mobility aspects of her new surroundings, her identity is re-moulded. This is an initial study that seeks to describe the journey towards some form of social cohesion and the fundamental changes in the personas of Zanzibari women as they integrate into British society.

Integration and identity

Swahili identity has been debated by various scholars[1] including Allen who argues that the Swahili do not form

> a tribe or any other group held together, even notionally, by links of blood or marriage, but a highly permeable population whose common factor is cultural in nature ... an identity which is neither tribal nor racial but an alternative socio-political structure which is more appropriate for urban living.[2]

This is echoed by Horton and Middleton, who point out that 'the Swahili have many identities and can select in different situations'.[3] Furthermore, Pat Caplan argues that 'an understanding of identity politics on the East African coast necessarily involves a consideration of its political and economic history'.[4] Around the twentieth century, Swahili laid claims to Arab status, although more recently, the stress has been on African identity.

The question of 'who is a Swahili' or who identifies themselves as Swahili continues to be contentious. When we think of identity as one's sense of self, one's feeling and ideas about oneself, we find that the people who live in the geographical area that is historically Swahili identify themselves with their place of origin. The term Swahili is the umbrella term for these various 'place identities'. For instance, all the three women in this study are from Zanzibar and identified themselves as *Wazanzibari* or using the local term, *Waunguja*. Therefore, depending on where one comes from, one would be, and would tend to remain *Mpemba*, if they are originally from the Pemba Island, *Mvita* if from Mombasa and *Mlamu* if from Lamu. It is rare to find someone who would claim that they are *Mswahili*. For purposes of this study, we will refer to the people who originate from the East African coast as Swahili, after all, they have historically been known as *Waswahili*.

In Britain, the people to whom Swahili is a mother tongue are generally either political or economic migrants. During the discussions held with numerous individuals including the participants in this study, it became clear that the exact number of Swahili-speaking people in Britain is unknown since several have adopted many and varying nationalities, largely for political reasons. Nevertheless, it seems that they still have some common factors: their language – *Kiswahili*; their culture – *Uswahili*; their place of origin, *Uswahilini*; and predominantly their religion – Islam, which is itself an identity group. Through this last factor, the Swahili share a common ground with adherents from other cultures.

Often the assumption is that identities stem from the expectations that are attached to internalized social roles. In this sense, identity is linked to the process of socialization; we construct our identities from what is presented to us during socialization, or in our various roles.[5] This then leads us to agree that identities are not fixed or given. Our identities change as we embrace and occupy various spaces and form new ties, in this sense, the identities of the Swahili would reflect the spaces that they occupy in regards to their families, the homeland, their adopted homes and so forth.

The term integration has become central in debates regarding the rights, settlement, adaptation and adjustment of groups of people such as refugees, asylum seekers and immigrants. And we find that various scholars have written extensively on the process itself linking it to migrant experiences.[6] Most academic work on integration highlights the conflicts between minority communities and the liberalism that is characteristic of mainstream western societies. One of the more idealist definitions of integration argues that 'integration means the ability to participate to the extent that a person needs and wishes in all of the major components of society, without having to relinquish his or her own cultural identity'.[7] In this light, a person settles and adapts into a given target culture through a process that does not annul what they see as their identity but rather, ideally, nourishes it. Discussing Muslims in Western Europe, Modood Tariq writes that there are four modes of integration—*assimilation*, where new immigrants become as much like their hosts as possible; *individualist-integration*, which deals with individual claimants; *multiculturalism*, where equality is central and the social significance of communities, not just individuals, is recognized; and *cosmopolitanism*, where 'difference' is positively appreciated. This means that the minorities and majority population mixes, borrows and learns from each other.[8]

Assimilation has been the dominant historical form of integration.[9] In Britain, however, there has been a lot of rhetoric on multiculturalism. Interestingly, a number of Swahili women who were interviewed thought of, in comparison with many European countries, Britain as a country where they are freer to conduct their lives. Of course, as immigrants, these women face a myriad of issues on a daily basis. These are no longer the traditional struggles against ignorance and poverty, but for many in the community key concerns include issues such as difficulties with immigration statuses, a balance between caring and raising a family in foreign lands and economic constraints. And yet other issues are relationships on and off social networks such as *Facebook* and *Instagram*. In order to understand this process, together with the perceptions and attitudes of these women on issues of integration and identity, this study will present a few case studies which would help bring out the settings in which women find themselves and how they have adapted to life as immigrants.

Case studies

Introducing the importance of personal life histories, Margaret Strobel, who authored a foundational study of three Swahili women in Mombasa, writes that 'in the hands of skilled scholars, these stories yield important insights about individuals, societies, and historical processes of change'.[10] Interestingly, this theme resonates well with this initial presentation which seeks to offer insights into the lives of three diverse Zanzibari women living in different English towns.

The present author held discussions with a good number of women; however, in-depth interviews for this initial study were conducted with three women. The selection criterion for the three case studies was based on their diverse social milieu, thus presenting their diversity. These women offer a window into the lives of Zanzibari women living in Britain. They are all recently arrived, with the earliest to have arrived in 1999. They have also adopted a spectrum of methods of integration into the English society.[11] They have all created their own identities in one way or another through what can be termed as a process of discovering, embracing and rejecting of new and old customs and traditions. Through them, we have a glimpse of the different Swahili husbands as well as a perceived 'deeper' understanding of their religion, Islam. Interestingly, when most of the respondents for this study accessed other ethnic groups on a personal level, Islam served as the common ground. Religion would therefore act as the catalyst for them to converge.

Ashura

Ashura was born in Zanzibar stone town in 1976 and moved to the UK in 2002. Her ancestors hail from Yemen. She holds a degree in Business Studies from Malaysia, but lives and works in Milton Keynes as a part-time care worker. She was married for two years to a fellow Zanzibari and has a 6-year-old daughter. Ashura is among a small number of women who had a registry wedding – most Swahili people marry through the *nikkah* (religious ceremony), which is not regarded as a legal form of marriage in Britain since it legalizes the union between one man and more than one woman. Ashura has been divorced in the religious sense but not legally – her ex-husband has re-married in Zanzibar but lives and works in London, visiting his new family annually and making rare visits to Ashura's daughter. He sometimes gives her a small amount of money for their child, especially during Ramadhan and Eid. She would have preferred this payment to be contracted and does therefore often threaten to report him to the authorities so he pays child support. Yet, the threats are empty since their families in Zanzibar have known each other for centuries; she would never follow through and take him to court; he knows that. We find here that, even thousands of miles away from the root of their familial ties, Ashura cannot shatter the links that are ages old. Some of her aunts are or had married into her ex-husbands family, which means that she shares some cousins with her ex-husband. There are therefore complex trans-local[12] links that somehow transcend the adopted home and the place of origin.

Ashura speaks English well and is very focused as a mother. She pays for private extracurricular activities for her child and makes sure that her daughter's life is part of the mainstream British society. Her daughter understands Swahili but responds in English. Ashura dresses modestly – trousers and long-sleeved shirts. While in Britain she does not habitually reveal her hair in public. She wears a small head scarf or a hat at all times, not the veil. She would only let her hair down at weddings, where she would also wear elegant evening gowns; most weddings are women-only affairs. When in Zanzibar, she prefers to leave her hair out wherever possible, or would don a scarf which hangs loosely on her head and shoulders, showing some hair.

The scarf seems to play an ambiguous role in her life. It is part of her Zanzibari identity in Britain since a large number of Zanzibaris in the UK wear the veil; she wears a small head scarf which is not really Islamic, but helps her to conform and fit in among Zanzibaris. It is not necessarily a symbol of any fundamental religious belief. In fact, there was a time when Ashura forsook her head scarf so as to attract employers, although following a number of failed attempts decided to take up care work and keep her small scarf on. On the other hand, when in Zanzibar, she adopts a personality that is linked to the prestige of living in Europe; the scarf then occupies a peripheral position. Living abroad has offered Ashura the possibility of climbing up the social ladder to embrace a new identity in her place of origin; she reinforces this perceived status by appearing Western when occupying the locale of her origins.

In keeping with this perceived status of prestige, Ashura tends to return to Zanzibar during her daughter's school summer holidays, which fall in the months of July and August; during the other holidays she travels to other European countries or North Africa. She is one of those who are referred to as 'June/July', which refers to those Zanzibaris who reside abroad and tend to return to the islands during the months of June, July and

August. They would then organize and finance huge weddings, attend a number of other June/July weddings and when the fasting month of Ramadhan happens to be during the June/July period they would organize ostentatious *futari*[13] where huge numbers of people would be invited to break the fast together. Ashura tends to save so as to purchase expensive garments, handbags and shoes, which she would wear during that period. She would also finance cultural events for family members, for instance, the previous year she had paid for the lunch ceremony of a young cousin. This is the lunch that is prepared by the bride's family the day after the wedding. This June/July concept is typically trans-local in its portrayal of the spaces that are occupied by the Zanzibari women living abroad. All the women interviewed for this study partake in it; the most religious would portray how morally upright they are and finance trips to Mecca for the Hajj pilgrimage as opposed to worldly ceremonies.

When one enters Ashura's home, as is customary in Zanzibar and similar to the majority of Swahili homes in Britain, they would remove their shoes. The shoe has remained the item that gathers dirt and must be left at the door. The symbolism of the shoe is also apparent in its link within the household where we find that the only place shoes are allowed are the toilet. Therefore, despite having mats in the toilet, a pair of flip flop sandals are always by the bathroom door. Interestingly, this was not the case for Ashura as it was in most homes. Once in the house, the guest is always offered something to consume – this aspect of Swahili hospitality is common among all the women encountered, it has never wavered. Similarly, food is cooked from scratch every day, and coal for burning the *udi* incense is lit daily. Ashura, like all other women, not only cooks for her immediate family members but also contributes to social events such as weddings, funerals or just to give a taste of home to their friends – these foods are eaten by hand, even by their westernized children.

One of Ashura's current preoccupation is finding a new husband. It took her more than a year after her divorce, and after her husband had moved out, to acknowledge that she had been divorced. She feared the stigma. In her words, 'there are just too many divorces in our society now'. She had not wanted to be 'like the rest'. Her initial fear of the stigma of divorce is somehow an illustration of the influence of Western ideologies as opposed to the Swahili. High divorce rate among Swahili is a historical fact. Strobel writes that 'first marriages frequently ended in divorce, contributing to an overall high divorce rate', and, according to the 1915–1950 statistics, one out of every two Kenyan Muslim marriages ended in divorce.[14] Although this statistic is old, divorce has continued to be extremely high among the Swahili and it is common place.

In the case of the Swahili communities in Britain, there are many reasons that lead to divorce. Finances play a big role, as happened to be one of the major reasons that led to Ashura's divorce. She believes that her husband felt threatened by her independence. It is therefore not surprising that his current wife has remained in Zanzibar. This is of course a very narrow window into the myriad reasons that lead to divorce. Ashura understands that individual responses to living far from the homeland play a big role in this. Initially, for many, living in Europe is a sign of prestige, every person that they know in the homeland wishes they too could live abroad. People tend to arrive in Britain with very high expectations, only to become disillusioned very quickly. They have to then find ways of adapting to change and accommodating it; these are the catalyst to disputes.

Men tend to feel that their wives have suddenly become too independent, forming their own networks and offering the husband a position in the household which is below the norm. Men therefore find that they are no longer the heads of their homes and need to accommodate women who for instance, suddenly develop busy diaries, needing to be out and about, leaving the children in the care of men. In one of our conversations, Ashura explained that back home children are the domain of the woman, and men are used to having their women ask for their permission for everything, even visiting one's parents. Then suddenly in Britain they have to deal with women who inform them of social events that require their attendance and for which they depend on the husbands to babysit. For most women, events such as weddings are the main form of social outing and they are also the link to home. At weddings, women can socialize freely, network, dance to Taarab music, eat Swahili food and reconnect with friends. But one finds that husbands would refuse to babysit, creating friction. The woman may seek a friend's support or take the child to the wedding, ignoring the fact that most weddings take place at night and do not allow children. The man would then complain that his wife is 'too much to handle'. Given the frequency of Zanzibari weddings – one could easily attend two weddings a month, and more in the months prior to Ramadhan – the woman therefore has to select her 'fights' carefully. But inevitable disagreements about babysitting, what is worn at the wedding and the cost or selection of the woman's chosen dress all lead to friction within couples. According to Ashura, a number of Swahili men tend to accommodate their wives, but there is also a large number that would refuse to babysit, largely because they too want to go out and meet their own friends or chat up ladies on social networks.

Ashura is also a member of a number of online social networks including *Whatsapp*, *Facebook* and *Instagram*. These offer a trans-local virtual ground on which she can interact. She has a smartphone, which she checks every now and then – eagerly discussing her friend's instant messages to her, their Facebook statuses and their Instagram pictures. All the women take part in social media using phones, tabs or laptops. A lot is shared online; interestingly, a highly western integrated familial image is portrayed. For example, Ashura's Instagram photos include those of her recent holiday to Morocco, her daughter's after-school activities, both of them playing in the snow, Ashura at parties, at cafes and so forth. On Facebook, similar to most of her friends, she enjoys reading and commenting on sensational statuses; some of these include:

> Aliyekunong'oneza yangu, na yako kanambia!
> The one who whispered to you about my affairs, also told me about yours!
> Kuna watu wanajifanya mashekhe kumbe hakuna firauni kama wao!
> There are people who pretend to be sheikhs (saintly) but there couldn't be bigger devils (like the Pharaohs).
> Kuna watu humu ndani unyagoni walichungulia tu maana hawafahamiki!
> There are people in here who just peeped at *unyago* (female rite) because they make no sense.

Ashura's Facebook friends list includes a number of people that she has never met. There are people with whom she shares a number of common friends, people from Zanzibar whose siblings or cousins she knows and so feels that, by default, she knows them. And there are also men who she has never met who have requested to be her virtual friend. She reveals that it is her search for that elusive man who would take her out of what she perceives as the stigma of being a divorcee that has led her to accept friendship requests from people who show potential. She is wary of married men pretending to be single or just lie; but Facebook has opened doors through which she can't be lonely, as she is surrounded by virtual friends. Through it, she can reach different spaces at once, transcending the traditional localities.

Ashura sighs at the fact that married friends deal with her with caution, as soon as one is divorced – one is seen as a husband predator. She has seen the number of married friends inviting her to their homes diminished, although she has also found deep friendships with other divorcees. This network of friends passes on tips on relationships, helping each other with child care and organizing social events. A recent well-attended event was the 'Eid Red Carpet', held in a well-known London night club. Ashura's individual integration is quite strong. She can make small talk with her Irish neighbour, updating her on her daughter's ballet progress; she can also proudly reveal to other Zanzibaris the latter's progress in Qur'anic classes and has also bonded well with her colleagues. She enjoys driving herself to work and taking her daughter on holiday. Despite this seeming assimilated integration, Ashura revealed to her daughter the first time that the latter talked of Father Christmas that there is no such thing. Christmas was easy to brush off, she had known about it and had known how she would explain it away to her child, as was Easter; but not other English traditions.

She revealed that one day her daughter woke up crying that the tooth fairy had neither taken the little tooth she had left under her pillow nor left her a coin. Ashura had not known what to do, unaware that British children have a custom of placing fallen teeth under their pillows expecting coins in return. The following day, she decided to put two coins under her daughter's pillow. There are too many little things of which one has to get a grip, and it is a learning curve, she pointed out. She is happy to integrate some of these snippets of British culture into her child's life, but not all.

Ashura's life is that of a contemporary Zanzibari in Europe. She is a Muslim, believes in the religious monotheism but struggles with the practical aspects of the religion. She prays sometimes, but not five times a day. She does not want to wear the long *baibui* black veil and she enjoys going out, meeting friends, watching a movie – all the things that her religious peers frown upon. She finds intolerable that some Swahili women refuse to venture out of their communities claiming that it is religion that demands that of them.

She recounted a funny incident where one woman passed the word around that there was bacon in the flour bought at a well-known economical supermarket. The woman had made this discovery at around 10 am and by the time this news reached Ashura at noon, almost all those who had heard the rumour, had thrown their cooking flour in the bin. Ashura remembers reading the flour bag instructions and finding out that it simply contained a recipe for making a quiche. One of the ingredients for the quiche was bacon. She quickly called back the person who had called her and informed her that the given ingredients were for a quiche – not the flour ingredients. By then, damage had already been done.

Food is important among Swahili women. Most pass on their latest discoveries on the recipes – if you add some condensed milk and a little bit of custard to the sweet plantains they taste heavenly. If one does not have coconut milk – they can use single or even double cream! It tastes even better in *mchuzi*, curry. Some even post some of their recipes on al-hidaaya – a websites that offers Swahili recipes as well as religious doctrines.

Ashura acknowledges that many of her compatriots are devout Muslims. A large number belong to the Al-Imaan association. She is herself a member of the Milton Keynes women association which is an association of Swahili Muslim women in Milton Keynes. She attends the gatherings, often held in community halls such as the Netherfield community hall. She praises the fact that it is an association of women dealing with issues of religion, family and communal living. It is good to have such an organization, as one does not know what tomorrow brings; at worst, she says, she could drop down and die in this foreign land. At least she is assured that the association would act as her sisters, informing the family back home and transporting her body. At best, her daughter is growing up anahitaji wa kumbeba chooni asije anguka! – (she needs someone to carry her as a bride ought to be; she must not fall down when carried into the bathroom where she would normally be cleansed).

Apart from this role, community groups such as the Al-Imaan have also tried to recreate the Zanzibar Eid day celebrations held at Mnazi Mmoja. Ashura drives the 15 minutes to Northampton on Eid day, where her daughter can have a good time. She can then tell her little friends that her Christmas is called Eid; a day when she gets a new dress, new shoes, new hair ribbons and above all, she gets money instead of presents. She can spend as she pleases, starting at the al Imaan celebrations where she can purchase toys of her choice, as her mother had done years ago in Zanzibar.

Tuma

Tuma was born in 1974 and grew up at the Kisiwandui suburb of Unguja. This area is part of *ng'ambo*, meaning 'the other side', an area that was initially disadvantaged, although this is now changing. We find that Tuma's life from the onset has been characterized by mobility. Her father had moved to Kisiwandui from the rural Kitope ndani in the 1960s. He had joined a Taarab music group and, as the performances in town increased, it became more viable for him to move into town. Her mother had always lived at Kisiwandui; she earned an extra income as a food vendor, selling *maandazi* (buns) and *vitumbua* (rice cakes) from the home. Tuma remembers that during the planting season, her father would move to Kitope ndani for a month or two to help his family, and later on he would commute to Kitope ndani and return with food stuffs for sale, including rice, cassava and green bananas. She often tells me *mtoto wa nyoka ni nyoka* (the child of a snake is also a snake), since she also cooks and sells foodstuffs from her home in Dagenham, East London. The going prices are small – three *vitumbua* (rice flour pastries) or £2; samosas at 50 p each; and chapatti at £1 each. She makes most of her income during the fasting month of Ramadhan and also when there are special occasions such as weddings, the prophet's birthday (*maulid*) and recitations for the dead (*khitma*).

Dagenham and the nearby areas of Barking boast a large Muslim settlement in London; they are also home to the largest Swahili-speaking communities in Britain. Zanzibaris, similar to most immigrants, have tended to gravitate towards localities with an established community of compatriots. A number of people from Mombasa, Zanzibar, Lamu and other coastal towns have settled in the area and have made the area a home away from home for most Swahili speakers in London and Britain in general. All Swahili delicacies such as the mixture of potato and savouries – *mbatata za urojo* or meat skewers – *mishikaki*, are abundantly available at the Barking market and also in certain homes. This area of East London has played host and actually became a 'locality' for many Swahili speakers. When discussing tourist locations, Appadurai writes that such

> locations create complex conditions for the production and reproduction of locality, in which ties of marriage, work, business and leisure weave together various circulating populations with kinds of 'locals' to create neighbourhoods which belong in one sense to particular nation-states, but are, from another point of view, what we might call translocalities'.[15]

As a trans-locality, Barking is *Uswahilini* in London.

We find that, although her English is quite sparse, Tuma easily accesses markets and shops in her area. She prefers the Upton park market to buy fresh produce and meat and Barking market for readymade Swahili foods. Advertisements for East African goods such as Azam flour and phone cards act as her guide; she knows that the given shopkeeper would understand her. Upon closer inspection, we may infer that there are particular connections between the shops that she frequents, their signs and Swahili immigrants in East London. Tuma is guided by these outward placards and signs capes, which can themselves be seen as trans-local since they evoke material and embody links between the immigrant clientele and their locality.

Tuma's children are all from her first marriage – the youngest is seven. She moved to Britain in 1999 when her oldest child was only 2 years old. Although Tuma easily accesses the markets and buys what she needs, her sparse knowledge of English has acted as a barrier to her accessing health-related matters such as her Doctor (GP), or when she has to deal with the council or the Department of Works and Pension, who are the source of her state benefits. For official interactions, she has relied on her children; although sometimes a translator is offered, she prefers her oldest daughter to translate for her.

At home, Tuma has a telephone package that she was attracted into buying during a visit to Upton Park market, and is one of her best investments yet. Through a SKY telephone package, which offers unlimited telephone calling for a fixed rate, she can call her friends all over the UK, in most European countries, and in the USA, she can talk for as long as she wants. She simply has to hang up and call them again every 60 minutes, she explained – calls are apparently charged per minute after the initial hour. This has made bearable the fact that her new flat is located at a remote area of Dagenham. The telephone acts as a very important and vital tool in trans-local communication. Interestingly, every household with a woman visited in this research would have a similar telephone package, allowing them to communicate with others in Europe and America.

Initially, Tuma had occupied a one-bedroom flat in the Barking area. She has very fond memories of the block of flats where she had resided temporarily for almost five years – a lot of Zanzibaris lived in the block – it was cramped and truly felt like the cramped flats of *michenzani*. Whenever a neighbour made a delicacy, they would bring her a platter, sometimes. She didn't cook anything, but would feast on what her neighbours brought in; the spicy chicken wings, samosa, *pilau*, it was ideal. She often laughs remembering the lifts in the block during weekends when immigrants from other countries would go out until all hours and relieve themselves in the lifts, making Saturday and Sunday 'no-go to lift' days.

She moved out of her 10th-floor, one-bedroom flat in 2005 immediately after divorcing the father of her children. She has since re-married twice, and is now expecting her fourth child. Moving into a bigger accommodation was beneficial for her children – they now have space and seem to achieve better at school – but the move had initially made her immobile. She had to depend on a bus whose stop was located at a 10-minute walk from her home and proved unreliable. She soon realized that she could no longer do 'the school run' where she took her children to school, and then have enough time to do her shopping, make the family meals, drop at a friend's house for a chat before it was time to pick the children up at 3.15 pm. The bigger house therefore alienated her from her compatriots as most still live at Barking.

She jokes that she had married her second husband because he had a car and could take her around. He had, however, been a mistake from the word go she says. She met him through *Facebook*; they had common friends, virtual friends from all over the world. He had often 'commented' on the 'posts' that she had commented on, making her aware of his presence, before he decided to request her to be his friend. At the time he had told her that he was a stressed divorced man, living with a friend who never bothered to hide his irritation at having a houseguest – *ninamkera kama nini n'navo kaa hapa!* His ex-wife lived in Slough. Their virtual interaction developed into a real friendship; she gave him her telephone number. He would call her from time to time, and she had felt as though they had known each other for a long time, and he had not waited long to ask her to marry him. Although they had never met prior to the marriage, she had felt that it was right to say yes.

He moved into her house and not long after the marriage she learnt that a 'friend' in Belfast who called him often was actually another wife; herself a divorcee with one child. He was also unemployed with no intention of getting a job; at least her first husband whom she had divorced after discovering he had acquired a second wife in Zanzibar, used to work at a butcher's. Looking back, Tuma is now convinced that her second husband had married her because of her independence; a single mother whose house and taxes are paid for by the state while the latter also hands her a financial state benefit on a weekly basis. Interestingly, this is something that crops up quite often among the Swahili where men attach themselves to 'independent women'.

Tuma informed me that upon arriving from Belfast, he had applied for the job-seekers allowance, which had been refused because he had had a pending application in Slough. Things soured immediately after that refusal; he had asked Tuma to hand him her benefits so that he could handle some domestic finances. She had refused, and this became an item of constant tension between them until she asked him to leave. Tuma says that the final decision to ask for a divorce was very hard. She had almost wanted to let him handle the finances, it took a lot of courage but in the end, she decided that it was better to be a twice-divorced woman than a slave in her own home.

Her third and current husband is *mu-ansar suna*.[16] He is among a growing number of young strict Muslims. He has a long untrimmed beard, wears his *kanzu* (white robe) well above his ankles; since being married to him, she has had to wear the full Islamic clothing, covering herself fully. She tells me that initially the change in her attire had been met by applause. Tuma had always donned a scarf which either hung loosely on her head or dropped onto her shoulders, and her hair had always been visible. So when she started wearing the hijab, where she only showed her face and palms, her friends had all said *mashallah*. But, when she then adopted the full *niqab* where her face was veiled and only the eyes visible, and would not wear anything of colour except black and grey, eyebrows were raised. A friend once remarked – '*eh, ushakuwa kizoro! ndio nini unajizonga zonga hivyo?*' – (you have now become 'like Zorro' – why are you entangling yourself thus?).

Tuma's current husband is younger than her and is originally from Mombasa. He had never married prior to marrying her, and it was *sunna* for him to marry her, since the Prophet had married Khadija who was much older to him and among other widows. Their marriage is sanctioned by religion and not the state – an imam married them, not a registrar. He works as a taxi driver and caters for all of Tuma's needs. He treats her with respect and expects that from her too. Her mannerisms, the way she carries herself and her way of dress are expected to portray purity. She therefore would not shake men's hands, dress appropriately at all times and surround herself with friends who uphold similar beliefs to her. The latter was not difficult, as her friends are also her compatriots, and coincidentally, there has recently been an upsurge of Swahili women who observe strict Islamic decrees.

Tuma tells me that many women attend *madarasa ya dini* (religious classes) held at the Canning town mosque, which is the preferred mosque by most Swahili people; their children also attend *madrassa* Islamic classes at the mosque. Tuma's involvement and what she calls 'deeper understanding' of Islam has meant that she now no longer attends social events such as *maulidi ya mtume*[17] and *khitma,*[18] since these are *bidaa* – i.e. 'new inventions' and therefore non-Islamic and illegitimate.

Maulidi ya mtume is a festival that has occupied a position of great importance among the Swahili for many years. This carnival-like celebration remains very popular among Swahili, where homes are decorated with flags and people celebrate their prophet's birth by reciting the Qur'an and enjoying great feasts. Tuma remembers that, back home in Unguja on the day of Maulid, school children celebrated in their respective schools wearing new clothes, reciting the Qur'an and listening to their peers' presentations, consuming a multitude of sweet pop, sweets and *pilau*. The celebrations would continue in their homes where familial celebrations would be upheld. Tuma and a growing number of Swahili women in the UK insist that this festival is *bidaa*, as are the celebrations of birthdays and music. And on the day of *Maulid*, they no longer call their families in Zanzibar to wish them happy celebrations; they only do so for *Eid* festivals. This position is supported by religious organizations such as the Al-Imaan association of Swahili Muslims in Britain.[19] Similarly, they do not hold the *khitma*, or reading of the Quran for the dead.

When a death occurs within the UK, the Al-Imaan association and people from the deceased community join together to ensure that the burial goes smoothly. Many Swahili families make a small contribution to Al-Imaan on a monthly basis, and the money is used for funeral expenses. This contribution gives Zanzibaris the assurance they need that, should they die in Britain, proper prayers and Islamic procedures will be followed to ensure that one is buried appropriately. When death occurs back home in Zanzibar, for instance, the norm has been for the UK-based family members of the deceased to invite friends and compatriots and then to recite the Quran. At times, a hall is hired to accommodate the tens or hundreds who would show up for the recitation. A religious scholar is called upon to recite the Qur'an on the day; a number of dry food stuffs such as samosas, *katlesi* (fish cakes), *visheti* (dry sugar-coated biscuits), soft drinks and bottled water are offered to those who attend. Swahilis would travel from Scotland and beyond to attend a *khitma* in Milton Keynes for instance. The *khitma* is thus a social event, almost an outing of sorts where one would meet those they have not in a long time. The family of the deceased would occupy central stage, near the *chetezo* (burning incense), dressed correctly either in the black *baibui* (jilbab) or donning the khanga cloth. The rest would occupy an area of choice on the carpeted hall.

A growing number of Swahilis now deny the legitimacy of the auspicious prayers that make up the *khitma*; only the children and family members of the deceased can pray for the departed soul in privacy. Therefore, we find that, when one hears of a death, they contact the deceased family to pay their respects but do not ask – '*khitma itasomwa lini?*' (when will the *khitma* be read); instead, they wait for those concerned to initiate this. Those who do not attend the *khitma*, for instance Tuma in this case, are not frowned upon, but are understood to be *muansari*. Thus, Tuma would alienate herself from this event, but she would pay her respects to the deceased family before or after the *khitma*, quietly.

Tuma introduced me to Nassor Bachu and Othman Maalim, Swahili Islamic preachers from Zanzibar whose speeches range from Islamic decrees on birth control to the importance of education and the punishment of those who do not observe prayers. I would find in a number of Swahili homes in the form of DVDs, saved as favourites from websites such as YouTube and alhidaaya. She informs me that she used to enjoy listening to Othman Maalim's sermons, but he recently gave a talk where he aligned himself with those who celebrate *Maulidi ya mtume* as an expression of gratitude and communal awareness, making her doubt his authenticity. She also listens to most preachers from *Uamsho* (awakening), the controversial Islamic organization based in Zanzibar. As students of Nassor Bachu, most of these preachers uphold a reformist kind of Islam.[20]

Tuma points out that, with hindsight, she is the happiest she has ever been especially since her husband supports her financially and emotionally. This relationship is quite common among the Swahili. Tuma's husband is recognized by all the Swahili as her husband, but not so by the state. It is common practice among the Swahili in Britain to marry in the religious sense but not legally with state sanction; thus, Tuma has always had a 'social husband'. For many, the so-called social husband is to a large extent dependent on his wife. He may be employed or may be claiming some form of state financial benefit. But, as a man, the benefits due to him are meagre as compared to those handed out to the woman. As custodian of children, the wife receives financial support which enables her to support her children. This may include subsidized housing rent, council taxes and some form of income support. The woman therefore offers stability.

Having a social husband allows a woman to have all the state benefits as a single mother, and yet be socially recognized as a married woman. For the husband, it allows him to have a partner, a home, security and a small window that would allow him to have an extra income. When I asked Tuma about this situation, her response was similar to that of many Swahili women in her situation – *ninayajuaje ya kesho*? (who knows what tomorrow brings?). She cannot let go of her single-mother status just because she has found a new partner. Indeed, divorce is still extremely high and commonplace among the Swahili. The reality is that she may need to re-apply to the state for her benefits sooner rather than later. And so, in Britain, husbands come and go, but the state benefits, council house and children are the woman's to keep; they are her independence.

Looked at superficially, one may deduct that Swahili women are simply maximizing on the benefits of the welfare state. This is not true. The Swahili women are dependent on the state as part of their integration into Britain. It helps them overcome some male-dominated practices such as second marriages and financial abuse. This dependence has actually re-defined and empowered them.

Zahra

Zahra was born in 1970 in Zanzibar. Her ancestors came from the Comoros, about which Zahra is very proud, and tries to instil the importance of her origins to her children. She has been married for more than 17 years. Her four children go to school in Northampton where she is an active member of the Al-Imaan association, which has helped her secure a place so she is currently training to be a child minder. She became religious once in Britain and argues that people back home in Zanzibar, and in most African societies in general, do not really understand religion – *ni uswahili tu* – meaning that they have incorporated traditions, sorcery and everything around them in their beliefs.

Zahra's husband used to commute to Milton Keynes everyday where he had worked at a factory involved in packaging chicken for freezing. The entire family naturalized and became British three years ago. Passport in hand, her husband had the freedom to travel to Zanzibar and Dar es Salaam, where he discovered that there was a large demand for second-hand white goods, such as refrigerators, cookers, washing machines, irons and microwaves. He became an export-import businessman. A year after starting this business he decided that life was better back home, where he could do business, have a big home, be surrounded by family and enjoy a quality of life superior to that in the UK. Zahra disagrees. The education that her children receive in Britain is equivalent to international schools in Zanzibar, where one has to pay thousands of dollars per child annually. Since they do not have that kind of money, she prefers to remain in the UK and forsake being 'someone' back home; she would rather remain a 'no one' away from home where her children are receiving a good education. She also points out that, even if she had that money, she believes that international schools spoil and disengage children. She enjoys the convenience of living in the UK and having financial independence, as well as the freedom of not having in-laws drop in every now and then, bringing in tension. In the end, they came to the agreement that, while the children are attending school she will remain in the UK with them, while her husband can live in Zanzibar, where they would visit him during the holidays; he also visits them. This arrangement puts her on a pedestal in the eyes of her friends, for she is offered more financial security by her husband as he sends her money from 'Africa'.

Zahra has surrounded herself with a large network of friends who, in one way or another, help in the running of her household. This includes help with child care, shopping and mobility. Similarly, she also helps her friends. She often has her friends' children spending the night at her home, because their mother has to leave very early to attend college or has just gone to another town for a funeral or a wedding. She sometimes goes through two or three schools to pick up children, because their parents are occupied elsewhere. Similarly, her friends take her shopping in their cars since she does not drive. She has become very prominent socially, always being among the first to be consulted for any event, be it a wedding or a funeral.

Her biggest fear is that her husband would acquire a second wife; this she talks about candidly, saying that she would not be able to accept that. Interestingly, a rumour was circulating at the time that her husband had actually taken a second wife. It is possible that Zahra was unaware of this, or she may have known but pretended not to know so as not to face this problem. There had been cases when only once confronted did husbands want to fully practice polygamy. Zahra mentioned that her husband had informed her that business was not as well as it had been, and he was not sending back amounts that he initially did. As an immediate effect of this, Zahra will most probably need to depend on the state for financial support.

When discussing polygamy, Zahra explained that men do complain that women in Britain are arrogant, expecting their men to help in the domestic setting and, in the process, to 'feminize' them and that women have no respect for their husbands, whereas in the homeland women are supposedly docile and respectful. But according to Zahra, men acquire extra spouses out of selfishness, and the girls they marry back home are only interested in them because they want financial stability, or they think that such men will take them to Europe.

Zahra continues to live in Britain because of her children. Her children are Muslim first, and then British, but they are also East African. They are all fluent in Swahili, although they all have a distinct British accent. The youngest is struggling with Swahili and has gone as far as banning Zahra from speaking to her in Swahili when she goes to pick her up at school. Zahra laughs at the idea of her child being embarrassed of being Swahili – but she recognizes that it is a situation that she will have to deal with. When asked about Zanzibar, the children remembered that they had enjoyed living in their father's big house and being driven in a big car. They also enjoyed not having to make their beds since there were maids. The heat, the sea and the walks had also been a lot of fun, but the dust, heat, mosquitoes, intermittent electricity and water had soured their stay. In the end, they could not wait to return 'home' to Britain. It is this generation of children that will shed more light on the identities, integration and experiences of the Zanzibaris, as they occupy different spaces in Britain and in their place of origin, Zanzibar.

Conclusion

To a large extent, the Swahili women have integrated into the British society since they have been able to participate in a number of social-economic and cultural activities in the country while retaining their Swahili identity. The integration is not uniform, since they inhabit different spaces as individuals and react differently to life in Britain. Similarly, while embracing what is actually foreign, especially in a secular host society, certain aspects of Swahili culture have had to be compromised. This has mainly happened in regards to religious rituals and beliefs. Brickell and Datta (2011) point out that the experiences of migrants are not straightforward articulations centred on any one scale, but rather consist of a multi-scalar repertoire of connections.

The Swahili women create identities that are distinct from the British society, and they maintain some cultural links with Zanzibar. They tend to retain their individuality in various ways, such as by retaining their maiden names. This has enabled them to not only keep their heritage but also keep their identities through divorces and find a type of independence in state dependence. They are the de facto heads of their households. These identities have religion as a primary identifier, playing a very important role socially and even economically. There is a sharp increase in the number of Swahili who engage in and observe strict Muslim rituals. This is the effect of the varying spaces that the Swahili have had to occupy. The children of these women are British Swahili of Zanzibari origin. They are the ones who have the greatest contact with other ethnicities, especially in public areas such as schools and parks. This is different in families where parents are fully integrated in the labour market, because their pattern of life tends to coincide with that of the mainstream. In this sense, there is a specific pattern in Swahili immigrant integration.

Through these women, we have had a glimpse of the multiple forms of spatial connectedness. The women are all struggling to locate themselves in multiple networks of communication and imagination. There is a social network that spans continents, an upsurge in virtual networks and a strong relationship with religion. Their lives occupy the 'here' and 'there' which are 'Britain' and 'Zanzibar'. These case studies have only offered us a firsthand glimpse and contributed towards our understanding of the Swahili in Britain, yet there remains a need to carry out more in-depth research into this subject, involving a larger sample.

Disclosure statement

No potential conflict of interest was reported by the author.

Notes

1. From Eastman, "Who Are the Waswahili", to Fair, *Pastimes and Politics*, and also Caplan and Topan, *Swahili Modernities*.
2. de Vere Allen, *Swahili Origins*, 5.
3. Horton and Middleton, *The Swahili*, 185.
4. Caplan, "But the Coast", 8.
5. See Scott and Marshall (2005).
6. See Saggar (1995); Favell (1998).
7. Interdepartmental Working Group on the Integration of Refugees in Ireland, *Integration: A Two Way Process*, 9.

8. Modood, "Post-immigration 'Difference' and 'Integration'," 2012.
9. Ibid.
10. Mirza and Strobel, *Three Swahili Women*, 1.
11. There is a great difference between the Swahili who immigrated to Britain in the 60s and those who did so within the last decade or so. One finds, for instance, that the majority of those who emigrated in the 1960s did so under the duress of Zanzibar's political situation, whereas the majority of current immigrants are motivated by economics.
12. This term has been used in this study to describe phenomena involving mobility, migration, circulation and spatial interconnectedness that are not limited to national boundaries.
13. Breaking the fast where all types of dishes are prepared.
14. Mirza and Strobel, *Three Swahili Women*, 10.
15. Appadurai, "The Production of Locality," 216.
16. The Swahili *wa-ansar sunna* are a group of Sunni Muslims who claim to be leading their lives as did the prophet – as demands the sunna – and are therefore often in opposition to other Swahili Muslims. For instance, they believe events such as the maulid (prophet's birthday), the *khitma* (praying for the dead on the third day) are all un-Islamic – they are new inventions (*bidaa*). One of the most famous Swahili *ansar sunna* is called Bachu. The term is derived from the Ansar al-Sunna, or Army of the Protectors of the Prophet Mohammad's *sunna*.
17. According to the Al Hidaaya, Swahili Muslim authority in Britain, upholding the Maulid means one will burn in hell since the Prophet never celebrated his birthday. http://www.alhidaaya.com/sw/node/3766
18. According to the Al Hidaaya, Swahili Muslim authority in Britain reading the Quran for the dead is forbidden unless it is by the child of the deceased or family. http://www.alhidaaya.com/sw/node/219
19. In my conversation with Swahili women, the Al-Imaan association sprung up every now and then. It is a religious association managed from Northampton. According to Zahra (third case study), the Al-Imaan has approximately 800 members, the majority being Swahili speakers from Tanzania, Kenya and Somalia and living around Milton Keynes and Northampton. It also has a few Jamaican and English converts as members – these are people with links to the Swahili either through marriage or friendships. The initial aim of this organization was to give support in times of death and marriage – therefore, the members of this association enjoyed what can loosely be referred to as an extended family. For its survival, every Swahili home contributes £5 a month (initially it had been £3). The organization offers Quranic lessons to approximately 200 Swahili children who pay £18 a month for weekend classes. This money is used in the running of the *madrassa* and also in paying a stipend of about £100 a month to 16 religious teachers. All the teachers are Swahili, apart from one who is English. The Al-Imaan offers guidance to the Swahili and directs them towards proper Islamic conduct and ritual observation. It is involved in reconciling prospective divorces, holding networking meetings for its members, conducting religious classes and has recently initiated a project that aims at reducing Swahili women's dependency on benefits. To this end, it has linked with colleges in Northampton and Milton Keynes and has been able to register a number of Swahili women into courses such as hair dressing, cake decoration and even ESOL.
20. The reformists preach a return to an original form of Islam as was practiced by the prophet Mohammad. They tend to refute most 'traditional' practices that Swahili observe.

References

Appadurai, Arjun. "The Production of Locality." In *Counterworks: Managing the Diversity of Knowledge*, edited by R. Fardon, 204–225. London: Routledge, 1995.
Brickell, K., and A. Datta, eds. *Translocal Geographies: Spaces, Places, Connections*. Farnham: Ashgate, 2011.
Caplan, Pat. "'But the Coast, of Course, Is Quite Different': Academic and Local Ideas about the East African Littoral." *Journal of Eastern African Studies* 1, no. 2 (2007): 305–320. doi:10.1080/17531050701452663, 2007.
Caplan, Pat, and Farouk Topan. *Swahili Modernities: Identity, Development and Power on the Coast of East Africa*. Trenton, NJ: Africa World Press, 2004.
de Vere Allen, J. *Swahili Origins: Swahili Culture and the Shungwaya Phenomenon*. London: James Currey, 1993.
Eastman, C. "Who Are the Waswahili." *Africa* 41 (1971): 228–236.

Fair, Laura. *Pastimes and Politics: Culture, Community, and Identity in Post-Abolition Zanzibar, 1890–1945*. Oxford: James Currey, 2001.

Favell, A. *Philosophy of Integration: Immigration and the Idea of Citizenship in France and Britain*. Basingstoke: Macmillan, 1998.

Horton, Mark, and John Middleton. *The Swahili: The Social Landscape of a Mercantile Society*. Oxford: Blackwell, 2000.

Interdepartmental Working Group on the Integration of Refugees in Ireland. *Integration: A Two Way Process*. Dublin: Department for Justice, Equality and Law Reform, 2001. Accessed December 27, 2014. http://www.irlgov.ie/justice/Publications/Asylum/integration.pdf.

Marcel, C., et al. *Migration and Public Perception*. BEPA: European Commission. 2015. Accessed December 27, 2014. http://ec.europa.eu/dgs/policy_advisers/publications/docs/bepa_migration_final_09_10_006_en.pdf.

Mirza, Sarah, and Margareth Strobel, eds. and trans. *Three Swahili Women: Life Histories from Mombasa, Kenya*. Bloomington: Indiana University Press, 1989.

Modood, Tariq. *Post-immigration 'Difference' and 'Integration': The Case of Muslims in Western Europe*. London: The British Academy, 2012.

Saggar, S. "Integration and Adjustment: Britain's Liberal Settlement Revisited." In *Immigration and Integration: Australia and Britain*, 105–131, edited by D. Lowe. London: Bureau of Immigration, Multicultural and Population Research and Sir Robert Menzies Centre for Australian Studies, 1995.

Scott, John, and Gordon Marshall. *A Dictionary of Sociology*. Oxford: Oxford University Press, 2005.

Waters, Maya. "Comparing Immigrant Integration in Britain and the US." 2015. Accessed January 6, 2015. http://www.ageofobamabook.com/papers/waters.pdf.

Beyond 'Great Marriage': collective involvement, personal achievement and social change in Ngazidja (Comoros)

Sophie Blanchy

Laboratoire d'ethnologie et de sociologie comparative, CNRS – Université de Paris Ouest Nanterre, Nanterre, France

The sumptuous 'Great Marriage' celebration in Ngazidja, Comoros, is a very dynamic social practice, but it is difficult to comprehend its attraction given the increasing cost. This paper argues that the 'Great Marriage' is the most salient part of an age system that should be carefully examined. The framework, in which collective commitment and individual achievement are managed simultaneously, and gendered conception of personhood and of human temporality are put into action, has no equivalent in Western life. Grounded in historical hierarchies, these institutions change under various influences without abandoning the core values on which they are based, which explains their enduring success.

Introduction

A man wearing an Omani-style embroidered robe and a splendid, coloured turban goes through the village of Dembeni, from his sister's (and mother's) house to the house of his new wife. His sister, dressed in beautiful, traditional striped and fringed fabrics, opens an umbrella over him. The sister's husband walks besides them. Students from the Koranic school sing and play flutes to announce the arrival of the three protagonists followed by family and neighbours. They are greeted at the door of the bride's house by her father and uncles. One of them chants the Islamic call to prayer, and the sister's husband gives the sum of 2 million Comorian francs from the bridegroom.[1] It is the payment for 'foot washing', which was in the past the purification of the groom's feet with perfume by a kinswoman to protect the integrity of the house. The groom is then led into the bride's bedroom to the sound of women ululating.[2]

This is one of the sumptuous celebrations and ostentatious exchanges of the 'Great Marriage', which have made the Comoros archipelago famous in Zanzibar, Madagascar and France, where many migrants live, as well as in tourists' imaginations. Zanzibari wedding festivities are also very lavish occasions,[3] but in Ngazidja, one of the Comoros islands, this life cycle celebration is linked to specific social and political institutions: the age and rank system and matrilineal descent groups, which form the backbone of the community-level specific polity, the city (*mdji*). Time in the city is punctuated by *ãda na mila*[4] events. However, the excessive expense is criticized by external observers as well as young Comorians studying abroad as counterproductive for development and a burden on individual life. According to the Human Development Index, a Western concept measuring life expectancy, literacy and living standards, Comoros ranks 163 out of 187 countries.[5] However, this standardized evaluation tool ignores local conceptions of temporality, personhood and accomplishment, and undervalues corporate groups' affiliations and collective agency.[6] How can the success of Great Marriage be explained in an era of monetization, migration, Western education, Islamic contestation and globalization?[7] A close examination of what lies beyond this enduring social practice is needed to understand its individual and social meaning.

In previous works I have described the complex relations linking institutions and framing collective and personal agency.[8] The most puzzling fact is the variability of age patterns. I argue here that the variability reveals both the persistence of core values and the system's ability to adapt to economic and social change. Adaptability concerns issues that are central for this society but whose relevance is broader. These issues are: gendered representation of personhood; temporality of human life; the local conception of equality in light of historical hierarchies and Western definitions of equality; tension between individual and collective agency; and citizenship concepts depending on affiliation to different political entities. Identifying the changing trends in social practices in Ngazidja will enable us to document the Comorian response to more general social concerns.

I shall first underline the uniqueness of Ngazidja from a sociological perspective and then present how people deal with ascribed positions depending on various criteria, and what range of personal agency remains to achieve both collective and individual goals. Next, I shall provide a historical summary of 20th-century political and economic changes to explain how some social rules have been challenged while others have been adopted even by former outsiders. I hope to account for the effectiveness of this social device, which would explain the reasons for its resilience.

Ngazidja's sociological uniqueness

The four Comoros islands, Ngazidja, Mwali, Ndzwani and Maore, in the Mozambique Channel were first inhabited (from at least the eighth century) by Bantu-speaking Africans. Islam was soon introduced by traders.[9] Muslims from Arabia and the Persian Gulf migrated along the African coast, reached the Comoros and Madagascar and married into the leading families, following the uxorilocal residence rule.[10] In the 15th century, the archipelago contained several small kingdoms. Under French colonial rule in the 19th century, it attained independence in 1975, although Maore remained French. Emigrants, mainly Wangazidja settled in France, maintain close ties with the archipelago.[11] A common life style and institutions in the four islands give an impression of cultural unity (uxorimatrilocal residence, the age and exchange system and Sunni Shafi'i Islam), but Maore's partition and the state's failure reveal the tension between this sense of socio-cultural unity and its denial by highlighting differences between the islands, and principally the *ãda* of Ngazidja.[12]

We owe the first anthropological study of Ngazidja to Shepherd,[13] who clearly showed the centrality of *ãda* payments for every Mngazidja, even for migrants keeping ties with their city. She identified Great Marriage as one matrimonial system in Ngazidja, besides the union without exchanges.[14] She recognized matrifiliation as an abiding principle in Ngazidja (with the exception of a drift towards patrilaterality among *sharifs* claiming to descend from the Prophet).[15] In the 1980s, the description of matrilineal land and property transmission (*manyahuli*)[16] and matrilineal transmission of political power within kings' lineages[17] revealed genuinely cognitive models of the relations between kin in the matrilineal logic, such as the rotation of uterine brothers and nephews to the position of power. Comorian scholars stressed the value of honour (*sheo*) in *ãda* practices.[18] Recently, the Comorian age system has received increasing attention.[19] Other works have reported Comorians' commitment in regional and international networks through intellectual exchanges or more global mimetic social strategies.[20] Although wedding celebrations are similar in many ways throughout the archipelago, exchanges in the age system are strictly egalitarian outside Ngazidja; the island of Mwali has a matrilineal structure,[21] and in Ndzwani and Maore, kinship is bilateral, and the age system is disappearing, giving way to more flexible associations. In Ndzwani, there is great discrepancy between the urban Arabic society of landowners and rural society made up of descendants of the free population and former slaves, who are landless and survive by migrating.[22] In the 1960s, Robineau described loosely formed age-sets (*hirimu*) of young adults attending the same mosque, showing the salient role of Islam in social organization.[23] In Maore, rapid demographic growth and development are causing a new social stratification to emerge, but hierarchy is still a negative idea and it is claimed that the Great Marriage (*arusi*) does not confer any special status.[24]

Having observed the islands' kinship systems and *ãda* events in the 1980s,[25] I then studied the political life of the 'cities' and the individual careers it offers.[26] In each city, a government of 'Accomplished Men' (*wandru wadzima*) controls men's progression in the age and rank system, matrimonial alliances between matrilineal houses, and life cycle exchanges, using the set of social rules called *ãda na mila*. At first glance, the wide variety of age and rank system arrangements I highlighted in the various cities appeared confusing, but in fact this demonstrates the two main forms and intermediary models, providing evidence of the institution's dynamic evolution.

City, house and personhood[27]

Today, every locality of the island is organized as a political city, with an assembly of Accomplished Men, matrilineal houses and Friday mosque. This is the result of the gradual weakening of ancient hierarchies. At the time of the kingdoms (15th–19th centuries), localities were distinguished as 'city of power' *mdji wa yezi* (king residence), 'big city' *midji mihuu* and 'outside locality' *mdji pvondze* (rural village); slave hamlets *zitreya* were not even mentioned.[28] In the 'cities of power', the three social divisions still live in separate districts (*wandru wa ntsi* landowners and farmers, *walozi* fishermen and *warumwa* people of slave descent), and thus form distinct assemblies – distinct 'cities' – with tacit hierarchical relations creating a serious obstacle to collective projects.[29] Hierarchies remain but are gradually evolving in different ways, making it possible for every man to obtain the local citizenship of Accomplished Man, although this is still limited by rules of commensality.

Matriliny, observed in many East and Central African societies,[30] should be considered, according to Peters' formula, as 'a set of characteristics rather than a totality or "system"'.[31] In Ngazidja, matrilineage *hinya* is a descent group localized in the town or village. According to myths heard repeatedly, the female ancestor made her home in the place she became pregnant. The lineages of the city are ranked, and their ranking is expressed by attributing pieces of meat from cattle supplied for *ãda*, according to their historical precedence and the exploits of its champions during past wars. Present-day *ãda* payments are also valued as actions performed by the lineages for the city and are claimed in ranking negotiations.

The age system, a classic issue in anthropology, should be considered with regard to its sociological efficiency insofar as it organizes polities;[32] its military role has been stressed in North-East Africa.[33] Using an earlier presentation of the Ngazidja age system[34] and participating in comparative collective research,[35] I have described age system models and the polity of which they form the basis.[36] The age system is made of two generational sets, Sons of the City (*wanamdji*) and Fathers (*wandru wababa*), and of grades of age and status that follow various patterns. Through Great Marriage, men leave the Sons category and obtain the right to sit on the assembly of Fathers, also called Accomplished Men (*wandru wadzima*): political fathering is thus linked to wedding festivities. The idea of accomplishment in the title of *mdzima* (complete, one) is an ideal to be achieved in a man's lifetime. In the same way, a woman obtains the status of mother of *ãda* through two successive Great Marriages, her own and her daughter's, making the temporal process of this achievement very explicit. Two key events occur simultaneously in Great Marriage: the husband becomes a political father and the house is transmitted from mother to daughter.

Marriage means the entry of a man into a woman's house, but the union, contracted by the Islamic ritual of *nikāh*, can easily be dissolved according to *sharia*, and men circulate between houses, villages and even islands. Every married woman is given a house (sometimes a very basic one) by her kin, and may be married by anybody whose social status is not inferior to her own. However, marrying 'by *ãda*' (Great Marriage) reduces the choice to the eldest daughter of a house of the city ready to pay *ãda*, and the series of payments must benefit the city. This requires substantial financial means, which men and women accumulate with the help of their relatives and from subscriptions from various groups; the goods exchanged – bullocks, rice, jewellery, money and various services – circulate between the houses of the bride and groom and between the male and female groups of the city. The criterion of birthright among siblings plays a role for both men and women. The firstborn daughter must be married in *ãda* for her first marriage. Today, all men attempt to pay for this ritual to have a voice in the city, but in the past, they were represented by their elder brother. The eldest son continues to enjoy his family's greater and earlier mobilization.

Although people think and talk about these social situations from the different perspectives of gender and generation, the main perspective adopted is that of the house. Both men and women often speak and act for it in *ãda* circumstances. The matrilineal 'house' (*daho*) is composed of several generations of siblings and headed by the elder married women and their brothers (maternal uncles: *wadjomba*, sing. *mdjomba*). Acting for the house is a collective task shared by siblings. The eldest daughter and eldest son assume the first two roles, and younger ones help them and may benefit from the house's prestige and resources. This creates a division between the houses of *ãda* and the others, between the wives of *ãda* and the others, the younger sisters thus forming a somewhat distinct and lesser society.

Once married by *ãda*, the elder sister has to achieve two tasks: to marry her brother and then to marry her daughter, giving and taking husbands on behalf of the house. As a person, she must prove her ability to organize ceremonies and supervise exchanges between women's groups. Her Great Marriage precedes that of her brother, so that as a woman of *ãda*, she is entitled to bring him to his bride's mother's house accompanied by her husband, an Accomplished Man. Her husband is the *shimedji* (brother-in-law) of her siblings, but during the brother's Great Marriage he assumes a broader role.

Let us return to first scene described in this paper (Figure 1). A man explained to me the role of the *shimedji* next to the groom in the ritual of 'entering the house' by arguing 'Who will be his father? There is a father on the bride's side, so there must be one on the

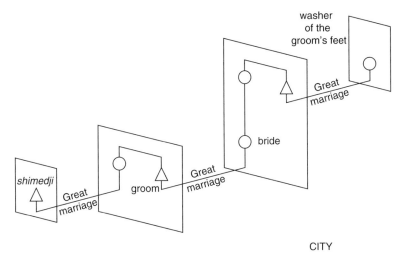

Figure 1. Foot-washing ritual on entering the house in Dembeni.

groom's side!'[37] Far from thinking of them as brothers-in-law, he was stressing the Father–Son relationship between the *shimedji* and his wife's brother. This evidently refers to their generational status and political fathering, since the *shimedji* is neither the groom's genitor nor his maternal uncle. Indeed, as the elder sister's husband, he is called 'the father of the house' (*mbaba daho*), representing the house in the city and with a duty to give it children. This does not prevent the *shimedji* from introducing the groom, once in the Fathers' category, into his own commensality group in the *mdji* assembly, as a strategy to optimize his access to the concrete resources of this *ãda* …

Another key point was highlighted when a man told me that when he celebrated the *ãda* for his son's circumcision, he was finally able to tell his wife 'Now I have completely married you [by *ãda*]!' meaning that this was the final stage of his commitment in the Great Marriage, since a circumcised young man is a marriageable one. A man who enters the house through marriage, and is called *mbaba* (father), is mainly considered in this matrilineal logic both as an affine and a genitor – which does not minimize his value, on the contrary. In parallel to the woman's two tasks (marrying her brother and her daughter), the man must be an initiator for his wife's brother during the latter's marriage, and must give a marriageable man to his wife's house.

Men's engagement consolidates links between each house and the city; uncles and fathers, brothers and husbands, all represent the house at several levels in the political institution, and a man's progression in grades of age and rank reflects his house's activity (Figure 2).

In this configuration, *sharifs*' patrilineages appear as an additional source of social distinction. As Shepherd observed, marriages with *sharif* men allowed a double descent system to develop among the elite.[38] Many *sharifs* from the urban aristocracy of Nzwani have entered Ngazidja ruling houses, and the aristocracy of these two islands is highly endogamous despite sociological differences. *Sharifs* also married into other social classes, and for offspring from modest matrilineal origins, inheriting this quality is a factor in social reclassification. However, the relevance of these patrilineages in the city as a polity is limited to the respect due to the noble and sacred Arabic origin of the *sharifs*, whose *baraka* (the power to transmit Allah's blessing) is sought after for many

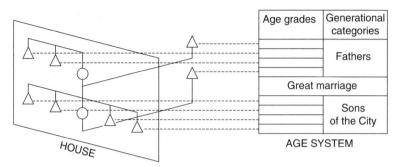

Figure 2. House and age system links.

private and public religious events. The *ãda* celebrations are placed under divine protection and most of them include Islamic prayers and benedictions. *Ãda* and Islam are usually experienced in a balanced and unitary mode. Religious leaders are brothers and uncles in their own matrilineal houses, and fathers in their wife's house. In recent decades, Comorian religious scholars, *ulama*, returning from Arab Muslim universities, have tried to stop *ãda* practices, as well as some Islamic local celebrations, but were expelled from the mosque by the Accomplished Men. A social banishment imposed upon their families was resolved by paying a fee, and the scholars who challenged it could not avoid being indirectly involved in the *ãda* activities of their house.

The first sign of the constant shift in the age-and-rank system is revealed by the variety of coexisting models. The *Wangazidja* are very fond of discussing and comparing this variety, although they do not know many details, given the autonomous organization of each city.

The evolution of the age and rank system: from collective to individual[39]

What makes a man's career in the age and rank system very attractive is the fact that collective advancement through age-grades does not exclude the possibility of individual progress thanks to a system of titles; Accomplished Men operate on both registers in terms of ascribed and achieved positions. Beyond the categories of Fathers and Sons established by the Great Marriage, several combinations link age-grades and ranks or titles.

In what appears to be the oldest model identified in the south, particularly in Dembeni, the age-set (*beya*) is a well-established institution (see Table A1 in Appendix). Bwanaidi Youssouf, whose uncle was a great connoisseur of *ãda*, presented it to me by saying 'The age-set lasts as long as we are all married [by *ãda*] and all dead.'[40] This suggests assurance of age equality and class unity throughout one's life (although one can acquire titles and gain some distinction). As men marry by *ãda* and become Fathers one by one, the class records their change in status without excluding anyone (the last ones are allowed to pay a global sum to obtain the status of Father). The age-set is given a name in a ritual ceremony as soon as two or three members have celebrated their Great Marriage, indicating that everyone in the age-set will succeed in doing so. A new age-set is founded by representatives of each lineage (Figure 3), the hierarchy of which is applied as a ranking order for all sharing of resources between members. Among young men of the age-set who are members of the same lineage, first place is given to the one whose Great Marriage is being prepared. He receives a share according to the rank of his lineage. This power position is accessed by rotation, like that of the king in the past.

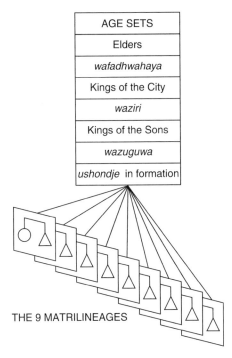

Figure 3. Matrilineal groups and age-sets in Dembeni.

The progression of all the age-sets in age-grades (*hirimu*) is collective. The age-grade of Kings of the Sons, as well as that of Kings of the City, is taken by a coup, prepared with the tacit acceptance of the elders, causing all the higher classes to rise in the grades.[41] In parallel to this collective progression, individual titles may be obtained by making payments to the titleholders. The name of the higher one, *ufukare ya handa* (seven of the first [degree]), suggests that, in the past, this payment was not disconnected from age, since the title had several degrees. Only those with the title of *mfukare wa handa* are qualified to create a group called *trengwe la daho*, 'assembly of house', which receives a significant share of the oxen during *ãda*. This group is not a kin group but a social one, as two *wafukare wa handa* have to found the group together and enrol their brothers and nephews, members of their two houses. Most of the younger men are Sons of the City, or have not yet entered the age system. In this way, and by sharing *ãda* gains with them, they urge them and their mothers to a greater and quicker involvement.

The model gaining ground today is characterized by a break that occurs with Great Marriage (see Table A2 in Appendix); the groom leaves his age-mates (thus the age-set progressively disintegrates) and enters an age and rank-grade in the Fathers' category where he is recruited by one of the commensal subgroups. He then rises to the upper grade of Kings of the City by marrying his daughter or niece, or by paying a special *ãda* to the city. This progression can be compared with obtaining titles in the first model. In the second model, a series of changes has gradually occurred:

- Age-sets are no longer structured by the hierarchy of lineages.
- They are limited to the category of Sons and gradually disintegrate when members marry by *ãda*, entering into rank groups of the Fathers category.

- In some cities, age-sets are losing their hold and individuals can move up through the grades alone, or they may pay to enter the age group at a later stage.
- In Moroni, the capital (an extreme case), classes of Sons were quite simply done away with voluntarily in the 1950s, when several Sons took on modern political roles.
- In the Fathers' category, rank-grades are attained individually.
- The hierarchy of lineages remains a criterion of distribution in the commensal groups of Fathers, although in some places it is strongly contested.

There are intermediate variants between these contrasting models of complexity and simplification.[42] In two of them, I observed that the age-set is reconstituted under another name after its members' Great Marriage. However, the general trend shows the fragility of age-set progression compared with individual progression, giving rise to a more competitive way of acting. Comparing variants reveals that a solution is always found to ensure that all the city's lineages and all ages are represented in the same group or in distinct ones. Everyone's position in the city is defined by one's affiliation to lineage and age group, but this is easily challenged and must be confirmed by achievements. 'So-and-so? Who is he? What has he done [for the city]?!' is a frequent formula for challenging a lack of commitment in *ãda*.[43] It is considered a public insult, which is the usual manner to force people to pay to avoid dishonour. 'Your brother is in the kitchen, wiping cooking-pots' was a direct insult addressed during a public dispute to a woman whose brothers had not yet married by *ãda* (in this case, the sister–brother pair is taken for the house).[44]

There have been many changes and other sociological transformations to the age system's and city's organization over the last century. Historical data contributes to understanding this dynamic of social and moral change.

From the end of the kingdoms to the Marxist revolution

There is little direct data on the age system and Great Marriage before colonization.[45] We know that married men were taxed, that Sons and Fathers wore distinguishing clothing,[46] and that kings could offer bullocks by the dozen for their marriage.[47] At the end of the 19th century, a number of Wangazidja migrated along routes that had been open for centuries. There were various reasons for this exodus: wars between the island's last kings, oppression by the newly arrived colonial planter, Léon Humblot,[48] the elite's impoverishment due to the abolition of slavery in 1904 and the revolution in farm production. Many people were compelled to sell or pawn their land to Humblot, on unfavourable terms, to raise money for *ãda* or for travelling.[49] Comorian landowners set up new plantations in Zanzibar or worked as literate employees for Omani sultan or Europeans; small freeholders and former slaves became porters, soldiers, dhow sailors or labourers. The two social classes of public employees and poor workers were only ever on an equal footing in football matches where they played against each other.[50] British archives in Zanzibar show that *ãda* were celebrated and at the same time contested in this migrant community. Fair records that young Comorians were accused of engaging in a dubious pastime called *shambe* where they danced in an effeminate manner, or even dressed as women, which was acutely embarrassing to the progressive leaders of this minority community. Did the poorest ridicule the spending on *ãda* that was so inaccessible to them, as they do today by holding the organizers to ransom?[51] By their disavowal of this dance, the Comorians leaders seemed to express the desire to do away with the *ãda*, and their active promotion of football was intended to divert the young away from it. However, other testimonies show that men practised both football and dance, and that the latter did not threaten masculine values. Instead the anecdote reveals the tension between rich and poor, who lived closer to each other in a migrant community.

In Ngazidja, by celebrating Great Marriages, the inhabitants of slave hamlets or districts were gradually taken into consideration by the free society, without, however, becoming fully integrated.[52] These Great Marriages required houses of *ãda* and a ruling assembly, and they founded both of these at the same time in a complex and fragile construction process of their own polity, the 'city'. In Irungudjani, formerly the slave district of Moroni, older people remember the first Great Marriage with slaughter of bullocks, dating back to 1912, followed, in the 1920s, by the founding of the assembly of Accomplished Men, mainly composed of low-paid employees of the colony. Monumental gates were eventually built at the entrance to the public square (*bangwe*) in 1931.[53] This architectural symbol of the existence of an assembly of Accomplished Men in the public space marks a turning-point in relations between social classes. In the 2000s, I witnessed and documented a similar process that had been ongoing for thirty years in Magodjuu, a district outside the city walls of Moroni, which has led to the progressive recognition of this political assembly by the Accomplished Men of the town's central districts.[54]

Reformist trends for social equality including criticism of *ãda* also came from the expanding Islamic Sufi brotherhoods. The popular Qādiriyya and Shadhiliyya were efficient instruments of conversion on the African continent, and there were many Comorians among Zanzibar's religious masters, along with the patrician Arab elite, Hadhramis and Somalis.[55] Like other Sufi masters in Africa, in Ngazidja, Said bin Sheikh (1851–1904)[56] of *sharif* descent and the grandson of a king, championed Islamic equality. Born in Moroni, he joined the Qādiriyya brotherhood in Zanzibar, studied in Arabia, and returned to Ngazidja where he was received into the Shadhiliyya-Yashrutiyya.[57] He developed this brotherhood in the archipelago, Madagascar and Mozambique.[58] Questioning the established order in Comoros, he opposed the mosques' control by the socio-political hierarchy and called for the abolition of inequalities in the traditional system. He instituted the *darwesh* marriage which was supposed to draw the groom out of the Son category without putting him in that of the Fathers, since, as a Sufi, he was to sit in the brotherhood's mosque (*zawiya*) and not in the political public square. His followers, the *darwesh*, adopted a range of attitudes that evolved from challenging customs to compromise. These *kidarwesh* marriages are rare today; only six were recorded in 1995 in Mdjoyezi, the heartland of the brotherhood.[59] Said bin Sheikh wanted to do away with the hierarchy expressed by sharing meat from bullocks slaughtered for feasts. Instead of each cut of beef representing the lineage's rank, he recommended the fraternal drawing of lots (*kuriya*). In several cities, the *darwesh* participate in *ãda*, establishing an egalitarian sharing group among the Accomplished. However, not everyone who joined did so for religious reasons. In Itsandra, for example, a man who considered himself hard done by in a previous distribution preferred to be chief in the *darwesh* group. Foreigners, such as a men with high social position from Mwali who married in the city, also joined the group. Claiming to be a *darwesh* may therefore merely be a strategy for eating more. Sharing by drawing lots (*kuriya*) has also been adopted in Itsandra by a group of educated men in senior administrative jobs, whose outlook is more modern from having lived abroad.

Other Islamic reformist influence on *ãda* came from scholars such as Omar bin Sumayt. A *kadhi* in Zanzibar and influential in larger intellectual networks, he was of Comorian maternal origin and Hadhrami and *sharif* paternal origin.[60] Returning to

Ngazidja during the Zanzibar revolution in 1964, he focused on religious education. He successfully introduced the *madjilis*, a men's prayer meeting, into *ãda* ceremonies to replace secular concert.

Migration to Madagascar generated other changes in Ngazidja society during the 20th century. Comorian migrants, both the French-educated elite and the workers, experienced professional training and a generalized wage system. Already numerous in the 19th century in Majunga, Comorians were hired in huge numbers to work in the plantations of the north. In the 1970s, there were around 60,000 Comorians in Madagascar, many of them labourers, dockers, cooks and caretakers, as well as civil servants, especially in the police. Two mass returns took place: in 1972, when the French Navy left the naval base in Diego Suarez where many Comorians were employed, and in 1976 when some 17,000 people were repatriated after the massacre of Comorians in Majunga. This tragic event put a brutal end to a well-established migratory flow. Some returnees left for Reunion and then France. The others, with little formal education but possessing manual skills that were scarce in Ngazidja, and above all freed from many constraints of behaviour, transformed the society, notably in terms of women's work, autonomy and organizational abilities; they now had their own system of subscription for Great Marriages. Comorian migrants who returned voluntarily with their savings, better educated and more progressive than their fellow-citizens, put the education of their children before the payment of *ãda*. However, those with political ambitions garner little support if they fail to respect the rules of their city.

Ãda exchanges were totally forbidden under Ali Soilihi's Marxist government from 1975 to 1978. I was told by middle-aged men in Itsandzeni how they were arrested in 1976 and accused of *ãda* activities. As Sons of the City at the time, they were preparing a coup to rise to the Kings of the Sons grade (*ufomanamdji*). They all denied the charge and upon release, immediately continued raising money to buy a goat, the required *ãda* payment ....[61]

Challenging the hierarchy

This brief revolutionary period profoundly affected public consciousness and transformed social relations.[62] The inhabitants of *zitreya* (the former slave hamlets) remember it as a period when there were no masters, everyone had to work the land, and prices were low.[63] Women worked like men in any job, even as builders. In the villages, power was in the hands of committees composed of young people aged from 20 to 40 (corresponding to the Sons of the City category). Each village had its own prison, and the deeds punished ranged from celebrating *ãda* of marriage or age-set feasts to *ugangi* 'witchcraft' rituals, theft and rape. Despite appearing to have returned to their previous form, the island's institutions were changed by this short-lived regime: the age system, social divisions, differences between the women of *ãda* and the others, and behaviours had all been called into question. The subsequent president, Ahmed Abdallah Abderemane, encouraged those with a high political position to celebrate their Great Marriage. Most politicians choose to engage in *ãda* payments for themselves and their families, displaying the wealth earned from their position, thus adopting the logic of patronage inherent in relations between the State and the cities (ministers used to invite the president for Friday prayer in their city, and it is prestigious for the city to have one of its members in a government position). Friends told me in 2012 how they felt uneasy seeing the former president Azali Assoumani (1999–2006), who had never celebrated his Great Marriage and remained *mnamdji*, given a second row seat in *ãda* circumstances.

Hierarchies gradually became less influential throughout the 20th century in Ngazidja, and this can be seen in the multiplication of central mosques. Holding the communal Friday prayer requires the presence of at least 40 literate Muslims, free and native to the village, from whom a muezzin is chosen for the call to prayer, an imam to direct the prayer and a *hatwibu* to give the sermon in Arabic (*hutba*) from a special book,[64] followed by a speech in Comorian. Establishing a central mosque requires the authorization of the literate men of the nearest dominant city, who thus grant a degree of religious and political independence. Previously, small communities would send their most titled Accomplished Men to the Friday prayer of the nearby town, who, after prayer, would gather information about the region's political and social life.[65] The spread of Friday mosques has enabled all villages to become 'cities' in the full sense of the term. The movement started after the First World War when many Comorians who had received a good religious education in Zanzibar opened Koranic schools in their villages and sent their best students to perfect their training in 'towns of knowledge' such as Moroni or Mbeni. The competition between communities each to have their own Friday mosque grew stronger (and they now compete by expanding them). Before it was banned in 2004, I observed the Islamic foundation Al Haramayn building large mosques in the last remaining villages without one, as well as providing a water supply.[66] Dynamic communities also encourage young people to emigrate to France from where they help families pay for Great Marriages and send money for public facilities, so that the village gradually gains recognition. One village in the south even organized subscriptions to pay for young people's tickets to France. Villages that do not send their young people abroad (e.g. Djumwashongo, a colonial workers' hamlet) are unable to build mosques and reconstruct the public square, and are thus unable to compete.[67]

Many migrants enjoy a new capacity in *ãda* exchanges because their financial resources make them less dependent on the position of their lineage in the city and the country. They introduce innovations during their brief returns to the island, which the city tolerates for fear of losing their *ãda*. They obtain rapidly, but generally at great cost, the status of Accomplished Man. These arrangements appear to be of little consequence, since the migrants do not stay on the island and, despite the payments they make, they do not really sit on the city assembly. The huge houses they build, which often remain unoccupied after their departure, stir the villagers' desire for success and encourage them to imitate, accentuating the negative effects of migration, such as young people's disaffection with farming. The danger of potential anomie caused by massive migration is offset by organizing Comorian 'cities' in France, where village associations are a projection of the political structure operating in Ngazidja. However, political authority has not shifted outside the country, despite migrants' economic power. Videotaping assemblies held at home and in France enables them to be seen by the other party: in France, regular meetings between cities and subscriptions for infrastructure are organized by an island-level committee.

The dynamic of *ãda* practices: enduring and adapting

Becoming an Accomplished Man remains a goal for both residents and migrants. Marrying one's brother and then one's daughter is still a major achievement for women. These careers have no equivalent in Western life, and their attraction lies in the way they combine collective commitment and individual progression. It is therefore important to recognize these underlying values in the modern forms Comorian society adopts to adapt to external opportunities and global standards. Changes in *ãda* practices correspond to global sociological trends as can been seen in the following examples.

Members of the Sons category (*unamdji*) are responsible for music and dances and organize 'bands' which, in the past, were indistinguishable from *unamdji* itself. Through migrants' travels, these bands, like the female dance groups, have been influenced by the *beni* bands of Swahili towns.[68] The *twarab* was introduced to Moroni in 1913 from Zanzibar.[69] The *unamdji* band has continued to evolve, calling itself a 'cultural association' in the 1970s, a period of independence and students' migration, and a 'development organization' today, adopting a legal form to receive government and agencies' grants. Membership rules have become more flexible, but the band's name still reflects the imagined community of *unamdji*.

Relations between Sons and Fathers are no longer dictated by the agricultural economy that used to be the framework for power and exploitation between generations. Over the last few decades, under the influence of Sons who are students or managers and migrants, the city's 'coffers' are no longer in the hands of the Fathers, but deposited in bank accounts with several signatories in Ngazidja or France. Consequently, Fathers with the grade of Kings and Elders, who used to take sums for their own needs, now depend on help from their migrant children to survive. An equivalent amount, from 5% to 10% of expenses, is now officially allocated to public projects. Only *ãda* subscriptions can be collected effectively, because this social investment prevents any other use of the money under pressure from the family, and this is why *ãda* subscriptions are more popular than bank deposits. *Ãda* expenses are now partly channelled by the city assembly into funding development. The moral force expressed by the verb *huhima*, 'to stand up', (the mainstay of participation in collective exchange), is now used to manage modern communities. A renewed conception of the city's public goods is emerging, increasing the scope of *ãda* rather than threatening it.

The definitive rejection of the hierarchy of lineages has been observed in some old cities such as Male. To escape a static order in which they remained trapped in the lower ranks, Accomplished Men of lower lineages have created intra-lineage sharing groups, contrary to the rule of lineage representation. This manoeuvre was only possible because of the demographic increase of the lineages in question, and soon revealed its limitations when applied to the sets of Sons: in Male, these sets no longer function. To avoid this in other cities, the historical hierarchy of lineages has lost its relevance and is negotiated or balanced by modifying the sharing of meat.

Great Marriage is becoming more accessible for both former dependents and younger siblings. Houses of *ãda* appear and disappear rapidly, and houses 'of today', *madjalelo*, founded recently, are numerous. The rule of firstborn remains, but is adapted to reality when necessary. For example, when, in the 1970s, Hulia left Madagascar where she had spent much of her life, and returned to her hometown Dembeni, she married her fourth daughter by *ãda*, since the others were already married (without exchanges). This daughter's children all settled in France, and her eldest daughter comes every summer to renovate the house for her own Great Marriage, which she and her husband will mostly pay for.[70] Another example is provided by Bacar, a university lecturer in Moroni born in Infundihe. He is not the elder sibling, but his regular income gave him the authority of an elder. However, it is not considered 'nice' (*ndzuzuri*) if the eldest does not marry first, if possible. Similarly, in Chezani, although his elder brother cared little about *ãda* and preferred religious studies, Ismael, also an employee, gave his family financial help to organize his brother's wedding first.

International development organizations encouraged the creation of local councils to bypass the predatory oligarchy of the State, and despite the Comorian Government's slow response to this, many cities formed their own councils. Their leaders stressed that they would need support not only from 'resident natives' (*wakavavo*) but also from 'migrants' (*wakandziani*), as the president of the mayors' association put it.[71] Some migrants with dual citizenship also play a role in French town councils. However, as polities, cities are facing a new political entity: the two conceptions of citizenship compete with regard to hierarchy and origin. Not every village will have its own town hall as it has its own Friday mosque. For the non-native resident or 'foreigner', marrying in the city is the only way to be granted a place on it. This poses a serious organizational problem for towns such as Moroni, the capital, where affiliation to a recognized matrilineal house was a condition to be eligible on the council.[72]

Conclusion

The city provides the framework for the interplay between matriliny, age and rank, and Great Marriage is the cornerstone of the device. The two fundamental values inherent in the age system still serve as a reference: membership of a local matrilineage, reflecting the collective temporality of the city, and the ages of life reflecting individual temporality, both shared with peers and punctuated by life cycle rituals. Personal achievement is validated by relatives as well as by society. The arena of the city allows for personal initiative while assuring (and sometimes coercing) solidarity and emulation, generating an unusual degree of social cohesion not found on the other islands.

The city has become more autonomous since the kingdoms ended, and previously dominated people's appropriation of this model polity has led to greater equality. However, this framework for personal fulfilment and collective action seems to be unavoidable. Even those *Wangazidja* who have dual citizenship and social security benefits in their adopted country find no equivalent abroad to what they obtain through Great Marriage in Ngazidja, and nothing else generates such a collective mobilization for the public good. Despite the negative effects of constant challenge, honour remains a driving force for this personal and collective mobilization.

Over time, the system has tacitly tolerated the relative integration of those previously excluded as well as dissenters. The actors are trying to adapt to other current pressures such as development and Islamic reformist trends. Change is slow but effective, which probably explains why individuals still find in it unparalleled conditions for personal achievement whilst fulfilling their collective moral commitments.

Acknowledgements

A first version of this paper was presented in the European Swahili Workshop, 'Contemporary Issues in Swahili Ethnography', organized by Iain Walker in Oxford, UK, 2010. The author thanks the participants for their comments; and the anonymous referees of this journal for their numerous suggestions.

Funding

Fieldwork conducted from 1995 to 2006 was funded by the French Centre National de Recherche Scientifique (CNRS) with a total amount of €25,000.

Notes

1. Equivalent to €4000.
2. Video-registered observation, Dembeni, Ngazidja, 2003.
3. Ivanov, "Constructing Translocal Socioscapes," 637.
4. These words of Arabic origin both mean tradition, custom. *Ãda* means customary payment, and *mila*, customary rank. *Ada* or *adat* is also used in Southeast Asia, *mila* in Eastern Africa;

Caplan, "Boys' Circumcision and Girls' Puberty Rituals," 30–2 and Junod, "Life of a South African Tribe." The Comorian language, which has different forms on each island, is a Bantu language related to Swahili with many Arabic words.

5. See http://hdr.undp.org/.
6. It also underestimates positive effects on the informal economy analysed by Walker, "Les aspects économiques du Grand Mariage."
7. Migrants, 99% from Ngazidja, sent back €93 million in 2011, used for living expenses, education, health and Great Marriages expenses estimated at between €25,000 and €40,000; Bourenane *et al.*, *Réduire les coûts*, 15. See also Vivier, "Les migrations comoriennes" and Blanchy, "Les Comoriens, une immigration méconnue."
8. For a summary, see Blanchy, *Maisons des femmes, cités des hommes*.
9. Wright, "Early Islam, Oceanic Trade."
10. Martin, "Arab Migrations to East Africa."
11. The population of the Union of the Comoros was 717,500 in 2012 (http://www.diplomatie. gouv.fr/fr/dossiers-pays/comores/), according to The World Bank (http://www.banquemondiale. org/). Comorians living in France are estimated at around 260,000, half of whom have dual citizenship; Al Watwan, Interview of Soulaimana Mohamed Ahmed, ambassador of Comoros in Paris, 2008.
12. Walker, "What Came First?," 599.
13. Shepherd, "Two Marriage Forms"; Shepherd, "Comorians in Kenya."
14. Shepherd, "Two marriage forms in the Comoros."
15. Shepherd, "Comorians in Kenya," 173. *Sharif* is said in Comorian language *sharifu* pl. *mazarifu*.
16. Guy, *Trois études*; Le Guennec-Coppens, "Le manyahuli grand-comorien."
17. Ben Ali *et al.*, *Traditions d'une lignée royale*.
18. Abdourahim, "Mariage à Ngazidja"; Abdourahim, "Echanges des biens"; Chouzour, *Pouvoir de l'honneur*.
19. Le Guennec-Coppens, "Influence from the Mainland"; Blanchy, "Partage des boeufs"; Blanchy, "Seul ou ensemble?"; Blanchy and Youssouf, "Hiérarchie et égalité."
20. Alpers, "A Complex Relationship: Mozambique and the Comoro Islands"; Bang, *Sufis and Scholars*; Walker, "Mimetic Structuration"; Walker, *Becoming the Other*.
21. Nansour-Riziki, *L'évolution des institutions sociales mohéliennes*.
22. Robineau, *Société et économie d'Anjouan*; Sidi, *Anjouan*.
23. Robineau, *Société et économie d'Anjouan*; Robineau, "L'Islam aux Comores"; Ottenheimer, *Marriage in Domoni*, does not describe *hirimu*.
24. Lambek, "Exchange, Time, and Person"; Blanchy, "Matrilocalité et système d'âge."
25. Blanchy and Said Islam, *Le statut et la situation*; Blanchy, "Famille et parenté."
26. Blanchy, "Cité, citoyenneté et territoire."
27. The matrilineal descent group is called *hinya*, or *daho* ('house') or *mba* ('belly') depending on the context; Blanchy, *Maisons des femmes, cités des hommes*.
28. Ben Ali, "Approche historiques des structures administratives," 25; Blanchy, "Cité, citoyenneté et territoire."
29. Walker, "Is Social Capital Fungible?," analyses the failure of a microcredit project.
30. Schneider and Gough, *Matrilineal Kinship*; Richards, "Some Types of Family Structure"; Beidelman, *Matrilineal Peoples of Eastern Tanzania*; Douglas, "Is Matrilinearity Doomed in Africa?"
31. Peters, "Revisiting the Puzzle of Matrilinearity," 137.
32. Bernardi, *Age Class Systems*.
33. Simonse and Kurimoto, *Conflict, Age and Power*.
34. Le Guennec-Coppens, "Influence from the Mainland"; Le Guennec-Coppens, "Les Hommes accomplis."
35. Directed by A. M. Peatrik and published in 2003 in *L'Homme*, a special issue entitled "Passages à l'âge d'homme"; Peatrik, "La règle et le nombre"; Peatrik, *La vie à pas contés*; Peatrik, "L'océan des âges."
36. Blanchy, "Seul ou ensemble?"; Blanchy, "Cité, citoyenneté et territoire."
37. Interview with Ali Chanfi, Djomani, 2004.
38. Shepherd, "Comorians in Kenya," 173, 417.

39. Fieldwork was conducted from 1995 to 2006 in more than 30 cities. Regular meetings occurred with the men who had a good knowledge of their age system rules; Blanchy, "Seul ou ensemble?"; Blanchy, *Maisons des femmes, cités des hommes*, 157–211.
40. Interview with Boinaidi Youssouf, Dembeni, 1996.
41. An additional grade cleverly allows adjustment between the Son's coup and that of the Fathers.
42. Blanchy, *Maisons des femmes, cités des hommes*, 191–4.
43. Interview with Naesha Youssouf Abdulalik in Moroni, 1998.
44. Interview with Yahaya Ibrahim in Mdjoyezi, 1999.
45. J. Martin's history of Comoros is central but does not mention local institutions. I used Henri Pobéguin's photograph collection (1897–1899) with its precise captions during fieldwork. It helped people remember old practices and explicitly talk about hierarchies in everyday life; Blanchy, *Grande Comore en 1898*; Blanchy, "Une expérience de retour d'archives."
46. Interview with Moussa Issihaka, Ikoni, 1995; information was confirmed by photographs from Pobéguin's collection.
47. Archives d'Outremer (AOM), Aix en Provence, 6 (8) D15; Kari-Ngama, *Flamme vive* (editing the manuscript of the Mdombozi royal matrilineage in Fumbuni).
48. Martin, *Comores, quatre îles*.
49. AOM, D 6(8) 15; AOM, 3D3, 49.
50. Saleh, "Communauté zanzibari d'origine comorienne."
51. Fair, *Pastimes & Politics*, 260–1. Fair bases this on both Saleh, "Comoro Islands" and British archives. The *shambe* probably designated the elegant and gracious dance still performed during *ãda* feasts.
52. Blanchy, "Esclavage et commensalité à Ngazidja." Romero-Curtin observes the same facts in Lamu where, despite different kinship and residence rules, former slaves 'have continued copying their former owners and have placed less emphasis on rising economically and more on emulating rituals"; Romero-Curtin, "Lamu Weddings," 152.
53. Interview with Ali 'Shioni' Moussa (born 1912) and Abdallah Himidi in Irungudjani, Moroni, 2005.
54. Interviews with Kassim Abdallah in Magodjuu, Moroni, 2005 and 2006.
55. Glassman, *Feasts and Riots*, 140.
56. Said Muhammad bin Sheikh Ahmed known as Al Maaruf.
57. Penrad, "Shadhiliyyah-Yashrutiyyah."
58. Alpers, "A Complex Relationship: Mozambique and the Comoro Islands."
59. Interview with Said Nassuir Said in Mdjoyezi, 1995. Blanchy, "Les Darwesh aux Comores."
60. Bang, *Sufis and Scholars*; Loimeier, "Patterns and Peculiarities of Islamic Reform."
61. This class of Kings of the Sons kept the power from 1976 to 1986, when the *wazuguwa* took it through a coup; Interview with Ahmed Ali by Moussa Said-Ahmed, Itsandzeni, 1986.
62. Very few studies have been done thus far about it; Mattoir, *Comores de 1975 à 1990*.
63. Interview with Msa Bwana, Mlali, 2004.
64. Collection of sermons written by Ibn an-Nubâta (946–984); Ahmed, *Islam et politique aux Comores*, 37, 79.
65. Blanchy, "Pouvoir et différenciation sociale."
66. About Al Haramayn and other agencies in Comoros, see Ahmed, "Networks of Islamic NGOs."
67. Interview with a man who had worked at the colonial sawmill established by Humblot near Djumwashongo, 2004.
68. Ranger, *Dance and Society in Eastern Africa*, viii, 18. The *beni* (from the English 'band') is derived from old dance companies from the Kenyan coast, which had an elaborate hierarchy and organized dancing and singing competitions between local factions in the towns.
69. Said-Ahmed, *Guerriers, princes et poètes*, 261–2; Graebner, "Twarab," 42.
70. Blanchy, *Maisons des femmes, cités des hommes*, 65–6.
71. *La Tribune des Comores* no. 9 (15 November to 10 December, 2006); Interview with Mohamed Said Abdallah Mchangama. He was using a very well-known formula. *Mkavavo*, "the one who is there," also designates the one who is actively committed to *ãda* and city life; *mkandziani*, "the one who is on the path," also means he who makes an effort to achieve *ãda* goals.
72. Preparatory documents communicated by Chamsidine Turqi in 2005.

References

Abdourahim, Said. "Echanges des biens lors des festivités matrimoniales, Le mariage coutumier dans l'île de Ngazidja." *Ya Nkobe* no. 2 (1984): 3–6.

Abdourahim, Said. "Mariage à Ngazidja, fondement d'un pouvoir." Doctoral diss., Université de Bordeaux III, 1983.

Ahmed, Chanfi. "Networks of Islamic NGOs in Sub-Saharan Africa: Bilal Muslim Mission, African Muslim Agency (Direct Aid), and al-Haramayn." *Journal of Eastern African Studies* 3, no. 3 (2009): 426–437. doi:10.1080/17531050903273727

Ahmed, Chanfi. *Islam et politique aux Comores*. Paris: L'Harmattan, 1999.

Alpers, Edward A. "A Complex Relationship: Mozambique and the Comoro Islands in the 19th and 20th Centuries." *Cahier d'Etudes africaines* 41-1, no. 161 (2001): 73–95. doi:10.4000/etudesafricaines.67

Bang, Anne K. *Sufis and Scholars of the Sea. Family Networks in East-Africa, 1860–1925*. London: Routledge Curzon, 2003.

Beidelman, Thomas O. *The Matrilineal Peoples of Eastern Tanzania*. London: International African Institute, 1967.

Ben Ali, Damir. "Approche historiques des structures administratives des Comores." *APOI (Annuaire des Pays de l'Océan Indien) 1986–1989* 11 (1989): 17–42.

Ben Ali, Damir, George Boulinier, and Paul Ottino. *Traditions d'une lignée royale des Comores*. Paris: L'Harmattan, 1985.

Bernardi, Bernardo. *Age Class Systems: Social Institutions and Polities Based on Age*. Cambridge: Cambridge University Press, 1985.

Blanchy, Sophie. "Cité, citoyenneté et territoire à Ngazidja (Comores)." *Journal des Africanistes* 74, no. 1–2 (2004): 341–380.

Blanchy, Sophie. "Esclavage et commensalité à Ngazidja, Comores." *Cahiers d'Etudes Africaines* 45, no. 3–4 (2005): 905–935. doi:10.4000/etudesafricaines.5693

Blanchy, Sophie. "Famille et parenté dans l'archipel des Comores." *Journal des Africanistes* 62, no. 1 (1992): 7–53. doi:10.3406/jafr.1992.2333

Blanchy, Sophie. *La Grande Comore en 1898. Photos de Henri Pobéguin, textes de Sophie Blanchy*. Paris: KomEdit, 2007.

Blanchy, Sophie. "Le partage des boeufs dans les rituels sociaux du grand mariage à Ngazidja (Comores)." *Journal des Africanistes* 66, no. 1–2 (1996): 169–203. doi:10.3406/jafr.1996.1100

Blanchy, Sophie. "Les Comoriens, une immigration méconnue." *Hommes et Migrations* 1215, October (1998): 5–21.

Blanchy, Sophie. "Les Darwesh aux Comores (île de Ngazidja). Systèmes de valeurs et stratégie: de l'idéal islamique à la réalité sociale." In *L'extraordinaire et le quotidien. Variations anthropologiques, Hommage au Professeur Pierre Vérin*, edited by Cl. Allibert and N. Rajaonarimanana, 217–241. Paris: Karthala, 2000.

Blanchy, Sophie. *Maisons des femmes, cités des hommes. Filiation, âge et pouvoir à Ngazidja (Comores)*. Nanterre: Société d'Ethnologie, 2010.

Blanchy, Sophie. "Matrilocalité et système d'âge à Mayotte. Notes pour une étude comparative de l'organisation sociale dans l'archipel des Comores." *Taarifa, Revue des Archives départementales de Mayotte* no. 3 (2012): 9–21.

Blanchy, Sophie. "Pouvoir et différenciation sociale à Ngazidja. Les mosquées du vendredi." *Tarehi* 10 (2004): 16–23.

Blanchy, Sophie. "Seul ou ensemble? Dynamique des classes d'âge à Ngazidja (Comores)." *L'Homme* 167–168 (2003): 153–186. doi:10.4000/lhomme.238

Blanchy, Sophie. "Une expérience de retour d'archives: la collection photographique Henri Pobéguin à Ngazidja, Comores." *Terrain et archive*, August 21, 2006. http://lodel.imageson.org/terrainarchive/document195.html/.

Blanchy, Sophie, and Moinesha Said Islam. *Le statut et la situation de la femme aux Comores*. New York, NY: United Nations Development Programme (UNDP), 1989.

Blanchy, Sophie, and Boinaidi Yousouf. "Hiérarchie et égalité dans l'organisation sociale à Ngazidja. Le cas de Dembeni." *Ya Mkobe (Comores)* 10 (2003): 28–46.

Bourenane, Naceur, Said Bourjij, and Laurent Lhériau. *Réduire les coûts des transferts d'argent des migrants et optimiser leur impact sur le développement. Rapport à diffusion restreinte*. Paris: Agence Française de Développement, Epargne Sans Frontière, Banque Africaine de Développement, 2011.

Caplan, Pat Ann. "Boys' Circumcision and Girls' Puberty Rituals among the Swahili of Mafia Island, Tanzania." *Africa* 46, no. 1 (1976): 21–33. doi:10.2307/1159090

Chouzour, Sultan. *Le pouvoir de l'honneur; essai sur l'organisation sociale traditionnelle de Ngazidja et sa contestation*. Paris: L'Harmattan, 1994.

Douglas, Mary. "Is Matrilinearity Doomed in Africa?' In *Man in Africa*, edited by Mary Douglas and P. Kaberry, 123–137. London: Tavistock, 1969.

Fair, Laura. *Pastimes & Politics. Culture, Community and Identity in Post-Abolition Urban Zanzibar, 1890–1945*. Athens, OH: Ohio University Press and Oxford: James Currey, 2001.

Glassman, Jonathon. *Feasts and Riots. Revelry, Rebellion, and Popular Consciousness on the Swahili Coast, 1856–1888*. Portsmouth, NH: Heinemann, London: James Currey, Nairobi E.A.E.P., and Dar es Salam: Mkuki wa Nyota, 1995.

Graebner, Werner. "Twarab: a comorian music between two worlds." *Kabaro* 2, no. 2–3 (2004): 41–67.

Guy, Paul. *Trois études sur une immobilisation foncière en faveur des femmes de la ligne maternelle à la grande-Comore ou 'maniahoulé'*. Paris: Centre d'Etudes Juridiques Comparatives de l'Université de Paris 1, 1982.

Ivanov, Paola. "Constructing Translocal Socioscapes: Consumerism, Aesthetics, and Visuality in Zanzibar Town." *Journal of Eastern African Studies* 6, no. 4 (2012): 631–654. doi:10.1080/17531055.2012.735418

Junod, Henri. *Life of a South African Tribe*, Vol. 2. London, 1927.

Kari-Ngama. *Flamme vive éblouit mais ne dure. Histoire de Ngazidja, du Mbadjini et du matriclan royal Mdo'mbozi, contée par Tabibou Ahamadi, rédigée par Abdourahim Moussa*. Peymeynade: Djahazi, 2002.

Lambek, Michael. "Exchange, Time, and Person in Mayotte: The Structure and Destructuring of a Cultural System." *American Anthropologist* 92, no. 3 (1990): 647–661. doi:10.1525/aa.1990.92.3.02a00060

Le Guennec-Coppens, Françoise. "An Influence from the Mainland: The Age-Grade System in Greater Comoro." In *Continuity and Autonomy in Swahili Communities*, edited by David Parkin. Beitrage zur Afrikanistik, Band 48. London: London School of Oriental and African Studies, 1994.

Le Guennec-Coppens, Françoise. "Le manyahuli grand-comorien: un système de transmission des biens peu orthodoxe en pays musulman." In *Hériter en pays musulman, habus, lait vivant, manyahuli*, edited by M. Gast, 257–268. Paris: CNRS, 1987.

Le Guennec-Coppens, Françoise. "Les Hommes accomplis." In *Autorité et pouvoir chez les Swahili*, edited by Françoise Le Guennec-Coppens and David Parkin, 131–153. Paris: Karthala, 1998.

Loimeier, Roman. "Patterns and Peculiarities of Islamic Reform in Africa." *Journal of Religion in Africa* 33, no. 3 (2003): 237–262. doi:10.1163/157006603322663497

Martin, Bradford. G. "Arab Migrations to East Africa in Medieval Times." *International Journal of African Historical Studies* 7, no. 3 (1975): 367–389. doi:10.2307/217250

Martin, Jean. *Comores, quatre îles entre pirates et planteurs*, 2 vols. Paris: L'Harmattan, 1983.

Mattoir, Nakidine. *Les Comores de 1975 à 1990. Une histoire politique mouvementée*. Paris: L'Harmattan, 2004.

Nansour-Riziki, Mohamadi. *L'évolution des institutions sociales mohéliennes*. Mémoire de maîtrise. Université de Bordeaux II, 1986.

Ottenheimer, Martin. *Marriage in Domoni, Husbands and Wives in an Indian Ocean Community*. Prospect Heights, IL: Waveland, 1985.

Peatrik, Anne-Marie. "L'océan des âges." *L'Homme* 167–168 (2003): 7–25.

Peatrik, Anne-Marie. "La règle et le nombre: les systèmes d'âge et de génération d'Afrique orientale." *L'Homme* 134 (1995): 13–49. doi:10.3406/hom.1995.369906

Peatrik, Anne-Marie, ed. *Passages à l'âge d'homme*, L'Homme 167–168 (2003).

Peatrik, Anne-Marie. *La vie à pas contés*. Nanterre: Société d'Ethnologie, 1999.

Penrad, Jean-Claude 'La Shadhiliyyah-Yashrutiyyah en Afrique orientale et dans l'Océan indien occidental." In *Une voie Soufie dans le Monde*, edited by Eric Geoffroy, 379–398. Paris: Maisonneuve & Larose, 2006.

Peters, Pauline E. "Revisiting the Puzzle of Matrilinearity in South-Central Africa. Introduction." *Critique of Anthropology* 17, no. 2 (1997): 125–146. doi:10.1177/0308275X9701700202

Ranger, T. O. *Dance and Society in Eastern Africa*. Berkeley, CA: 1975.

Richards, Audrey. "Some Types of Family Structure Amongst the Central Bantu." In *African Systems of Kinship and Marriage*, edited by A. R. Radcliffe-Brown and D. Forde, 207–251. Oxford: Oxford University Press, 1950.

Robineau, Claude. "L'Islam aux Comores. Une étude d'histoire culturelle de l'île d'Anjouan." *Revue de Madagascar* 35 (1966): 17–34.

Robineau, Claude. *Société et économie d'Anjouan (Océan Indien)*. Paris: ORSTOM, 1966.

Romero-Curtin, Patricia W. "Lamu Weddings as an Example of Social and Economical Change." *Cahier d'Etudes africaines*, no. 24 (1984): 131–155. doi:10.3406/cea.1984.2214

Said-Ahmed, Moussa. *Guerriers, princes et poètes aux Comores (littérature orale)*. Paris: L'Harmattan, 2000.

Saleh, Ibuni. "The Comoro Islands. Note of a Lecture Delivered at the Zanzibar Museum." *Tanganyika Notes and Records* 12 (1941): 51–61.

Saleh, Mohammed A. "La communauté zanzibari d'origine comorienne. Premiers jalons d'une recherche en cours." *Islam et Société au Sud du Sahara* 9 (1995): 203–210.

Schneider, David M., and Kathleen Gough (eds). *Matrilineal Kinship*. Berkeley, CA: University of California Press, 1961.

Shepherd, Gillian. "The Comorians in Kenya: The Establishment and Loss of an Economic Niche." Doctoral diss., London School of Economics, 1982.

Shepherd, Gillian. "Two Marriage Forms in the Comoro Islands: An Investigation." *Africa* 44, no. 4 (1977): 344–359. doi:10.2307/1158341

Sidi, Ainoudine. *Anjouan, l'histoire d'une crise foncière*. Paris: L'Harmattan, 1998.

Simonse, Simon, and Eisei Kurimoto (eds). *Conflict, Age and Power in North East Africa: Age Systems in Transition*. Nairobi: James Currey, 1998.

Vivier, Géraldine. *Les migrations comoriennes en France: Histoire de migrations coutumières*. Dossiers du CEPED, no. 35 (1996): 38pp.

Walker, Iain. *Becoming the Other, Becoming Oneself. Constructing Identities in a Connected World*. Newcastle upon Tyne: Cambridge Scholars, 2010.

Walker, Iain. "Is Social Capital Fungible? The Rise and Fall of the Sanduk Microcredit Project in Ngazidja." *Journal of Eastern African Studies* 6, no. 4 (2012): 709–726. doi:10.1080/17531055.2012.729779

Walker, Iain. "Les aspects économiques du Grand Mariage de Ngazidja." *Autrepart* 23 (2002): 157–171. doi:10.3917/autr.023.0157

Walker, Iain. "Mimetic Structuration: Or, Easy Steps to Building an Acceptable Identity." *History and Anthropology* 16, no. 2 (2005): 187–210. doi:10.1080/02757200500116147

Walker, Iain. "What Came First, the Nation or the State? Political Process in the Comoro Islands." *Africa* 77, no. 4 (2007): 582–605. doi:10.3366/afr.2007.77.4.582

Wright, Henry T. "Early Islam, Oceanic Trade and Town Development on Nzwani: The Comorian Archipelago in the XIth–XVth Centuries A.D." *Azania* 27 (1992): 81–128. doi:10.1080/00672709209511432

Appendix

Table A1. Age system, continuous development model (example of Dembeni).

Generational categories	Grades	Proper name of age-sets (and their position in 2000)
FATHERS		
wandru wababa	Elders *wazee*	*Wamhizi*
or	Elders *wazee*	*Wadjadidi*
ACCOMPLISHED MEN	Elders *wazee*	*Washami*
wandru wadzima	*wafadhwahaya*	*Wamadina*
Majority of FATHERS	Kings of the City *wafomamdji*	*Waswafa* (came to power in 1998)
	and 'them' *wandru tsawo* (not married by *ãda*)	
SONS and FATHERS	*mawaziri* (married by *ãda*) and *maguzi* (not married by *ãda*) Position of the set outside grades	*Wa'arafa*
Majority of SONS	'Kings of Sons of the City' *wafomanamdji* (some married by *ãda*)	*Wamakka* (named in 2000)
SONS OF THE CITY	*wazuguwa*	(No proper name yet)
wanamdji	*washondje*	(No proper name yet)

Table A2. Age system, discontinuous model.

Grades	Generational categories
FATHERS	Elders *wazee*
wandru wababa	Elders *wazee*
or	Elders *wazee*
ACCOMPLISHED MEN	*wafadhwahaya*
wandru wadzima	'Kings of the City' *wafomamdji*
	'Sons with the Cap' *wanazikofia*
(Great marriage)	
	maguzi
SONS OF THE CITY	'Kings of Sons of the City' *wafomanamdji*
wanamdji	*wazuguwa*
	washondje

Is social capital fungible? The rise and fall of the Sanduk microcredit project in Ngazidja

Iain Walker

University of Oxford, Oxford, UK

In 1993 the Sanduk, a French microcredit project that was explicitly modelled on the Bangladeshi Grameen Bank, was established on Ngazidja. Reasoning that in order to succeed the project would need to adapt to local conditions, the project operators drew up a blueprint for the project that was inspired by the Grameen Bank but attentive to the specific social and cultural context, thus merging Bangladeshi principles of social solidarity with a Ngazidja cultural context. The concept of social capital was invoked and oversight of the bank conferred upon customary authority figures, the assumption being that men who had acquired status in a ritual context would be able to exercise authority over the banks debtors. This proved not to be the case; many of the banks found themselves operating without effective control and were chronically dysfunctional. This paper looks at how the concept of social capital framed thinking within the project management, and suggests why this led to failure.

Introduction

"Social capital" refers to the internal social and cultural coherence of society, the norms and values that govern interactions among people and the institutions in which they are embedded. "Social capital" is the glue that holds societies together and without which there can be no economic growth or human well-being. Without "social capital", society at large will collapse.[1]

Over the past 15 years or so the term "social capital" has become part of everyman and woman's toolkit in the development industry. Following Robert Putnam's influential *Making Democracy Work*,[2] the World Bank took up the idea, enthusiastically harnessing it to its own agenda and ensuring the rapid spread of the concept in development circles.[3] But if the idea of "social capital" has subsequently "expanded in all directions like a swamp in wet weather",[4] someone seems to have forgotten to tell the anthropologists. A keyword search for "social capital" in a major bibliographic database returns 2985 articles published since 2000; and while 37 of these articles were analysed as "anthropological", only five were both published in anthropological journals and concerned with non-Western societies. This is hardly the publication pattern that one would expect of a cutting edge theoretical concept.[5] Why, one might ask, should a term that would appear to have relevance for the anthropologist (and is widely used in development anthropology) be so comprehensively ignored by mainstream anthropology?

Part of the answer, and perhaps the most obvious one is that, as Fisher points out, "social capital is everything psychological and sociological about a person,"[6] and thus as an anthropological tool it would appear to be an exceptionally blunt one. This is implicit in much of the development literature, which, with its strongly positivist bias, grasps eagerly at the prospect of socio-anthropological input if there is any suggestion that it might be quantifiable, gathering together "everything psychological and sociological", calling it social capital and, if at all possible, giving it a number.

Even if the seemingly boundless character of the concept (and its doubtful utility) has caused concern,[7] reflection remains inscribed within the paradigm itself: there has yet to be a serious rethinking of the concept, either within development circles or elsewhere. And, indeed, for the anthropologist, "social capital" in its development incarnation would appear to be far too vague to be of use, since it effectively refers to anything an anthropologist might care to study. If the concept is to be of any value to the anthropologist it therefore seems essential that it be reconsidered; the question I wish to ask, through a specific case study in which the concept was explicitly invoked, is whether a reconsideration of the term is indeed likely to produce anything that might be of analytic value or whether anthropology is right to ignore it.

The forms of capital

Although he was not the first to invoke the idea of social capital,[8] Pierre Bourdieu's elucidation of the concept, part of his general science of the economy of practices, was the most influential in anthropology. Extending the concept of capital beyond the formal economic domain, he identified four forms of capital – economic, symbolic, cultural and social – and insisted that each needed to be taken into consideration in any attempt at an analysis of practice.[9] Before discussing social capital, I will briefly outline the other forms as they appear to Bourdieu. Economic capital should require no explanation: it refers to money, commodities, land and other material means of production; economic capital is reasonably clearly delimited in capitalist societies, although in pre-capitalist societies the lines between economic and other forms of capital may become blurred.

Cultural capital has three aspects: the embodied state, the objectified state and the institutionalised state. The embodied state, acquired over time and inherited for the most part (imperceptibly, almost invisibly) from the family, inheres in the individual as "durable disposition": it is a habitus. The objectified state refers to material appurtenances of cultural significance (books, paintings, monuments, tools), while the institutionalised state (in the educational context with which Bourdieu was specifically concerned) includes diplomas and degrees, but more widely any institutionalised cultural marker.[10]

Bourdieu's final form of capital, symbolic capital, is manifested in the respect accorded to individuals or groups by virtue of their identity *ipso facto*: family names, tribal affiliation, aristocratic titles. Symbolic capital is perhaps the least useful of Bourdieu's four forms of capital since, although more durable than other forms, it seems in many cases, to be subsumable within the categories of cultural or social capital.

Bourdieu's definition of social capital is straightforward, almost intuitive:

> "Social capital" is the whole of the actual or potential resources that are linked to the possession of a *durable network of relationships*, more or less institutionalised, of mutual acquaintance and of mutual recognition; or in other words, to *the membership of a group*, as a collection of actors who are not only endowed with common properties... but who are also united by permanent and useful *connections*.[11]

Social capital, like other forms of capital, is therefore *possessed by* individuals. It is not – and usefully not – a vague all-purpose "glue" holding society together; it does not "[refer to] friends, colleagues, and more general contacts",[12] nor to "naturally occurring social relationships between persons".[13] Even Coleman's assertion that social capital "inheres in the structures of relations between actors and among actors"[14] seems vague and not particularly useful: social capital is not the networks of relationships themselves, but the resources that produce and are produced by those relationships. The implication of this is that, while exercises in quantifying relationships and networks may be indicative of the presence of social capital, they are not measuring social capital itself but the putative effects of social capital: they are measuring a "proxy for social capital".[15] In other words, quantitative surveys of formal group membership fail to recognise the nuances underlying group membership or lack thereof: levels of participation, reasons for participation, sanctions on non-participants or even the possibilities for refusing membership. This explains the difficulties inherent in measuring and correlating social capital and project success and failure: direct measurements of social capital are extremely difficult and thus measurements must be indirect. Hence attempts to identify the relationship between project success and levels of social capital can reveal either a widespread lack of correlation or a high degree of correlation.[16] The diversity of results – social capital causes association membership vs. social capital results from association membership – casts doubt on the very idea of a quantifiable social capital. Indeed, it suggests, as Bourdieu recognised, that social capital is culturally defined and thus not amenable to the sort of analysis to which it is generally subjected. The problem with such analyses is that the definition of "better outcomes" (undoubtedly more flexible than "higher incomes") is nevertheless highly subjective. If the outcome is financial debt, legal action, and prison is this a "better outcome"? In the Comoros, when accompanied by the saving of honour, the answer might be "yes"; for a World Bank economist the answer is more likely to be "no" regardless of the honour saved.

The objections to the use of the term "social capital" are numerous; two of them particularly concern me here. The first is the fact that in contexts within which the term social capital is applied is that there is the underlying assumption that the goal of human activity is to maximise profit/income or, more generally to increase economic capital. That is, that social capital is subsidiary to economic capital, something along the lines of a form of economic capital that can't quite be quantified and is thus given a different label that nevertheless allows it to be dealt with. Contrary therefore to Bourdieu's establishment of different types of capital as being conceptually equivalent, contemporary development dogma (driven of course by mainstream economics) is that all is economic capital; that all activity is aimed at maximising profits, and that a value can be ascribed to all our forms of capital, economic, social, cultural or symbolic.

Also worrying, and an implication of this, is the suggestion that social capital is fungible; that is, that social capital can be acquired in one sphere of activity, stored or even invested, and later "spent" in another context. This is a characteristic imputed by analogy with economic capital but is entirely contrary to what might be expected by a concept qualified as "social": the context-dependent quality of social capital (assuming for the moment that there is indeed such a thing at all) must surely inhibit the transformation of capital acquired socially into some form of social "cash" that can then be used elsewhere at will. And, as I shall demonstrate below, social capital can only be context dependent: individuals who acquire or possess social capital in specific contexts may well find themselves capital-free in other contexts. This context-dependency is worth insisting upon, since some analysts are somewhat dismissive of the culturally inscribed value of social capital.[17]

This is not to suggest that there is no relationship between, nor interconvertibility of different forms of capital. All forms of capital are interrelated: economic capital can produce the material manifestations of cultural capital; cultural capital is predisposed to function as symbolic capital; symbolic capital may be converted into economic capital; and, by implication, cultural capital is a pre-requisite for the acquisition of social capital: the individual requires an understanding of the relevant cultural mores and values before being able to apply them in establishing relationships and subsequently acquiring social attributes such as power, honour, status (or shame, impotence, disgrace).[18]

Finally, in what follows, I am circumspect about the importance of membership of formal associations. This may seem minor, but in many analyses the urge for quantification sees memberships of associations seized upon as indicators of levels of social capital. In Ngazidja, somewhat perversely, the membership of (or "ownership of") an association is more usually seen as a prerequisite to a request for funds from an NGO or other funding body rather than indicative of any sort of cooperative activity on the part of the association's members, if indeed there are any. This, I believe, reflects Bourdieu's reference to "membership of a group" – he was, of course, referring to social groups, networks of closely associated individuals established on criteria such as kin, spatial and residential criteria, and so on, and not formal groups such as farmer's associations or sewing clubs.

It should be clear from the preceding, somewhat cursory overview of social capital and its applications, that I am not particularly concerned with the more mainstream definitions and uses of the term – what I might call the Putnam-Coleman (PC) definition of social capital, and which has of course evolved over the years, but which I believe is of so little utility that to use it as a basis for critical discussion would be analytically unproductive; rather I wish to draw on a more culturally inflected use of the term social capital and ask whether it is not possible to salvage something of the tool for analytical purposes.

Ngazidja and the Sanduk Project

In the 1980s, and in an understandable and not untimely reaction to the large budget infrastructure projects that characterised development programmes in the late colonial and immediate post-colonial era, microcredit increasingly came to be viewed as a panacea for all manner of problems faced by the poor in developing countries. Briefly, microcredit philosophy holds that access to capital will enable the poor to escape from the closed cycle within which lack of capital restrains production which impedes the constitution of capital: given access to capital, the poor will escape from their poverty. This somewhat formalist economic approach to development met with widespread approval and as a result there are currently more than three thousand microcredit institutions worldwide sharing more than 92 million clients and an equally voluminous literature.[19]

Although there are a variety of models for microcredit institutions, the general consensus is that a move away from the formal sector is a pre-requisite for success in targeting the poor. Collective responsibility, peer monitoring and, generally, the close involvement of the beneficiaries themselves in projects that concern them are principles based on institutions such as the Grameen Bank of Bangladesh, the classic success story (although success is a relative term: Woolcock points out that it is practically impossible for a Grameen Bank to fail.[20] The Grameen Bank holds that development and economic growth are socially determined and not simply financially defined, and the loans they provide do not require formal collateral (since borrowers are rarely have the assets to provide collateral), but instead require the formation of solidarity groups, members acting as guarantors for one another.

The Grameen Bank model has been replicated both in Bangladesh and elsewhere,[21] not always successfully. The problems of cross-cultural replication of the Grameen Bank are certainly in part due to the fact that the bank was not an externally conceived development project but a locally developed initiative, thus specific to the Bangladeshi context; and so in an effort to smooth the path for Grameen Bank imitators, the Grameen Bank itself produced a manual for the replication of the bank in other cultural contexts.[22] More generally, the ability to replicate the Grameen bank has been the subject of much discussion.[23]

Microfinance institutions now exist throughout the world, both in developing countries and in the West but if success is frequently reported from South Asia, results elsewhere are sometimes equivocal. This is particularly true of Africa, where the success of microcredit programmes has been mitigated for numerous reasons: economic, cultural and political.[24] There is a recognition of a need for close analyses of the social contexts in which microcredit projects operate and the extent to which they have adapted to those contexts, and this particularly in view of the failures; using an example from the Comorian island of Ngazidja, in the rest of this article I explore the context-specific (as they must invariably be) reasons for the failure of one village bank.

The Union of the Comoros is an insular state in the western Indian Ocean. The country's current underdeveloped status is the result of many decades of social, economic and political marginalisation within the French colonial empire and, subsequently, within the global order, generally accompanied by political instability and a weak and undiversified economy. The latter is based largely on a small handful of (increasingly unprofitable) niche-market cash crops (vanilla, ylang ylang), remittances from emigrants in France and development aid; industry is virtually non-existent and tourism undeveloped, both through lack of infrastructure and through lack of transport to the islands. Politically, the state is effectively absent from daily life: a lack of involvement of customary powerholders in the formal state structure, a rupture between these customary systems of power and the formal, Western sector, and the superficial nature of the colonial power structures themselves impeded the establishment of a effective Western-style state in the Comoros. The islands remain strongly dependent, both economically and politically, on the former colonial power although there has in recent years been a rapprochement with the Arab world. The nominal annual per capita GNP is approximately US$800.

As elsewhere, donors have turned to credit in an attempt to reach the needy and the country has seen the implementation of a number of credit projects over the years, ranging from the Banque de Développement des Comores, a parastatal body that offers medium to large loans targeted at all sectors of the economy, to smaller rural credit schemes often linked to agricultural development projects. Most of these projects have met with limited success. In particular, the size of the loans on offer, the requirement that borrowers provided collateral, the daunting paperwork involved and the poor management of these projects, implied that not only were the poor excluded, but that the loans were frequently considered to be gifts and therefore repayment rates were low: often below 50 per cent and in one case as low as 28 per cent.[25] State implication in the management of these projects has frequently been cited as a factor in their failure.

The Projet Sanduk was established in the Comoros in 1993 by two French NGOs, Institut de Recherches et d'Applications de Méthodes de Développement (IRAM) and Groupe de Recherches et d'Echanges Technologiques (GRET), and financed by the French government through the Caisse Française de Dévelopment (CFD[26]). Drawing on the Grameen Bank model, it aimed to distribute small loans to the poor via a network of village banks (Sanduk[27]) linked through an overseeing body (the Sanduk Union, Umoja wa Masanduku) that would eventually replace the project, thus endowing the network with a degree of perennity. The principles of the project implied the establishment of some general basic rules.[28] The banks' capital would, at least in part, be constituted by the villagers themselves, thus conferring collective ownership on the community and removing the banks from the control of the state. Each Sanduk would be responsible for the drawing up of its rules (within certain limits laid down by the project operators); each Sanduk was to be registered as an association under Comorian law and members were to be organised into solidarity groups of five. Loan requests were to be discussed within each group and the request approved before being submitted to the Sanduk by the group leader. Loans, which were small (initially limited to 50 000F [€100] in rural Sanduk, 80 000F [€160] in urban Sanduk), were to be for productive use and repayments were to be made at regular intervals at a fixed rate of interest. The solidarity groups, copied from the Grameen Bank, were seen as being particularly important, since, in the absence of material collateral, they effectively constituted the borrower's guarantee. If a group member defaulted, the remaining members of the group would be held responsible until such time as the situation was regularised.

Three different bodies were established to manage each Sanduk, conveniently corresponding to the Western separation of function into legislative, executive and judiciary. The members of the Sanduk formed, by delegation or election, the management committee, responsible for decisions regarding the granting of loans, the application of penalties and the establishment of rules; at the annual general assembly they voted for an executive committee, usually of three members (president, secretary and treasurer) and charged with executing the decisions of the management committee; and, at the moment of the formation of the association, an elders' council was named. This latter group was responsible for overseeing requests for membership, the constitution of groups and the imposition of penalties and sanctions.

The existence of the elders' council owes much to the specificities of Ngazidja society and is a result of the project's desire to be socially acceptable; it drew quite explicitly on the concept of social capital. The age system is a salient feature of Ngazidja social organisation; the men's age system is comprised of two sequences of age grades that of youths (*wanamdji*) and that of the elders (the *wandrwadzima*). Entry into the system, as well as movement between grades is affected upon the payment of a prestation, usually in the form of a meal or, increasingly, a cash payment for the individual's coevals. The passage between the two sequences of *wanamdji* and *wandrwadzima* is effected on the occasion of a marriage and gives rise to a particularly onerous and lengthy series of events known as *aada*.[29] Ostensibly the most important effect of the *aada* is to confer status and access to power upon the individual. Having performed his *aada*, an elder has certain rights and obligations, some symbolic (the wearing of certain types of clothing, for example, or the right to enter the mosque through the door reserved for the *wandrwadzima*), others very real: the right to eat at subsequent *aada*; the right to receive payments in certain situations; and, above all, the right to speak in public, to represent the community and hence to participate in the political process in the local community and beyond.

Power at the local level in Ngazidja is, in the absence of any functioning form of Western-style local government, based on custom. Authority is sedimented in the age grade system; the *wandrwadzima* are the senior decision-makers: they resolve disputes, inflict punishments and establish rules. Their authority is not inflexible, however. Judgement is reached after discussion and is characterised as being by consensus; the parties concerned are usually permitted to express their opinion, be it in public or in private, and the final decision is held to be fair or, at least, acceptable.

It is, then, the *wandrwadzima* who composed the elders' council in the Sanduk. As the senior men in the village, they were intended to accord a social acceptability to the project, moving it out of the state domain and into the domain of custom. Their knowledge of the local community would in theory prevent disreputable or dishonest individuals from obtaining credits that they were unlikely to repay, and they had the authority to inflict customary punishments on defaulters which would, again in principle, encourage prompt and regular repayments. They possessed, according to the project operators, the requisite social capital.

In the following section I turn to one Sanduk, Sanduk Itsandra, which consistently failed to operate correctly. Despite the expressed policy of the project to encourage the appropriation of the bank by the local community, and the recognition of local social and cultural specificities, the failure of the bank was ultimately due to the conflicts that arose between Western logic and local strategies and the perceived failure of local actors to effectively employ their social capital.

Sanduk Itsandra

The town of Itsandramdjini, the commercial centre and erstwhile port of the *ntsi* ("region") of Itsandra, has a population of about 2500. It is divided into three quarters: Harumwamdji, the free (or noble) quarter; Befuni, the fishermen's quarter; and Mirereni, formerly the slaves' quarter. Each quarter is socially autonomous: each has its own *aada*, with a distinct age system and sequence of ceremonies; *aada* marriages between quarters are rare and the quarters do not eat together in the context of the *aada*. The three quarters are thus, from a social point of view, three separate villages. Itsandramdjini is five kilometres north of Moroni and the suburbs of the capital threaten to encroach upon the town. As a result the town emphasises its identity and social contacts with Moroni are sometimes restrained.

The inhabitants of Harmuwamdji are renowned for their pride, their religious leadership (a number of religious figures prominent throughout the East African region were from Itsandramdjini) and their status (to a degree self-accorded). They are generally well educated, a landowning class whose members are frequently in public service or politics, although some own businesses. Pressure on land and social status preclude agricultural activities of any scale. Befuni, the fishermen's quarter, although of lower status than Harumwamdji, is nevertheless a free quarter. Some inhabitants run small businesses, but the dominant economic activity is fishing. The third quarter, Mirereni, was home to the slaves of Harumwamdji and its inhabitants continue to suffer from the low status of their ancestors. The inhabitants of Mirereni are frequently labourers and small business owners, often working in Moroni: outside Itsandramdjini it is easier for them to conceal their origins.

Aada marriages between Befuni and Harumwamdji are not unknown, but *aada* marriages between Harumwamdji and Mirereni are rare and disapproved of; social contacts between Befuni and Mirereni are stronger, partly because of their shared lower status and partly through lack of historical constraints on links between the two quarters since fishermen rarely possessed slaves. The quarter of Harumwamdji represents the town in its contacts with other towns: it is synonymous with Itsandramdjini in the *mila na ntsi*,[30] the body of customary rules that governs social interaction on the island. A corollary of this is that it is structurally impossible for Befuni or Mirereni to interact with other towns as towns: they are "represented" by Harumwamdji, which rarely deigns to represent them.

Sanduk Itsandra,[31] one of the first Sanduk, was established in late 1993. The town was an unusual choice since it did not fit the profile sought by the project: neither an agricultural town with potential but lacking capital, nor an urban area with small businesses requiring finance. It seems, rather, that the choice was encouraged by a consultant to the project operators, who was herself from Harumwamdji and who wished to see the project benefit her own town. Attempts to set up a Sanduk open to the entire town failed, as did attempts to implant the bank in the quarter of Harumwamdji: the offer of loans of 80 000F (€160) was not calculated to entice individuals educated in France and employed in or seeking highly paid positions in the public sector – indeed, the sum was ridiculously small. Although the bank may have been more appropriate to the needs of the inhabitants of Mirereni, this option was considered socially inappropriate to the consultant, who favoured Befuni.

Befuni was slightly more enthusiastic than Harumwamdji, but the potential for success was similarly limited. The needs of fishermen far exceeded the 80 000F that was on offer: although outrigger canoes (*ngalawa*) are inexpensive (50 000F to 100 000F), not only are they less desirable (less "modern") than motorboats, but they are social objects and rarely purchased as such. More pressing needs are fibreglass or plastic hulled boats and outboard motors, each of which cost more than 10 times the sums on offer, as well as refrigeration facilities and access to markets, also needs less easily met by small personal loans. 80 000F might serve to purchase minor items, such as hooks, lines or spare parts, or meet daily expenses – fuel for a day's fishing costs 20 000F – but the demand was not sufficient to support a village bank.

As a result interest in the Sanduk was aleatory; member numbers were low and borrowers were generally not among the more economically productive residents of the quarter. The first year of operation was disastrous, loan repayment rates plummeted and the project announced that the Sanduk would be closed. Although this did not in fact happen, Sanduk Itsandra continued to function with poor results and was constantly under threat of closure.

The reasons for this failure are multiple. The solidarity groups did not function as planned. A prohibition on family members forming a group prevented individuals willing to guarantee one another from so doing. Kin-based relationships are the basis of Ngazidja society and to prevent these networks from functioning was to deny any real effectiveness to the solidarity groups. Furthermore, the 'vicious cycle of poverty' from which microcredit projects are intended to lift the beneficiaries does not exist in Ngazidja, and certainly not in Itsandramdjini. There is little poverty on the island: homelessness and hunger are largely unknown and most individuals are able to obtain money (gifts or loans) from family if required. In situations whereby a defaulter blocked loans to other members of his group, the expected peer pressure did not materialise: the other members of the group simply looked elsewhere for cash.

Most significantly, from a project policy perspective, was the failure of the elders' council. The *wandrwadzima* were largely uninterested in the functioning (or misfunctioning) of a bank and the elders' council (most of whose members were retired fishermen with little need for a loan and less knowledge of the banking system) was rarely convened. Indeed, from the very start, the elders' council effectively existed in name only and the much desired social acceptability of the bank was absent. The individuals responsible for the running of the Sanduk, members of the executive committee and the management committee, were all either youths or socially children, having yet to enter the age system.

Approximately one year after its establishment, Sanduk Itsandra opened its doors to residents of other quarters and initially attracted a number of new members, mostly from Mirereni, after which recruitment stalled. As a result of its poor performance and management (accompanied by an eight month ban on granting loans, imposed by the project), the Sanduk had a bad reputation. Nevertheless, as the Sanduk extended into other quarters of the town it attempted to shake off its reputation both as a failure and as "fishermen's business". Although Mirereni was the most obvious target quarter, individuals from Harumwamdji also joined, and, in an internal power struggle, lower status members from Harumwamdji gradually replaced those from Befuni on the two committees – but, significantly, not in the elder's council, which remained, nominally at least, composed of elders from Befuni.

Despite its expansion the Sanduk continued to be dogged by problems and five years after it opened the bank compared unfavourably with Sanduks barely a year old on every count: number of loans granted, total capital held, number of members and repayment rates. Defaulting on loans became a pattern. In the absence of a rigid policy regarding repayment, borrowers in difficulty realised that they would not be pursued: the solidarity groups remained ineffective and threatened seizures of goods offered as collateral were rarely carried out, ostensibly due to the difficulty (for social reasons) of selling seized goods but frequently also due to the status of the defaulters, either within the community or as members or kin of members of one of the committees. In particular, the elders' council always aleatory, ceased even to pretend to function once membership was opened to other quarters: quite simply, and despite any social capital they may have had, the elders had no authority outside Befuni. By August 1998 26 of the 28 debtors had fallen behind in their repayments and the late repayments amounted to more than 1.4 million francs (€2800), almost one third of the total of loans outstanding.

The Umoja wa Masanduku

Although the case of Itsandramdjini was particularly bad most Sanduks were suffering from repayment problems. Despite the fact that the national economy was in crisis the umbrella body, the Umoja wa Masanduku, the Sanduk Union, of which all banks were a member, decided that the Sanduks should nevertheless be held accountable and custom, in the form of the *wandrwadzima*, the elders, was called into play. The Union, financed by members' dues, had by then assumed most of the functions of the project and was composed of two individuals from each bank, usually the president and another committee member. All Sanduk presidents, with the exception of the president of Sanduk Itsandra, were elders; the expectation that all Sanduk presidents be elders was intended to indicate that the Sanduk was socially acceptable: it was not an affair of the young, the civil servants, development organisations, foreigners or the state: it fell within the customary domain and it was the village elders who were responsible. It was quite absurd therefore (for a project appealing to notions of social capital) that the president of Sanduk Itsandra was a youth from Mirereni.

The political influence of the elders has increased since the abolition of the pre-colonial sultanates into which the island was divided. Colonial policies, probably unintentionally, led to the development of a pyramidal system of customary government that saw the role of the elders extended from the quarter and the village to the region and, finally to the entire island. An assembly of the elders of the entire island is referred to as a *bunjileo wa Ngazidja*: a meeting of Ngazidja, Ngazidja or, simply, "the island". Although this group is constituted ad hoc and has a shifting membership, both it and other various but similar manifestations of elders' councils have consistently been conceptualised as corporate groups, leading to problems not only among the Sanduk but in Ngazidja generally.

In 1997 the Sanduk of the town of Dembeni was the object of a fraud: the four million francs provided by the project had been stolen by the president of the Sanduk. As the project attempted to retrieve its capital, the Umoja wa Masanduku was applying for recognition by the elders of Ngazidja. This was, after some negotiation, accorded, and almost immediately negotiations with Dembeni bore fruit. The Union requested that the island intervene and *mlapva* was applied. A *mlapva* bars the community concerned from participating in the *aada* until such time as they redeem themselves by (and Ngazidja accepts) payment of a fine: this is a particularly effective sanction in a society where custom is paramount. No longer did the affair concern an individual and a sum of stolen money: through his actions the entire town was banned from fulfilling its social obligations. The sum, and an additional fine, was swiftly repaid by the elders of Dembeni who took it upon themselves to deal with the defrauder themselves. However, it is salient that the Sanduk dispute occurred at the same time as another dispute that opposed Dembeni against another town in the *ntsi*: the conflation of the two disputes in the public imagination was certainly at least partly responsible for the success of this customary intervention.

Nevertheless, the event was widely commented upon; it featured in the national press and on the radio. Some days later members of the committees of Sanduk Itsandra, accompanied by one of Harumwamdji's senior elders, visited one of the bank's more recalcitrant defaulters and informed him that Itsandramdjini, too, would suffer the fate of Dembeni if he did not repay his loans. The individual, an elder from Harumwamdji himself who, as one of the most senior members of the bank, had consistently ignored vague threats and would have been unimpressed by the largely powerless elders' council, immediate repaid two thirds of his outstanding debt.

Although this episode reflects the power of the elders in customary contexts, it was an individual episode: it required a personal visit from a senior elder to obtain results and it was, effectively, a semi-private affair between two elders of the same quarter. Collectively the elders of Itsandramdjini remained largely uninterested, and did not of course compose Sanduk Itsandra's formal elders council. Indeed, the elders were even less involved than before: those of Harumwamdji still considered the bank to be "fishermen's business" and thus none of theirs, while the elders of Befuni, similarly, no longer concerned themselves with the bank, if indeed they ever had: the office had physically moved outside the quarter (it was now in Mirereni) and most of the committee members were also now from other quarters. As for Mirereni, the elders are effectively uninvolved in customary events outside the context of the quarter: they showed no interest in the bank either, which was, by now, dominated by junior elders from Harumwamdji. No quarter was prepared to accept social responsibility for the bank.

In January 2000 Sanduk Itsandra was expelled from the Union. In June 2000 the Union called upon the island, who met and decided that, in view of the refusal of Itsandramdjini to refund the bank's capital, the *ntsi* of Itsandra would be required to pay in their stead: having satisfied the Union, the matter would then become an affair between the *ntsi*, Itsandramdjini and the island. Negotiations continued between the Union, the island, the *ntsi* and the town, but the town, drawing on its particular status within the *ntsi*, consistently refused to accept responsibility for the Sanduk on the basis that, firstly, the affair was a development project (and, moreover, a gift from France) and thus outside the customary domain and, secondly, the affair did not concern Itsandramdjini, but was rather an internal matter for the Befuni quarter. This latter claim took advantage of the fact that Befuni, being a quarter and not a town, had no distinct identity in the *mila na ntsi* outside the town as a whole and thus could not interact either with the *ntsi* or with the island.

The inability of the *ntsi* to impose its authority on the town led to the *ntsi* also declining responsibility: the *ntsi* were well aware that their attempts to recover the money from Itsandramdjini would be met with failure and were not willing to assume the debt themselves. A stalemate was reached, in which the various actors consistently refused either to bow to custom or, quite simply, to appear at meetings[32] and the attempt to invoke custom finally ended when, in October 2000, the Union decided that they would instead appeal to the formal judicial system and brought a legal action against Sanduk Itsandra. This would avoid the humiliation that would naturally follow the failure of the island's customary powerholders to resolve the dispute; it also admitted not only that the attempt to insert a development project into the customary sphere had in this case failed, but that the fluidity of customary structures was inadequate to resolve such disputes.

Conclusion: wherefore social capital?

It is clear from the above that the project's expectations that the elders would draw on their reserves of social capital to manage Sanduk Itsandra were not met. The elders of Befuni played no role overseeing the bank, either when it was purely a Befuni organisation or, more understandably, when it was opened to the rest of the town. In the latter period of the Sanduk's operations, the elders of Harumwamdji were equally negligent; and when the dispute escalated to involve the entire island, custom still failed to operate. And yet, by the all measuring sticks in the World Bank's panoply, surely these men had significant stocks of social capital: high status, political powerholders, they were firmly embedded in local, regional and island-wide networks – these are men who spend the marriage season in taxis travelling from village to village, participating in ceremony after ceremony, sometimes in great haste lest their absence be remarked upon. Their names are, in many cases, renowned across the island, their faces familiar to all; their right to the exercise of power, in the relevant spheres, is uncontested and their decisions are often binding. How, then, could they have failed to discipline a somewhat undistinguished group of young men and women, most of whom were unemployed and of low social status? This failure is all the more ironic given the role of cyclical debts and reciprocal obligations in a ritual context. The entire *aada* system is maintained through the continuing and ongoing establishment, renewal and acquittal of debts, all of which are carefully noted in exercise books and in many cases maintained from generation to generation. Indeed, Wangazidja are extremely adept at managing debt and making repayments; the failure to repay customary debts invokes social sanctions of the highest order as, no doubt, elders bring their social capital into play.

Sanduk's elder's council has striking parallels both in the (utterly unsuccessful) Ouatou Akouba, or Conseil des Notables, established by the French colonial government in 1915,[33] and in President Mohammed Taki's similar attempt (in the mid-1990s) to establish a Ngazidja elders' council, formally nominated and complete with an elders' president. Both attempts to formally constitute an elders' council failed completely because the elders' councils (at village, regional or island level) are not corporate groups with fixed members or a fixed identity; rather they are groups constituted in response to specific events or circumstances and composed of those elders who claim and are accorded the status to participate, and who have an interest in doing so. The fact that the members are generally the same individuals each time is irrelevant to the character of the group itself and accords the group neither permanence nor identity as a corporate group. These individuals may well – indeed, almost certainly do – possess social capital, but the value of this capital is entirely context dependent. If their arbitration is uncontested in disputes over the distribution of meat in ritual contexts, it is likely to be ignored in disputes over repayments of a loan to a bank.

Thus, not only was the elders' council in Itsandramdjini doomed to failure even as it was formed, but its existence permitted the other elders of the town to allow the formal council responsibility for the Sanduk and ignore it themselves. This was clearly demonstrated in those other towns where the council, recognised as meaningless, was disbanded and responsibility confided in the customary power holders, collectively, the elders of the town. In these latter cases, the abolition of the elders' council was a sign of social acceptance of the bank and although many of these banks also failed, the elders nevertheless played a real role. In Itsandramdjini, the elders' council, intended to facilitate appropriation, was instead an obstacle to appropriation. Conceived as a means of involving customary powerholders in the management of the Sanduk, the elders' council in Itsandramdjini ensured exactly the opposite: the very existence of the elders' council was contrary to custom, for any group constituted according to custom could not, by definition, cut across socially constructed boundaries. Even when the Sanduk extended its operations, and drew its elders from Harumwamdji, the elders selected were those who spent their days in the village, adjudicating on matters such as the quantity of rice to be cooked for an *aada*; the younger, more dynamic and better educated elders, who might well have been equipped, socially, to exercise authority over the Sanduk, were employed elsewhere, in the formal sector or running businesses in Moroni. They were not seen as sufficiently "traditional" to be able to exercise their authority in the village and were therefore not recruited. Ultimately, it seems that there could be no meeting of the two systems: customary elders, bearing customary authority ("social capital"), were unqualified to manage a bank; "modern" elders, with social capital accrued and potential in a formal sphere, were unqualified to exercise authority in what was intended to be a customary sphere.

The ultimate cause of the failure of Sanduk Itsandra was conflicting cultural expectations underpinned by misplaced faith in the fungibility of social capital. While the project continued to insist on the culturally appropriate nature of the Sanduk and its insertion into a customary space, the town were unable to understand why the project operators should want a bank to be housed in someone's back room and overseen by a group of old men who knew nothing of banking. There was a glaring (and oft-commented upon) contrast between the office of Sanduk Itsandra and that of a rival microcredit institution in nearby Moroni, the MECK[34]. Sanduk Itsandra sits in the front room in a private house, which contains a desk, a chair and a safe and is occupied, on a busy day, by not more half a dozen individuals, often arguing with the cashier, who is himself kin to many of them. On a similarly busy day the MECK's offices (which admittedly has a larger catchment area) is thronging with dozens of clients, the cashiers (unrelated to the majority of the clients) are behind a counter protected by a wire grille and, generally, the place has the feel of a bank. There is no appeal to custom, to solidarity groups or to elderly fishermen; it is a real bank and it inspires confidence. The fact that the "culturally appropriate" elements of the bank's operations were culturally quite inappropriate seemed to be irrelevant. The general belief was that, for reasons of their own, the project wanted it so, and so it should be.

Sanduk Itsandra failed not because the project was not appropriated by the local community; rather it failed because, as a bank, it was not sufficiently Western. In an anti-climactic post-script to the history of the failure of Sanduk Itsandra, therefore, the project office was finally obliged to file a lawsuit in the civil courts in order to retrieve its debt. Even in failure, the project had been unsuccessful. In the terminology of the World Bank (perhaps) the elders were unable to transfer social capital acquired in the customary sphere to the formal (Western) sphere. In other words, their social capital was not fungible.

What conclusions can be drawn from the Sanduk's failure for the relevance and utility of the concept of social capital within the academy, and within development practice? In the introduction I raised the question of whether the concept might be of use to anthropology; in what followed I suspect that, in this particular context, the question has been shown to be an irrelevant one since social capital, within the development paradigm, is a very different creature from anything that might have developed from the writings of Bourdieu. Much of the foregoing discussion has instead been about social capital as a tool of the development industry, a positivist interpretation of what is essentially a constructivist notion: context dependent, shifting and fluid, social capital in not, despite what might be assumed from Bourdieu, analogous to economic capital. The resources that an individual derives from his or her durable networks of social relationships are not fixed, tangible or quantifiable: they are not the social equivalent of cash and therefore cannot be treated as such. If they are, then concept becomes either insufficiently flexible to usefully be engaged, or so wide in its scope that it loses all acuity.

Acknowledgement

An early version of this article was presented at seminars in the anthropology departments at the University of Sydney and at Macquarie University in 1999 and 2002 respectively; it was extensively rewritten to be presented at the European Swahili Workshop held in Oxford in 2010. I wish to thank participants at all three events for their comments, and the usual anonymous referees. I would also like to thank Olivier Maes, former project manager of Sanduk, and others associated with Sanduk Ngazidja, for their assistance and for fruitful discussions.

Notes

1. World Bank, *The Initiative on Defining*, iii.
2. Cf. Putnam, "Bowling Alone: America's Declining"; Putnam, *Bowling Alone: The Collapse*.
3. World Bank, "'Social capital'"; World Bank, *World Development Report*; World Bank, *The Initiative on Defining*; World Bank, *Overview: Social Capital*.
4. Fischer, "Book Review," 157.
5. The five were Gardner, "Keeping Connected"; Gebremedhin and Theron, "Locating Community Participation"; Godoy et al., "On the Measure of Income"; Petit, "Rethinking Internal Migrations"; Virtanen "The Urban Machinery". This analysis, in ISI's Web of Science Arts and Humanities and Social Sciences citation indices, was the result of my quest for an anthropological grounding for this article, which was not as successful as I had hoped. Despite this absence from the anthropological sphere, the number of articles on "social capital" shows no signs of decreasing and had reached an annual total of 755 in 2011: "Social capital", useful or not, is still very much on someone's agenda.
6. Fischer, "Book Review", 157.
7. See Fine, "Social Capital: the World Bank's Fungible Friend"; Fine, "Social Capital"; Fine, *Theories*, for insistent criticism that nevertheless appears to fall on deaf ears.
8. See Portes, "Social Capital", for the history of the term.
9. Bourdieu, *Outline*; Bourdieu, "Les Trois Etats"; Bourdieu, "Le Capital Social", Bourdieu, "The Forms of Capital."
10. Bourdieu, "Les Trois Etats"; cf. Bourdieu, *Outline*.
11. Bourdieu, "Le Capital Social", 2; emphasis in original.
12. Burt, *Structural Holes*, 9, cited in Woolcock, "Social Capital", 189.
13. Loury, "The Economics of Discrimination", 100, cited in Woolcock, "Social Capital", 189.
14. Coleman, "'Social capital'", S98.
15. Narayan and Pritchett, "Cents and Sociability", 872. The implication of this, of course, is that they may be measuring something else altogether: the man who lives in a palace and rides in a Rolls Royce may be the king, but he may also be the king's chauffeur.
16. For example, Van Bastelaer and Leathers, "Trust in lending"; Widner and Mundt, "Researching Social Capital", for the former; Narayan and Pritchett, "Cents and Sociability", for the latter.
17. For example, Narayan and Pritchett, "Cents and Sociability".
18. Bourdieu, "Les Trois Etats", 4; Bourdieu, *Outline*, 171–83.
19. Daley-Harris, *State of the Microcredit Summit*. The literature is compendious but see, for example, Basu et al., *Microfinance in Africa*; Bateman, *Why Doesn't Microfinance Work?*; Fernando, *Microfinance*; La Torre and Vento, *Microfinance*; Roy, *Poverty Capital*;

Sengupta and Aubuchon, "The Microfinance Revolution", for various perspectives and overviews.

20. Woolcock, "Learning from Failures." See also Hossein, *Credit for Alleviation*; Khandker et al. *Grameen Bank*; Wahid, *The Grameen Bank*; Dyal-Chand, "Reflection in a Mirror", Parmar, "Micro-credit"; Selinger, "Does Microcredit 'Empower'?".

21. See, for example, Goenka and Henley, *Southeast Asia's Credit Revolution*; Robinson, *The Microfinance Revolution*; Yaron, *Successful Rural Finance Institutions*.

22. Gibbons, *The Grameen Reader*.

23. Auwal, "Promoting microcapitalism"; Bhatt, "Delivering microfinance"; Hulme, "Can the Grameen Bank be Replicated?"; Hulme and Mosley, *Finance Against Poverty*; McDonnell, *The Grameen Bank*; Rahman, "The General Replicability"; Schreiner and Woller, "Microenterprise development programs"; Woller and Woodworth, "Microcredit as a Grass-Roots Policy".

24. Bamfo, "A Grassroots Developmental Strategy"; Berhane et al., "Risk-matching Behavior"; Buckley, "Microfinance in Africa"; Copestake et al., "Assessing the Impact"; Hazarikaa and Sarangib, "Household access"; Hulme, "Can the Grameen Bank be Replicated?"; Masanjala, "Can the Grameen Bank be Replicated in Africa?"; Perry, "Microcredit and Women"; Snow and Buss, "Development"; Udry, "Credit Markets", Zeller, "Determinants".

25. Gentil and Lefèvre, *Crédit Rural*.

26. Until 1992 the Caisse Centrale de Coopération Économique (CCCE) and since 1998 the Agence Française de Développement (AFD); for the sake of consistency, it is referred to in this paper as the CFD.

27. In Shingazidja, *sanduku*, pl. *masanduku*. The word *sanduku* means chest or trunk.

28. Details of Sanduk philosophy and regulations from Gentil and Lefèvre, *Crédit Rural*; Kaiva, *Projet Sanduk*; Lefèvre, *Projet Sanduk*, various internal documents and Sanduk Itsandra association statutes. See also, Pierret "Entre Croissance et Crise".

29. The functions of the *aada* are multiple and touch all spheres of life: it establishes and confirms alliances between clans, rights over land, membership of a community and relationships between individuals; it acts as a mechanism for the redistribution of wealth and effectively acts as a social security system for the older members of the community. However, the *aada* is also costly: the smallest socially acceptable *aada* in a rural area requires at least 2mF (€4000); in an urban area an *aada* of 25mF (€50000) is not exceptional. See Chouzour, *Le Pouvoir de l''honneur*, Walker, *Becoming the Other*.

30. Literally, "tradition and land".

31. Initially called Sanduk Befuni, I refer to the bank as Sanduk Itsandra throughout for the sake of consistency.

32. A visit by the elders to a village is generally a ceremonial affair, both visiting and receiving elders dressing formally, the latter officially receiving the former in the public square or some other appropriate location. However, I recall one visit by the elders of the *ntsi* in connection with the Sanduk affair: they wandered around Itsandramdjini dressed in their finery, incensed that the elders of the town had completely ignored their visit and were nowhere to be found. They were forced to return home. This was a humiliating snub and it is indicative of the status of Itsandramdjini that it is perhaps the only town on the island that could have carried it off without risking further censure.

33. Walker, "What Came First."

34. Mutuelles d'Épargne et de Crédit ya Komor (sic).

References

Auwal, Mohammad. "Promoting Microcapitalism in the Service of the Poor: The Grameen Model and its Cross-Cultural Adaptation." *Journal of Business Communication* 33, no. 1 (1996): 27–49.

Bamfo, Napoleon. "A Grassroots Developmental Strategy for Africa: Towns as Agents of Growth Through Financial Credit." *Policy Studies Journal* 29, no. 2 (2001): 308–18.

Basu, Anupam, Rodolphe Blavy and Murat Yulek. *Microfinance in Africa: Experience and Lessons from Selected African Countries.* Washington: International Monetary Fund, African Dept., 2004.

Bateman, Milford. *Why Doesn't Microfinance Work? The Destructive Rise of Local Neoliberalism*. London: Zed, 2010.

Berhane, Guush, Cornelis Gardebroek and Henk A.J. Moll. "Risk-matching Behavior in Microcredit Group Formation: Evidence from Northern Ethiopia." *Agricultural Economics* 40, no. 4 (2009): 409–19.

Bhatt, Nitin. "Delivering Microfinance in Developing Countries: Controversies and Policy Perspectives." *Policy Studies Journal* 29, no. 2 (2001): 319–33.

Bourdieu, Pierre. *Outline of a Theory of Practice*. Cambridge: Cambridge University Press, 1977.

Bourdieu, Pierre. "Les Trois Etats du Capital Culturel." *Actes de la Recherche en Sciences Sociales* 30 (1979): 3–6.

Bourdieu, Pierre. "Le Capital Social. Notes Provisoires." *Actes de la Recherches en Sciences Sociales* 3 (1980): 2–3.

Bourdieu, Pierre. "The Forms of Capital." In *Handbook of Theory and Research for the Sociology of Education*, ed. John G. Richardson. Westport: Greenwood Press, 1986.

Buckley, Graeme. "Microfinance in Africa: Is it Either the Problem or the Solution?" *World Development* 25, no. 7 (1997): 1081–93.

Burt, Ronald. *Structural Holes*. Cambridge: Harvard University Press, 1992.

Chouzour, Sultan. *Le Pouvoir de l'honneur. Tradition et Contestation en Grande Comore*. Paris: L'Harmattan, 1994.

Coleman, James "'Social capital' in the creation of human capital." *American Journal of Sociology* 94, Supplement (1988): S95–120.

Copestake, James, Sonia Bhalotra and Susan Johnson. "Assessing the Impact of Microcredit: A Zambian Case Study." *Journal of Development Studies* 37, no. 4 (2001): 81–100.

Daley-Harris, Sam. *State of the Microcredit Summit Campaign Report 2005*. Washington: Microcredit Summit Campaign, 2005.

Dyal-Chand, Rashmi. "Reflection in a Distant Mirror: Why the West has Misperceived the Grameen Bank's Vision of Microcredit." *Stanford Journal of International Law* 41, no. 2 (2005): 217–306.

Fernando, Jude L. *Microfinance: Perils and Prospects*. London: Routledge, 2006.

Fine, Ben. "Social Capital: the World Bank's Fungible Friend." *Journal of Agrarian Change* 3, no. 4 (2003): 586–603.

Fine, Ben. "Social Capital." In *The Elgar Companion to Development Studies*, ed. Clark David. Cheltenham: Edward Elgar Publishing, 2006.

Fine, Ben. *Theories of Social Capital: Researchers Behaving Badly*. London: Pluto Press, 2010.

Fischer, C.S. "Book review. Bowling Alone: What's the Score?" *Social Networks* 27 (2005): 155–67.

Gardner, Katy. "Keeping Connected: Security, Place, and Social Capital in a 'Londoni' village in Sylhet." *Journal of the Royal Anthropological Institute* 14, no. 3 (2008): 477–95.

Gebremedhin, Solomon Haile and François Theron. "Locating Community Participation in a Water Supply Project: The Galanefhi Water Project (Eritrea)." *Anthropology Southern Africa* 30, nos. 1–2 (2007): 20–8.

Gentil, Dominic and Luc Lefèvre. *Crédit Rural et Micro-entreprises Urbaines aux Comores. Rapport de Mission*. Paris: GRET, IRAM, 1991.

Gibbons, David, ed. *The Grameen Reader: Training Materials for the International Replication of the Grameen Bank Financial System for Reduction of Rural Poverty*. Dhaka: Grameen Bank, 1994.

Godoy, Ricardo, Victoria Reyes-Garcia, Tomas Huanca, William R. Leonard, Thomas McDade, Susan Tanner, Craig Seyfried. "On the Measure of Income and the Economic Unimportance of Social Capital: Evidence from a Native Amazonian Society of Farmers and Foragers." *Journal of Anthropological Research* 63, no. 2 (2007): 239–60.

Goenka, Aditya, and David Henley, eds. *Southeast Asia's Credit Revolution: From Money-lenders to Microfinance*. London: Routledge, 2010.

Grootaert, Christiaan and Thierry van Bastelaer, eds. *The Role of Social Capital in Development: An Empirical Assessment*. Cambridge: Cambridge University Press, 2002.

Hazarikaa, Gautam, and Sudipta Sarangib. "Household Access to Microcredit and Child Work in Rural Malawi." *World Development* 36, no. 5 (2008): 843–59.

Hossein, Mahabub. *Credit for Alleviation of Rural Poverty: The Grameen Bank of Bangladesh.* Washington: International Food Policy Research Institute, 1988.

Hulme, David. "Can the Grameen Bank be Replicated? Recent Experiments in Malaysia, Malawi and Sri Lanka." *Development Policy Review* 8, no. 3 (1990): 287–300.

Hulme, David, and Paul Mosley. *Finance Against Poverty.* London: Routledge, 1996.

Kaiva, Moussa. *Projet Sanduk. Credit Rural et Urbain des Comores.* Moroni: Programme Regional Environnement Coordination Nationale des Comores Direction Générale de l'Environnement, Table Ronde Audit/Gouvernance Locale/ONG, 1998.

Khandker, Shahidur, Baqui Khalily and Zahed Khan. *Grameen Bank: Performance and Sustainability.* Washington: World Bank, 1995.

La Torre, Mario, and Gianfranco A. Vento. *Microfinance.* Basingstoke: Palgrave Macmillan, 2006.

Lefèvre, Luc. *Projet Sanduk: crédit rural et micro-entreprises urbaines aux Comores.* Paris: GRET, IRAM, 1993.

Loury, Glenn. "The economics of discrimination: getting to the core of the problem." *Harvard Journal for African American Public Policy* 1 (1992): 91–110.

Masanjala, Winford. "Can the Grameen Bank be Replicated in Africa? Evidence from Malawi." *Canadian Journal of Development Studies* 23, no. 1 (2002): 87–103.

McDonnell, Siobhan. *The Grameen Bank Micro-credit Model: Lessons for Australian Indigenous Economic Policy.* Canberra: CAEPR. CAEPR Discussion Paper No. 178/1999, 1999.

Narayan, Deepa, and Lant Pritchett. "Cents and Sociability: Household Income and Social Capital in Rural Tanzania." *Economic Development and Cultural Change* 47, no. 4 (1999): 871–97.

Parmar, Aradhana. "Micro-credit, Empowerment, and Agency: Re-evaluating the Discourse." *Canadian Journal of Development Studies* 24, no. 3 (2003): 461–76.

Perry, Donna. "Microcredit and Women Moneylenders: The Shifting Terrain of Credit in Rural Senegal." *Human Organization* 61, no. 1 (2002): 30–40.

Petit, Pierre. "Rethinking Internal Migrations in Lao PDR: The Resettlement Process Under Micro-analysis." *Anthropological Forum* 18, no. 2 (2008): 117–38.

Pierret, Dorothée. "Entre Croissance et Crise: Quel Avenir Pour le Reseau Sanduk aux Comores?" In *Viabilites et Impacts de la Microfinance. Bilan et Perspectives. Dossier Préparatoire des Journées d'études IRAM, 7 and 8 Septembre 2001.* Paris: IRAM, 2001.

Portes, Alejandro. "Social Capital: Its Origins and Applications in Modern Sociology." *Annual Review of Sociology* 24 (1988): 1–24.

Putnam, Robert. "Bowling Alone: America's Declining Social Capital." *Journal of Democracy* 6, no. 1 (1995): 65–78.

Putnam, Robert. *Bowling Alone: The Collapse and Revival of American Community.* New York: Simon and Schuster, 2000.

Putnam, Robert, with R. Leonardi and R. Nanetti. *Making Democracy Work. Civic Traditions in Modern Italy.* Princeton: Princeton University Press, 1993.

Rahman, Atiur. "The General Replicability of the Grameen Bank Model." In *The Grameen Bank: Poverty Relief in Bangladesh,* ed. A.N.M. Wahid. Boulder: Westview Press, 1993.

Robinson, Marguerite. *The Microfinance Revolution: Sustainable Finance for the Poor.* Washington: World Bank, 2001.

Roy, Ananya. *Poverty Capital: Microfinance and the Making of Development.* London: Routledge, 2010.

Schreiner, Mark, and Gary Woller. "Microenterprise Development Programs in the United States and in the Developing World." *World Development* 31, no. 9 (2003): 1567–80.

Selinger, Evan "Does Microcredit 'Empower'? Reflections on the Grameen Bank Debate." *Human Studies* 31, no. 1 (2008): 27–41.

Sengupta, Rajdeep, and Craig Aubuchon. "The Microfinance Revolution: An Overview." *Federal Reserve Bank of St Louis Review* 90, no. 1 (2008): 9–30.

Snow, Douglas, and Terry Buss. "Development and the Role of Microcredit." *Policy Studies Journal* 29, no. 2 (2001): 296–307.

Udry, Christopher. "Credit Markets in Northern Nigeria: Credit as Insurance in a Rural Economy." In *The Economics of Rural Organization: Theory, Practice, and Policy,* ed. Karla Hoff, Avishay Braverman, and Joseph E. Stiglitz. New York: Oxford University Press, 1993.

Van Bastelaer Thierry, and Howard Leathers. "Trust in Lending: Social Capital and Joint Liability Seed Loans in Southern Zambia." *World Development* 34(10) (2006): 1788–807.

Virtanen, Pekka. "The Urban Machinery Youth and Social Capital in Western Amazonian Contemporary Rituals." *Anthropos* 101, no. 1 (2006): 159–67.

Wahid, A.N.M., ed. *The Grameen Bank: Poverty Relief in Bangladesh*. Boulder: Westview Press, 1993.

Walker, Iain. "What Came First, the Nation or the State? Political Process in the Comoro Islands." *Africa* 77, no. 4 (2007): 582–605.

Walker, Iain. *Becoming the Other, Being Oneself: Constructing Identities in a Connected World*. Newcastle: Cambridge Scholars Publishing, 2010.

Widner, Jennifer, and Alexander Mundt. "Researching Social Capital in Africa." *Africa* 68, no. 1 (1998): 1–24.

Woller, Gary, and Warner Woodworth. "Microcredit as a Grass-roots Policy for International Development." *Policy Studies Journal* 29, no. 2 (2001): 267–82.

Woolcock, Michael. "Social Capital and Economic Development: Toward a Theoretical Synthesis and Policy Framework." *Theory and Society* 27, no. 2 (1998): 151–208.

Woolcock, Michael. "Learning from Failures in Microfinance: What Unsuccessful Cases Tell Us About How Group-based Programs Work." *American Journal of Economics and Sociology* 58, no. 1 (1999): 17–42.

World Bank. "'Social capital': the missing link?" In *Monitoring Environmental Progress – Expanding the Measure of Wealth*. World Bank, Indicators and Environmental Valuation Unit, 1997a.

World Bank. *World Development Report 1997. The State in a Changing World*. New York: Oxford University Press, 1997b.

World Bank. *The Initiative on Defining, Monitoring and Measuring "Social Capital" Overview and Program Description*. Washington: The World Bank, Social Development Family, Environmentally and Socially Sustainable Development Network. "Social capital" Initiative Working Paper No. 1, 1998.

World Bank. *Overview: Social Capital*. http://go.worldbank.org/C0QTRW4QF0 (accessed October 17, 2012).

Yaron, Jacob. *Successful Rural Finance Institutions*. Washington: World Bank, 1992.

Zeller, Manfred. "Determinants of Credit Rationing: A Study of Informal Lenders and Formal Credit Groups in Madagascar." *World Development* 22, no. 12 (1994): 1895–907.

Attempts at fusion of the Comorian educational systems: Religious education in Comorian and Arabic and secular education in French

Damir Ben Ali[a] and Iain Walker[b]

[a]CNDRS, Moroni, Comores; [b]Martin Luther University, Halle, Germany

The Comoros archipelago has two institutions to train its youth. The first is the Koran school, which teaches children to write their mother tongue in Arabic characters, instils the practice of religion, and transmits the models, values and symbols that underpin a sense of national identity. The second institution is the French school. Originally opened only to a small minority, the French school was focused on building the top of a social pyramid formed by a bureaucratic elite committed to the interests of the colonial power. After independence, the first government decided to give all youth an education that met the needs of the country. A Koranic education and a secular education were integrated into one community-based system, so that a predominantly rural population could participate actively in education and children would be integrated into the community and develop their personalities.

Introduction

Until the arrival of Europeans in the Indian Ocean in the sixteenth century, the inhabitants of the Comoros were embedded in a world dominated by Islam. The Comorian nation – four islands isolated by the ocean – defined itself not so much by a centralised political power but by a willingness to co-exist framed by rules both moral (*akhlaq*) and ethno-social (*mu'amalate*), parameters for social relations, provided in the first instance by the Koran. Islam generated an individual, familial and social "life code" which underpinned the solidarity and cohesion of the country's political institutions until the beginning of the nineteenth century. During this period the Koran school played a decisive role in the construction of society and the blossoming of a cultural identity.

Beginning in 1843, however, French colonialism imposed, first in Mayotte, 43 years later on the other three islands, a new societal model through the introduction of new economic needs and a new training institution to provide the administration and the colonial companies with the subaltern agents that they required. Since independence in 1975, the official secular school, closely based on the colonial model, has assumed responsibility for a growing number of children, from the age of 6 to 20 or older. However, successive governments have on a number of occasions attempted to integrate these two institutions that have long operated independently of one another – the Koran school, or *shioni*, with its communitarian character, and the secular school, with a more individualist programme – into a single educational system. These attempts, aimed at permitting a largely rural population to participate actively in the education of their children and to integrate them into their environment, better to attain their potential, have generally been marked by increasingly unsatisfactory levels of achievement among the students.

The educational policies of the Comorian state, like those of many other post-colonies, are constrained both by colonial heritage and by contemporary global definitions and expectations of what education should be. In this article we trace the history of education in the Comoros, from pre-colonial institutions to the schools of the contemporary state, with particular attention to the tensions between customary, Islamic and western conceptualisations of the educational process. As Dale Eickelman has pointed out, in the decolonized world, non-Western institutions of learning have largely ceded place to institutions constructed on the European model of education: other forms of education are often marginalised, both conceptually and practically (Eickelman 1978). While this is particularly true of "traditional" forms of education (eg Avoseh 2011, Merriam & Young 2008, Raum 1938), this observation also extends to the more formal schools that exist in the Islamic world, a particular point of encounter between coloniser and colonised. Indeed, for many observers, these were not schools either. The articles in a 1946 special issue of the *Journal of Negro Education* on the "Problem of Education in Dependent Territories" barely mentioned Koran schools: Jean de la Roche's comments, in his article on the French territories, were representative of perspectives on non-Western forms of education at the time: "a rapid glance at Africa's past history will show that no educational system of any kind existed prior to the establishment of the present French administration. The nearest approach to a school was the Koranic teaching provided for a select few in the areas of the north which had been overrun by Arab invaders." (1946: 399). This despite saying that "education in French Africa is naturally not limited to the work done by the schools, but is understood in the broader meaning of the word." (ibid.: 407). Observations of this kind were not limited to external observers – even those working within the colonial educational system were disparaging. Thus in 1928 a British colonial officer wrote of the Koran schools of Zanzibar that "a training more deadening to the intellect can hardly be imagined," (Hendry 1928: 343). Generally, many reports on education in the colonies barely mentioned local schools of any sort, and even then only to dismiss them as ineffectual at best.

Nevertheless, in some jurisdictions the importance of Koran schools was recognised. In Palestine religious education was seen as complementary to secular education and a basis for social stability, acting as an anchor against calls for reform (Schneider 2014). In the Anglo-Egyptian Sudan, despite (or perhaps because of) limited resources and in recognition of the fact that there was unlikely to be any alternative for many years to come, the government made salary grants to Koran school teachers who were willing to undertake basic training (Wieschhoff 1946). In Somaliland, somewhat unusually, a network of assisted Koran schools provided the first three years of education before feeding students into the public school system. This was facilitated by the fact that instruction in the government schools was in Arabic, so Koran schools provided useful groundwork; and all schools offered religious education and taught the Arabic language (Millman 2014). Indeed, administrators in most British colonies with a significant Muslim population rapidly realised that, for various reasons, religious education had to be incorporated into the public schooling curriculum. Roman Loimeier has described in some detail the development of Islamic education in Zanzibar and how the struggles of the British administration in the face of opposition both from Islamic scholars and parents finally saw an accommodation that led to the incorporation of Koran schools into the public schooling system and the teaching of religion in schools (Loimeier 2009, see also, Bang 2003 for religious education in the region).

There were, of course, significant differences between French and British perspectives and policies on education, most notably the implications of France's 1905 law on the separation of church and state, which generally precluded the possibility of religious teaching in publicly funded schools, a constant point of frustration for administrators in the colony of the Comoros who (and despite attempts to prevent them from doing so) saw a steady flow of Comorian children, particularly from Ngazidja, attending school in Zanzibar. Indeed, Zanzibar was a frequent point of reference for administrators in the Comoros since not only did the public schools of the protectorate include religious education in their curricula, but the Comorian School of Zanzibar – unusually, because although it was an independently run school it was funded by grants from the French government – also provided religious instruction for its pupils.

Furthermore, the aims of colonial education policies differed. While both powers intended that local subjects be educated in order to participate in the administration of the colony, in the British colonies education was, perhaps unsurprisingly, decentralised, often confided to missions and other local groups. French policy, on the other hand, was central-ised, aimed at the assimilation of colonial subjects: government schools were charged with the task producing good French subjects (Cogneau & Moradi 2014). In the French colo-nies Algeria was often held up as an example of successful integration, even if rather critical later assessments would challenge these perspectives. Indeed Pechmarty, adminis-trator of Grande Comore, wrote that the Algerian schools "produce excellent results" (1993: 112; see below),[1] although for whom he does not specify. It is true that in the early colonial period in Algeria both Arabic and religion were taught in schools, and a network of locally-run Islamic schools operated in parallel with (although more than three kilome-tres from) government schools; however, under the Third Republic Arabic was removed from the curriculum and the French subsequently deliberately undermined the Islamic schools in an attempt to push children into European schools (Heggoy 1973, Kateb 2004).

In many Islamic colonies (including both the Comoros and early twentieth century Zanzibar) parents refused to send their children to state schools for fear of Christian indoc-trination; colonial administrators were forced to recognise that Koran schools would have a role to play in the education of the colonised child, not only in view of the hostility with which many parents viewed the colonial schools but also through lack of funds. Moreover, the focus on Koran schools as religious schools (eg Eisemon & Wasi 1987) was often misleading. In both the British and the French systems the non-religious aspects of the Koran school were generally overlooked, if not dismissed altogether. The 1911 Zanzibar Annual Report on Education stated disapprovingly that "the teachers spend much of their time in attending to other matters and make use of their pupils as hewers of wood and drawers of water" (cited in Loimeier 2009: 274); rarely were the less formal aspects of an indigenous education viewed positively, even if the more perspicacious of colonial officers harboured doubts about the appropriateness of the colonial systems: "Formerly the child learned in school how to live, now he learns how to make a living." (Furnivall, 1943, cited in Watson, 1982: 40). Koran schools in many locations, were places of socio-cultural education as much as they were religious: in Burkina Faso they "combined Islamic educa-tion with functional learning" (Wodon 2015: 81), while Michael Lambek recounts how, when he said he wanted to learn about local culture in Mayotte he was told to report to the Koran school at dawn the next morning (1990).

The Koran school in the Comoros

From the third century of the Hegira (ninth–tenth centuries of the Christian era), numerous Arab and Persian families, fleeing politico-religious conflicts at home, settled in the Comoros.[2] Aujas (1911) dates the migrations of groups of Yemenis to 192 AH/807 AD, while according to Guillain the first Muslims to settle on the east coast of Africa were Zayidis (1856: 160). They were followed by adepts of a variety of different sects who had fought (and lost) wars in their homelands and who found themselves together several years later in the Comoros, where they co-existed, each practising Islam according to the rites of their own community. The original inhabitants of the islands therefore followed a syncretic Islam highly influenced by pre-Islamic traditions.

The importance of education, and specifically Islamic education, is indicated by its place in oral tradition. Thus, one narrative recounts how, towards the tenth century, a Sunni Arab sailing from Ndzuani was shipwrecked on the coast of Mayotte. He married the daughter of a local chief, a woman called Masingo, who gave her name to Ntsingoni, the future royal capital of the island of Mayotte. The couple brought an educated man from abroad and married him to their daughter. The son-in-law of Masingo expressed a desire to teach the Shafi'i rite to the locals: "'You others, come and instruct yourselves to emerge from your ignorance!' Thus they gathered people from Dzoumogne and as far as Saziley in order that they come and learn from the Arab" (Allibert 1976: 37). The students were adults, not children; they gathered together under the roof of the *paya la mdji*,[3] a shelter reserved for men, constructed on the public place (*shandza ya dago* or *mpangahari*).

In the fourteenth century teachers from Kilwa Kisiwani arrived in the islands (Allibert 1976, Damir & al., 1985, Gevrey 1870); their leader, Mohamed ben Isa, whose daughter married the *bedja* (chief) of Hamanvu, one of the chiefdoms of Ngazidja, settled in Ntsaweni. His son Hasane settled at Sima (Ndzuani). Another member of the family, Othmane ben Ahmed, gave his daughter, Mwanafatima Nyiladhahabu, in marriage to a *bedja* of Ndruani, on Ngazidja, named Ngoma Mrahafu, before settling in Mayotte. These scholars all not only taught the Koran and religious knowledge, but trained apprentices in agriculture, masonry, carpentry and ironworking trades, skills which the inhabitants of the islands had not realised could be exercised with such talent. All these *wasta'arabu* (literally "arabized people", colloquially "civilised people") married the children of local chiefs. Theologians and craftsmen, all received the prestigious title of *fundi* from the locals.

The Koran school is open to children of both genders

With time the *fundi*s, descendants of the first teachers, started teaching children, both boys and girls, moving the classes to a shelter modelled on the *paya la mdji*, close to the mosque. They were the founders of the Koran schools. These establishments rapidly became known as *paya la shio* ("kitchen of the book", or *palashio*), the *shio*, or *kitab*, being the sacred book, the Koran. The school is known as the *shioni* (the place of the book) and the pupil the *mnashioni* (literally "the child of the school, or of the place of the book", plural *wana-zioni*). The same term *mnashioni* is also used to designate a literate or learned person.

These *fundi*s, who possessed knowledge and skills, both religious and technical, contributed significantly to the development of the production of wealth as well as to the integration of the islands into ocean-wide maritime trading networks. Their prestige rivalled that of kings, if they were not themselves kings, as was Mhasi Fe Simayi, first king of Mbude, known as Mtswamuyindza. He was responsible for the construction of the first two stone houses in Ntsaweni (Ngazidja): Daradju, the functional residence of the kings of Mbude, and Darambwani, the residence of the princesses of the royal lineage, the Hinya Mwatwawuziwa. Likewise, Fani Othmani Kalishtupi of Domoni (Ndzuani) constructed the Darini Mwa Dari palace in 672 AH/1274 AD. Numerous mosques with finely sculptured coral *mihrabs* at Domoni, Mironstsi and Sima on Ndzuani, and Ntsaweni and Bangwakuni on Ngazidja are the work of these *fundi* kings, theologians and engineers.

Hatibu Ibrahim built what was the archipelago's largest mosque at the time, which he called "the Friday mosque of the Comorian people",[4] in Moroni. The foundation stone, to the right of the old *mihrab* and the wooden *mimbar* (chair), bears the date 830 AH/1426/27 AD (Gou 2000).

Towards the middle of the sixteenth century, as the state structures of the sultanates were put in place and the sultans, preoccupied with trade and dynastic rivalries, no longer engaged in teaching, scholars, both men and women, constructed shelters in the courtyards of their houses and opened Koran schools. The institution kept the name of *palashio*, doubtless both because it originally was held in the *paya la mdji* and because of the style of construction, which resembles the traditional Comorian kitchen (*paya*), a shelter constructed in the courtyard and detached from the main body of the house. Thus, the Koran school was, at least until the first half of the twentieth century, a shelter constructed close to the teacher's house, usually composed of a simple roof of dry grass or woven coconut fronds, supported on wooden poles. In the urban areas, the children were sometimes taught in the open air in a courtyard protected from the sun by the walls of two storey houses. More recently, many communities have added an upper floor to a mosque which is put at the disposition of the Koran teacher.

The Traditional Organisation Of Koranic Teaching[5]

Until the early twentieth century, the Koran school welcomed children from the age of five, from Saturday to Wednesday, morning and afternoon, and on Thursday mornings. The materials used were of local provenance. In the primary section the children learn to write the Arabic alphabet on slates with a type of chalk called *darasa*,[6] or using pens dipped in ink obtained from crushing the leaves of a shrub called *mlala*,[7] or, again, using a piece of bananas stem (*kwingwi*) mixed with soot. The ink was kept in a *ntsambu*[8] nut shell, which served as an ink-pot (*nyongo*). The pupils, seated cross-legged on mats spread on the ground, wrote on their slates with a pen (*kalam*) made from a reed. The manufacture of these items by an adult in front of the children, then by the children themselves as part of a group, contributed to the development of their mental and motor faculties. These activities were presented as religious acts imbued with moral values. As the teacher was often called away during the class, there was a system of monitors, and the pupils were divided into groups according to the levels of knowledge attained.

The pupils learned to pronounce correctly and to write the names of the 28 letters of the Arabic alphabet as well as certain characters borrowed from the Persian alphabet which are used to represent Comorian sounds not heard in Arabic. They learned to distinguish consonants and vowels, then to read syllables, words, and finally short phrases in the Comorian language. They then passed to the next stage, that of the *kurasa*, a small printed manual. The Arabic word *kurasa* means notebook or booklet; here it refers to a small work whose correct title is *The Baghdadi method, followed by the juz amma*,[9] the *juz amma* being thirtieth and last section of the Koran, which contains the shortest suras. The pupils progressively committed to memory the short suras and were thereby initiated into the reading of the Koran.

The passage from the stage of the *kurasa* to that of the reading of the Koran itself was marked by a ceremony, the *hunwa fwahamwe* (the awakening of the memory and of understanding, literally, "to drink the memory"). The name given to the ceremony emphasises intelligence. It is said that this prayer develops the faculty of memory (*beshelea*) and intelligence (*fwahamwe*). The *fundi* writes a number of prayers on a porcelain plate with the usual school ink. The text is then removed with some water, and curdled milk and honey, brought to the school by the parents, is poured onto the plate. The pupil drinks as much as he or she can, then gives the rest to other pupils. The family bring cakes and tea which are served to all, both pupils and guests, the latter including former pupils, family, and friends, both of the family and of the *fundi*. This event incorporates the children into the school environment, affirming their identity in the class and their religious awakening. They are taught to recognise and respect symbols of authority, the knowledge of the class leaders and the more advanced pupils.

The children then proceed to a full reading of the Koran. Each day the teacher reads a few verses, without translating them, and the next day the pupils read the same verses before the teacher, until the whole Koran has been read. Once a pupil has fully mastered the readings, he or she then reads the entire Koran in a ceremony in honour of the Prophet known as *hitima ya mtrume*.[10] The *hitima ya mtrume* is a large celebration that brings together the *fundi*s of the village and important local personalities, as well as both former and current pupils of the school, to celebrate the child's achievement. The pupil's family arrives bearing a great number of different varieties of cakes and an equally great number of teapots full of milky tea. The teacher reads the last part of the Koran, from sura 94 until the end of the holy text, then the pupil is installed in the middle of the classroom, seated facing the *qa'aba*; all present stand around the child and say a prayer. Once the religious ceremony is finished, the tea and cakes are served to the assembly.

This full reading of the Koran and the ceremony that commemorates the event marks the end of supervised reading in the presence of the *fundi*. The *hitima ya mtrume* is presented as a sort of diploma awarded at the end of the first cycle of the primary education, granting access to certain socio-religious functions and to leave the school before the *hitima ya mtrume* ceremony represents a scholastic failure. However, many Comorians attain adulthood having lost the capacity to read and write and only retain in their memories the texts learnt by heart and recited either during daily prayers or collectively during community events.

The second element of primary Koranic education is dedicated to learning the obligations that Islam imposes on the faithful. Drawing upon handbooks of religious education, children learn about the Koranic cleanliness of water, and the hygiene of the body, clothing and places (*twahara*), through the theme of ablutions, and the practice of prayer. Learning the five daily prayers allows them to start understanding their place in space and time, for example, the chronology of the day and the orientation of the *mihrab* of the mosque toward Mecca.

The passage of time is addressed by means of celebrations of events that occur throughout the Islamic lunar year: the anniversary of the birth of the prophet (*maulid*), his ascension (*miraj*), the holiday of Eid al Fitr at the end of Ramadan, and the *hajj*, the pilgrimage to Mecca. The new year in the Nairuzi calendar, with its seven-year cycle, offers an opportunity to discuss the agricultural calendar. The child discovers the natural rhythm of the days, the months, the seasons and the years, and the periods of agricultural work, scarcity and abundance of various products of the land and of the sea.

By teaching *fikhi* (jurisprudence), the *fundi* seeks to cast light on the eminently social character of religious duties. Religious rules permeate daily life, thereby underpinning a feeling of solidarity and interdependence among and between Comorians. These sentiments are based on a fundamental identity, that of commensality, of shared food, itself based on the distinction between *halal* and non-*halal* meat and the prohibition on fermented beverages, a distinction that has shaped the frameworks, both religious and customary, that render every daily act Islamic, even those traditions that are entirely of Bantu origin. Thus, even if principles of residence have remained uxor-matrilocal and properties are passed from mother to daughter, they are recorded by the cadis' courts which have, since the fourteenth century, officially applied the *Minhadj at Talibin* ("the guide of zealous Muslims").[11]

The teaching of *fikhi* consists in translating the Arabic text of the *Minhadj* into Comorian; the students memorise it and the following day, in front of the teacher, they must read the Arabic text and translate it into Comorian. At the same time as they learn their religious obligations, they learn the use of a specific Comorian lexicon and acquire a more complex syntax better suited to processes of reasoning. The convergence and encounter of the Comorian and Arabic languages were and remain a daily reality. The two languages are already mixed in both individual and collective practices. An education in the vernacular was essential in order for the student to acquire the knowledge appropriate to the different fields of their social, cultural and economic life.

Between the prayers of *maharibi* (sunset) and *isha* (night), all, young and old, gather for the *darasa*, the evening lesson, at the mosque, listening to the *fundi* lecturing on history, morality and Islamic doctrine. This moment of contact with adults teaches the children the rules of civility, in accordance with the precepts of religious morality and social tradition that they have already begun to discover at home. They gradually acquire the familiar signs and symbols of social relationships. They assimilate the words, gestures and norms that express the hierarchies of social status, and which make a tool of culture, orientating people with respect to the situations of daily life, indicating when to shake hands, what to say for introductions, how far from an elder they should sit, in what circumstances they should be present or absent, speak or be silent. The mastery of these words, gestures and practices is the main criterion for assessing the social value of the individual.

Life cycle rituals

The bath of the Nairuzi year (uyela mwaha)

On the first day of the *Nairuzi* agricultural year it was customary for the Koran school to organise a festival called uyela mwaha (literally "the bath of the year"), in which the whole village participated.[12] The entire population, men, women and children, gathered together for a ceremony in the public square, where the *fundi*, or the senior *fundi* if the village had several schools, recited a long prayer; this was followed by a collective recitation of certain suras of the Koran. In coastal areas, the children then bathed in the sea, hence the name of the festival *uyela mwaha* (bath of the year), and throughout the archipelago the children would often light a fire to warm themselves since the *Nairuzi* new year – *Nairuzi* is a solar year – falls in the cold season, July and August. Scholars trained in countries bordering the Arabian desert where this calendar is not used have assumed this practice to be a ritual worship of fire and have campaigned against the observation of the *Nairuzi* new year and as a result it has largely fallen into disuse. As a result, contemporary agricultural workers and fishermen no longer have a common unit of measurement of time and children no longer master the details of the cycle of agricultural production.

The annual school fete (maulida shiyo)

Maulida is the commemoration of the birth of the prophet Muhammad and one of the principal feasts of the Comoros. It takes place throughout *rabi' al Awwal*, the third month of the Islamic year and better known in the Comoros as *mwezi wa maulida* "the month of the nativity". During this third month of the lunar year each village and each mosque organises its own celebration, as do associations, government offices and state-owned companies, private businesses and even individuals born during the month. The government organises a national ceremony in the capital, Moroni, on the evening of the twelfth day of the month, the date of the birth of the Prophet in Mecca. Such celebrations include chanted or sung readings about the birth and life of the prophet. The Koran school invites parents, neighbours and other friends to the *maulida shiyo*. The *Barzandji*,[13] a collection of texts on the birth and life of the Prophet, is read.

The hitima *and the* hauli *for the dead*

Children join the adults for Koran readings on a variety of occasions. Before death, relatives recite the sura Ya Sin for the dying. Children are often told *"enda shiyoni udje uniswomeye yeyasin maudu eka tsifu"* ("go to *shioni*, so you can read the Ya Sin for me tomorrow when I'm dead"). To this end, children are carefully monitored in order that they master the reading of the Koran. This reading helps the deceased to expiate his sins.

The *hauli* is also a reading of the Koran, and thus a *hitima*, but one held annually on the anniversary of an individual's death, be it a relative or a religious scholar. *Hauli*s are widely celebrated for individuals either recently or long deceased. The ritual consists of a reading of the Kuran (*hitima*) at the mosque after the *laâswiri* (*asr* or afternoon) prayer, following which traditional pastries and tea or coffee are served. After the reading of the Koran, and as the refreshments are served, a speech is delivered. The speaker recounts the deeds of the deceased and exhorts the participants to be attentive in their religious practices.

Initiation to productive work

Until the early 1950s, every Comorian child passed through the mould of the *palashio* according to the traditions of the land. The Koran school drew the necessary resources for its teaching from its environment. It maintained the link between what was taught to children and what was lived by parents. The acquisition of fundamental skills, those of reading and writing, was transmitted in the language to which the student was the most heavily exposed. The institutionalised relations between the school and those who possessed the relevant knowledge and expertise permitted the initiation of children to the diversity of trades that met the demands of the local economy.

The *palashio* prepared the children to face all aspects of life and in particular to produce goods and services for their own well-being and that of their fellow citizens. Thus the children learned to work in the fields on their teachers' lands, their parents' lands, and, indeed, of any who requested their labour, on the condition that the children would be well fed after work. Any craftsman enjoying a good reputation could obtain the services of a pupil for the day, and would report both to the teacher and, on occasion, to the parents. The pupils participated in community works undertaken by the village such as the improvement of a street or road, or the construction of a water tank or a mosque. In this way, each child could in turn be a farmer, a mason labourer, a carpenter's apprentice or a manufacturer of lime, and was able to discover a calling for one or other of these trades. These opportunities were offered to children, regardless of the economic and social circumstances of their parents, thereby allowing them to learn about manual labour and to respect it as a noble and vital activity.

Children thus acquired a taste for group activities, learned the skills of cooperation and the taking of initiatives. Their education also dealt with language, emotional development and cognitive and motor skills. It offered the children an opportunity to broaden their experiences and helped them to share moments with their coevals, whether playing games or performing socially useful tasks that taught the children to express and communicate their emotions to their entourage. Whenever the opportunity arose the teacher would select children to participate in work that would enhance their expertise in trades that interested them. In due course, he advised the parents to send their children to be apprenticed to particular craftsmen. Similarly, students who fulfilled positions of responsibility during the teacher's absence to the satisfaction of the teacher and parents, were orientated towards a career as a *fundi*.

In the *palashio*, an apprenticeship was made through the intermediary of pedagogical processes which, at the same time as knowledge, know-how and social skills, aimed at transmitting a model of authority which underpinned an ideology. In the relationship between master and pupils, a distance is always maintained; the master is the sole source of authority and knowledge. There existed a code of relations between master and pupil to which the pupils gradually learned to submit themselves.[14] Recourse to physical sanctions was habitual, for discipline was believed to be at its most effective when it symbolically invoked a sense of culpability.[15]

An institution of fundamental importance, for over a millennium the *shioni* has provided for the socialisation of children by communicating, to all and on all the islands, a coherent system of values and symbols. In every village, and according to rules common to all islands, it has provided the national community with frameworks of thought, language and etiquette that form the backbone of the collective mentality of Comorians. Unity and social and religious solidarity were preserved and repeatedly revitalised by prestigious ulemas who were at the same time customary leaders who emerged with every generation and on all the islands. Their authority rested neither in coercion nor in persuasion, but simply by virtue of their position in a spiritual and social hierarchy whose places and functions were fixed by customary laws and recognised by the people.

The Official School (*Likoli Ya Kizungu*[16])

In the nineteenth century, French colonialism imposed a new societal model and introduced new economic obligations and a new structure for the education of children. The latter was established with the intention of training a bureaucratic elite intended to serve as intermediaries between the administration and the population. The first French schools in the archipelago were opened in Mayotte by Catholic missionaries as early as 1843. In 1859, there were two schools: one for boys in Mamoutzou, with 50 students, and another for girls in Dzaoudzi, with 34 pupils.[17] A public school opened its doors on Ndzuani in about 1887, shortly after the 1886 signatures of the various protectorate treaties between the sultans of Ngazidja (Grande Comore), Ndzuani (Anjouan), and a council of elders on Mwali, on the one hand, and the commander of Mayotte, Gerville Reach on the other.

The schools' objectives and personnel at the beginning of colonisation

In 1913, a year after the Comoros became a French colony, the archipelago had six primary schools ("*écoles des enfants indigènes du premier degré*"): two on Mayotte, one on Ndzwani and three on Ngazidja, each with one teacher. These schools nevertheless had to compete with the Koran school, of which there were of course a far greater number: a report by Pechmarty, *Chef de district* on Ngazidja, dated 6 January, 1917, provides the number of the Koran schools of Ngazidja by canton and the number of teachers and pupils by gender.[18]

SUMMARY

Canton	Schools by teacher		number of pupils	
	Men	Women	Boys	Girls
Bambao	29	29	811	402
Badjini	44	11	680	399
Mitsamihuli	32	14	575	317
Washili	34	20	456	475
Itsandra	22	12	358	265
Total	**161 (65%)**	**86 (35%)**	**2880 (61%)**	**1858 (39%)**

The French administrator distinguished two levels in the Koran school that he called *primaire* and *supérieur*, and although overall the numbers were significant, there were fewer women teachers than men and none at all at the higher level. Proportionally, there were slightly more girls in the schools than women teachers (*op. cit.*).

The resources allocated to the "native" schools were extremely limited. The colonial archives allow us to compare the numbers of teachers in the Koranic system and the French system during the first decades of the annexation.

1918

Island	Koran schools				French schools		
	Primary schools	Superior schools	Teachers	Pupils	Schools	Teachers	Pupils
Maore	93	15	93	925	2	2	38
Ndzuani	158	23	158	2650	1	1	36
Mwali	25	n/a	25	230	1	1	18
Ngazidja	306	32	306	4925	3	3	64
Total	**582**	**70**	**582**	**8730**	**7**	**7**	**156**

1921

Island	Koran schools				French schools		
	Primary schools	Superior schools	Teachers	Pupils	Schools	Teachers	Pupils
Maore	78	4	78	850	3	3	71
Ndzuani	125	16	125	4246	1	1	n/a
Mwali	30	n/a	30	248	1	1	20
Ngazidja	302	27	302	6239	2	2	51
Total	**535**	**47**	**535**	**11583**	**7**	**7**	**142**

From 1918 to 1921, the number of students at Koran schools increased from 8730 to 11,583 while numbers at the French school fell from 156 to 142.[19] This decline worried Pechmarty, and he wrote in his report: "It would be easier to attract more children and younger children to our official schools. To do so, it would be sufficient to introduce the teaching of Arabic in our schools. I am sure that parents appreciate that this organisation would respond to their wishes because it would give a better quality of education to their children. Franco-Arab schools operate in Algeria, where they produce excellent results".[20] And, indeed, following Pechmarty's recommendation, Arabic language teaching was introduced in the European school. Pechmarty's initiative launched a reflective discourse on the relationship between the Koranic school and European school which would endure through subsequent decades (Ahmed 1999).

Until 1950, the "native" school followed an original programme within which teaching was oriented towards local conditions and needs. It was particularly concerned with manual labour such as agriculture and wood- and iron-working. Those graduating from these schools thus possessed a French vocabulary that matched their employers' needs for the management of land and for a workforce in the colony, and for scientific knowledge and techniques that improved labour productivity. Education lasted four years.

An annual competition open to the entire archipelago allowed between three and five young Comorians to attend a Regional School in Madagascar for a three year secondary cycle, upon successful completion of which they were awarded a diploma, the CESD (*Certificat d'Études du Second Degré*). Holders of a CESD could then enter one of the specialised sections of the École Normale le Myre de Vilers in Antananarivo: a medical section, which prepared the student for medical school; a teacher training section; an administrative section; a financial section; or a technical section. This teaching did not isolate the students from their social and technological environment but it brought them scientific knowledge and an understanding that induced them to encourage their community towards material progress.

The school, instrument of a policy of assimilation to French citizenship

In 1946, the Fourth Republic granted French citizenship to all subjects of the French empire. The universal free school, according to the spirit of the founders of the Third Republic, became the main instrument for the policy of assimilation of new citizens. From 1950, a new official school replaced the former one. The programmes, methods and time-tables were thenceforth those which, as in France, were part of ten years' compulsory education given in the mother tongue and the culture of a traditional Judaeo-Christian industrial society.

The public primary school recruited Koran teachers to teach Arabic, but this decision was much more symbolic than effective. These teachers had not received any teacher training and their numbers were woefully inadequate. Schools of six or more classes were only provided with one or two teachers who generally read and wrote Arabic but did not speak it.[21] Arabic classes did not appear either on the official programmes or on the school timetable; classes were held either in the morning, an hour before the official start of school at 7am, or for an hour after the end of the school day at noon.

The use of Koranic teachers did not mean that the colonial school system intended to provide religious education. Teaching was limited to instruction in the Arabic language, which would give the French-speaking elites symbolic tools with which to usurp the position of the notables; but the lack of competence of the teachers failed to allow them to achieve this goal. There was no teaching of religion.

As long as numbers were deliberately kept very low and the pedagogic means relatively high, the standards of the 25 students admitted annually to secondary school was satisfactory. Overall schooling rates increased from 0.12% in 1912 to 11% in 1959. Nevertheless, these schools isolated children from their environment, killed their creative spirit, and debased and despised the peasantry and manual labourers. It pursued only one objective, entry into a secondary school which, at the time, offered the illusory hope of a position as an employee in the clerical services of the administration and the colonial companies.

In this political context, the Koran school became the shield against the colonial cultural invasion. It abandoned its social functions and initiation to manual labour and instead devoted itself exclusively to teaching Islamic doctrine. Any country, even a post-industrial one, that excludes from its curricula any reference to its own language, history, environment, be it natural or social, and any initiation to productive labour will very rapidly see its economy decline and even its very existence, as a permanent national community, called into question. The successive crises – economic, social, political and institutional – that the archipelago has been subjected to are fundamentally a product of these two educational systems, neither of which responded to the economic, social or cultural needs of the population.

Ali Mroudjae's reforms

The elections of 1972, for the first time in the colonial history of the Comoros, saw members of the opposition admitted to the territorial assembly.[22] The president of the territorial council formed a coalition government and gave the education portfolio to Ali Mroudjae, one of the leaders of the opposition. In view of his party's pro-independence stance, the minister called upon international expertise to undertake an evaluation of the territory's educational system in order to determine what might be achieved, given the limited means of a future independent state.

The territorial government lodged a request with the UNICEF regional office for Eastern Africa and the Indian Ocean. A joint UNICEF–UNESCO mission was established in 1974 and its report, by a UNICEF consultant by the name of Claude Chicot, recommended that the education of the young Comorian include a personal element based on Islamic values and a communitarian element aimed at the socio-economic development of the archipelago with rural development as an absolute priority (Chicot 1974). The author of the report highlighted that the seventh Comorian plan insisted, quite legitimately, on the necessity of increased agricultural production and it was felt that education should contribute to this effort. Nevertheless, he added that agricultural production should not be confused with rural development; the latter implied a rural transformation, that is, the transformation of the possibilities offered to the rural world

The basic education program was then broken down by age group. The mission identified three different "educational markets". The pre-primary group included children aged 4 to 7 who attended the Koran school. The primary age group, from 6 or 7 years old to 14 or 15, attended both the official school and the Koran school. Certain children attended them alternately. Most of those in the post-primary group, 14–19 years old, joined youth associations.

The seventh plan also made provision for a pedagogical institute. It was established and became the executive organ of government policy. It developed programmes adapted to the different "educational markets": private Koran schools, rural community primary schools, secondary schools and centres of professional training – men's associations and women's associations. It trained, and re-trained staff, be they government employees or volunteers; it produced and distributed educational material – manuals, teaching aids, rural newsletters, radio programmes. It monitored the system and made changes where necessary, according to the needs on the ground.

The Chicot report had taken note of the cultural and practical purposes of the precolonial *palashio*, which was well integrated into its social context and contributed to the active adaptation of children to their human and material environment, notably by the introduction of a practical component in its programme, and by the establishment of professional training courses adapted to development needs. Indeed, a number of schools were equipped with gardens.

Nevertheless, the effects of the colonial system continued to be felt. The report recommended limiting the integration of Koranic education program into the school curriculum to the preschool level, and only granting selective access to secondary and higher education. These strategies were intended to respond to the needs of a qualified labour force within both the private and public sectors, and not to the necessity of raising the level of knowledge of the nation and promoting the economic, social and cultural development of the country.

The reform of the system during the secular and social republic of Ali Soilihi (1975–1978)

Independence led to a rupture with the former colonial power, which immediately withdrew all technical and financial assistance. However, the administration had almost entirely been staffed by French civil servants. Secondary education was provided to 3,580 pupils on the four islands by 215 teachers of whom 200 were expatriates and only fifteen Comorian. Public sector costs amounted to some seven billion CFA francs while revenues were less than one billion.[23]

The government decided to establish a new educational system that was within the financial and human resources of the country and which met the real needs of the young state. It was decided that Koranic education and formal secular education were to be integrated into a single system, communitarian and rural, so that people perceived the new structure as an extension of those to which they were accustomed in everyday life. Parents could thus contribute financially to the educational system and encourage the personal development of their children.

The new system included a basic education of eight years and a secondary specialised education of four years. Basic education consisted of two cycles of five and three years each, during the first two years of which, as in the Koran school, the language of instruction was Shikomor.[24] The child was introduced to reading and writing Shikomor in the Arabic script and received religious training. From the third year, they began learning the Latin script used for transcription of the official national language. During the second cycle of primary education which lasted three years, French became the language of instruction. The specialised secondary education set up in January 1978 comprised two cycles of two years each, with streams in education, management, agricultural engineering, health and technology.

The demand for education increased sharply and was reflected in the numbers of pupils in the existing institutions, primary and secondary, which rose from 33,000 in 1975 to 57,000 in 1979; the enrolment rate among children aged 7 to 12 was 70%.[25] Each village had its school and the number of *collèges* (lower secondary schools) increased from 5 to 54. However, the programme aimed at integrating the Koranic and secular schools in a single educational system, initiated by President Ali Soilihi, only finally succeeded in reprising Pechmarty's 1917 proposal that the teaching of Arabic be introduced in the official schools in an attempt to attract pupils.

Under the Soilihi regime the public schools were renamed *madrasat*, the change of name emphasising their difference from the old Koran schools set up under a simple shelter, exposed to the wind. Indeed, in every village a new *paya la shiyo* was built of bricks and mortar. The system was highly centralised, the schools were no longer autonomous, as they had previously been, organised around and by a single teacher (*fundi*) or a single family or a married couple. They were no longer dependent for their management upon the willingness of the *fundi*s: the State, with financial and technical support from

UNICEF and UNESCO, was responsible for training the *fundi*s so they could teach using the new methods. The *fundi* was no longer responsible for the syllabus, for the teaching programme, for enrolments or for the school's operating procedures. The material conditions had changed: the children sat on chairs and wrote on slates and in exercise books, distributed for free.

The content and philosophy of education had also changed profoundly. The traditional method was used for learning the Arabic alphabet but children used more modern materials: the slate, the notebook, the blackboard. Arabic was taught in primary school. The children read and copied Arabic words written on the blackboard, with their translation into the Comorian language also written in Arabic script. This was followed by the reading of the Koran, beginning with the shorter suras (as in the traditional Koran school), and without any translation or explanation.

This renewed Koran school only operated from 7 to 9 in the morning, following which, in the same rooms, the children followed the courses of the French school given by the primary teacher. The time devoted to religious teaching was too short to be comprehensive, and the teaching programme therefore abridged. The study of *fikhi* was no longer part of the curriculum. Indeed, the revolutionary government, as part of its fight against idleness, had banned gatherings in mosques outside of prayer times, thereby abolishing the *darasa*s or evening *fikhi* courses which had formerly been held there. The "revolutionary youth committees" justified their decision with a Koranic verse: "And when the Prayer is finished, then may ye disperse through the land, and seek of the Bounty of God and celebrate the Praises of God often (and without stint): that ye may prosper".[26] Students could no longer study in the mosques three times a day, morning, afternoon and evening. This evening class had been the most effective because they learned much more than was contained in their textbooks; students could also listen to the lectures aimed at adults. Once these lessons had been banned they remained in the state schools, which did not teach *fikhi*, but only Arabic literacy.

The revolutionary authorities similarly abolished other religious events, such as the sufi *daira*, the *hauli* and the *hitima*.[27] All the social and educational activities organised by the Koran school, in which not only parents but the entire community participated, and which embedded the institution in social life, were banned.

The counter-reform under the Federal Islamic Republic of the Comoros

In May, 1978 a coup d'état led to the establishment of a new regime, which proclaimed a Federal Islamic Republic in the Comoros. They encountered a highly democratised educational system, but one which was under-equipped compared to the standards of the small number of French schools which had been built and equipped by the French Fonds d'Investissement pour le Développement Economique et Social (FIDES) during the colonial period. The short-term solution was to attempt to re-create the conditions of the elitist educational system of the quarter century prior to independence (1950–1975).[28]

All the teachers recruited and trained to teach in the Comorian language in public schools were dismissed; the teaching of the Koran was abandoned. There was a massive exodus of students from secondary education, the school recruitment process was abolished, boarding schools were closed, and a reduction in the number of rural schools obliged the poorer children, and especially those from rural areas, to abandon their studies. However, Comorian society is fundamentally egalitarian and local communities responded by engaging in self-organisation and engaging the solidarity of their citizens in the diaspora. They undertook the construction of numerous primary school classrooms, and later secondary schools, and private schools have been opened in towns and villages across the country.

Nevertheless, the post-independence social elite is no longer capable of defining and imposing upon the political and religious elites a coherent project for social reproduction. The inadequacy of teaching programmes is one of the principal reasons for the inability of these schools – whether they be French language or Arabic language institutions – to carry out their tasks regarding the cognitive development of the children and raise school attendance rates that are reflected in the national examinations.

Beginning in the 1980s the French language public school suffered – somewhat paradoxically – from an influx of large numbers of graduates of universities in Europe, capitalist and socialist, Africa and North America, who were employed as teachers. However, these young graduates had not received a professional training that would prepare them to exercise a profession that was not straightforward. Teachers by necessity and not by vocation and with inappropriate professional qualifications, found themselves faced with a student body of very low levels of achievement and exposed to difficult, even delinquent behaviour. Teaching, once a noble profession, had become a stop-gap job in the expectation of a better position in the public service or in political office.

The teaching of Arabic and the Koran suffered less than other subjects, since some of the teachers trained under the revolutionary regime opened their own schools. In the 1980s new educational institutions dedicated to teaching Arabic and Islam were created in the context of educational development programmes sponsored by the Arab states and the Islamic World League. The teachers were trained in the more conservative countries of the Islamic world and they have seen it as their duty to undertake a campaign of "re-Islamisation" of society. With this in mind, they target women, whose "indecent" modes of dress are judged to be against Islamic values; burial rituals; sufi practices;[29] and indeed, the state itself, specifically its legal system, which is nominally based on shari'a but in practice draws significantly on the colonial legal legacy as well as incorporating elements of customary law.

Conclusion: a legal framework for a unified educational system

According to the census all Comorian children between 3 and 6 years of age attend an educational institution of some sort.[30] The preschool educational institutions have various names: *jardin d'enfants* (kindergarten) or *école maternelle* (nursery school) for the structures inherited from the colonial French, *palashio* and *madrasat* for traditional and Arabic structures. In 2013 legislation establishing the *palashio* in law defined it as "a religious institution commonly called 'Koran school', intended principally to dispense Koranic education and to respond to the fundamental needs of Muslim and traditional education."[31] Article 4 of the same law states that "the *palashio*, as a pre-elementary school, is created by the commune, the village community, or by the associations of the parents of the pupils, as well as by individuals, if the circumstance fall with the remit of the present law."

For officials in the ministry of education, the concept of a basic education that began at the Nairobi Conference in 1974[32] should be the cornerstone upon which a new unified education system would be built. The aim is for all Comorian children to be equipped with a common minimum portfolio of knowledge, skills and attitudes that would prepare them to serve the national community. These principles prompted the management of pre- and elementary schools to rehabilitate, upgrade and modernise the village Koran school. This modernisation programme would not only introduce new teaching methods and contemporary materials, it would also provide for modern socio-educational activities that would stimulate a child's spirit of initiative and synthesis while instilling a sense of collective work and capacity for expression.

Despite these intentions, a document entitled "Paquet minimum pour l'Enseignement préélémentaire coranique" signed by the Ministère de l'éducation nationale and UNICEF notes that "it is important at this stage to be able to respect a decisive moment, that is, the entrance of the child into the primary system, as established by law. It is absolutely necessary to ensure that the transition to primary school does not lead to a brusque change that risks disturbing the child, affectively or psychologically." However, rather than establishing a primary school curriculum that follows on naturally, only one hour per week is devoted to the teaching of Islam and the Koran school, now relegated to the status of a preschool, has lost its plurisecular mission, that is, the reproduction of a Muslim society that preserved Comorian social values. Its mission today is limited to preparing the child for entry to the secular primary school.

This gap between ideology and practice is characteristic of the dilemmas faced by states that attempt to fuse religious and Western educational programmes, particularly since secular educational programmes are, and often despite protestations to the contrary, the product of Judaeo-Christian pedagogies. The articulation with Islamic curricula is doomed almost by definition. But even in contexts where Koran schools remain vital and flourish, they are often trapped between the westernising influence of an educational programme tailored towards Western outcomes – diplomas, certificates, degrees – and the pressures of an increasingly vocal Islamising minority that is equally disparaging towards such schools (eg Loimeier 2002). Whether the Comoros can trace a path between the two remains to be seen.

Notes

1. All translations from French sources are our own. Under the *Loi du 30 octobre 1886 sur l'organisation de l'enseignement primaire* Algeria was an exception to the rule that prohibited state funding of religious teaching.
2. One oral tradition, collected in Ndzwani in 1976, tells how, towards 884AD, a group of Ibadis led by one Muhammad Ben Ahamad Ben Huseyini al Abadiya arrived in the Nyumakele peninsula in Ndzwani.
3. Literally the "kitchen of the village", the *paya la mdji* is a covered space, generally in the social centre of a village, where items required for ritual and celebratory events were formerly kept, suspended from a roof beam: the *ngoma* (tambourines) and the *shanda* or *shandaruwa*, a white or multicoloured velum that covered the area reserved for gathering and dancing.
4. It has undergone numerous modifications including the addition of the side rooms across the width of the building; an upper floor was added in the early twentieth century. The old part is recognisable by its painted ceiling beams and polygonal columns.
5. This description is from the personal experience of the primary author. His father was a Koran teacher prior to the author's birth. At the age of 50 he closed his school. The author's mother had a Koran school at home. The school that the author attended in the late 1940s was the only Koran school that used exercise books and a blackboard instead of slates. Nevertheless, all the ceremonies descibed below, such as the *unwafwahamwe* were still current practice. They have today largely been abandoned, although slates are still used in certain villages in rural Mwali and Ndzuani.
6. Although *darasa* means lesson, in this case it is a form of chalk made from coral, a by-product of the production of lime. Coral is burnt in wood-fired kilns, often for several weeks; at the end of this process, in addition to the lime there remain solid pieces which can be used as writing chalk.
7. *Mlala* (*Noronhia sp.*), an Oleacea, see Adjanohoun et al., 1982: 108–109) is a tree that grows both close to the sea and further inland on the lava flows. Comorian women use the root to make lipstick.
8. A cycad, *Cycas thouarsii*. The nuts are a quintessentially Comorian foodstuff (Walker 2012).

9. *Qaida baghdadi ma juz amma*. This is widely used as an introductory text to the study of the Koran.
10. The word *hitima* has its roots in the Arabic word *khatama*, to seal, achieve, finish, and refers both to a complete reading of the Koran as well as to the ceremony or meal to celebrate the reading.
11. A guide to jurisprudence written in Damascus by Abu Zakaria al-Nawawi (1233–1278). This was recognised as the legal code in the Comoros by the colonial government's decrees of 29 March 1934 and 1 June 1939.
12. This festival was still being held as late as the mid-twentieth century in certain regions of Ngazidja.
13. This book – *Iqd al-Jawhar fi Mawlid al-Nabiy al-Azhar*, ("the Jewelled Necklace of the Resplendent Prophet's Birth") is generally known as Maulid al Barzandji, for its author Ja'far b. Hasan al-Barzanji, who lived in the twelfth century of the Hegira (eighteenth century of the Christian era).
14. See Mercier-Tremblay 1982.
15. See Perrenoud 1970.
16. Literally, "the European school".
17. Boudou (1940: 143, 323) cited in Mohamed (2001).
18. From Vérin, 1993: 123.
19. Figures for 1918 and 1921 are from Sultan Chouzour, *Enseignement et développement*, unpublished text communicated to the primary author.
20. Vérin 1993: 112.
21. In 1950 there were 19 Koranic teachers for 34 schools and 2216 pupils. ("Comores: L'enseignement officiel 1947–1950, caractéristiques générales", Dépôt des archives d'outre mer BN 1951).
22. Ibrahime 2000.
23. Approximately US$35m and US$5m respectively at the time.
24. The Comorian language, although the diversity of the dialects means Shikomor as such does not exist. See Ahmed Chamanga & Gueunier 1979 and Rombi & Alexandre 1982, on the Comorian languages.
25. *Rapport général du 1er Séminaire de réflexion et d'orientation en matière d'éducation*, Institut national d'éducation, Moroni, Août 1981.
26. Koran, sura 62, verse 10.
27. Ironically, the anniversary of the death of President Ali Soilihi is now celebrated with a *hauli*, which is simultaneously a holiday. *Fundi*s and notables, as well as government officials, travel to his village for the celebration, which is preceded by a *hitima*. Yet during his lifetime, Ali Soilihi was hostile to such ceremonies, and had banned them.
28. See Bouvet 1985, on the problems facing post-socialist education in the Comoros.
29. Attacks on sufi practices by Islamicists are something of a paradox, since the adepts of the sufi brotherhoods in the Comoros are among the most erudite of Comorian Muslims. See Ahmed 2002, Toibibou 2008, on *da'wa* in the Comoros.
30. Source: Direction de l'enseignement préscolaire, Commissariat à l'éducation de l'île de Ngazidja, 2001 report.
31. "'Un palachiyo' s'entend au sens de la présente loi comme une institution religieuse communément appelée 'école coranique' destinée à dispenser, principalement l'enseignement coranique et à répondre aux besoins fondamentaux de l'éducation musulmane et traditionnelle" Article 1 of *Décret n° 13 – 140/PR du 14 décembre 2013 portant promulgation de la loi n° 13–009/AU du 21 novembre 2013, portant statut du « palachiyo »*.
32. See UNESCO/UNICEF 1974.

References

Adjanohoun, E.J., L. Aké Assi, Ali Ahmed, J. Eymé, S. Guinko, A. Kayonga, A. Keita, M. Lebras, eds., *Médecine traditionnelle et la pharmacopée: contribution aux études ethnobotaniques et floristiques aux Comores*. Paris: Agence de Coopération Culturelle et Technique, 1982.

Ahmed Chamanga, Mohamed, & Noël Gueunier. *Le Dictionnaire comorien-français et français-comorien du RP Sacleux*. Paris: SELAF; Louvain: Peeters, 1979.

Ahmed, Chanfi. *Islam et Poltique aux Comores. Évolution de l'autorité spirituelle depuis le protec-torat français (1886) jusqu'à nos jours*. Paris: L'Harmattan, 1999.

Ahmed, Chanfi. *Ngoma et Mission islamique (da'wa) aux Comores et en Afrique orientale. Une ap-proche anthropologique*. Paris: L'Harmattan, 2002.

Allibert, Claude. "Le manuscrit de Chingoni (Mayotte)." *Asie du Sud-Est et du Monde Insulindien*, 7, no 2–3 (1976): 119–122.

Aujas, L. "Notes historiques et ethnographiques sur les Comores." *Bulletin de l'Académie Mal-gache*, 9 (1911): 125–141.

Avoseh, Mejai. "Informal community learning in traditional Africa," in Sue Jackson, ed., *Innova-tions in Lifelong Learning*. London: Routledge, 2011.

Bang, Anne. *Sufis and Scholars of the Sea. Family Networks in East Africa, 1860–1925*. London: Routledge Curzon, 2003.

Bouvet, Henri. "Les problèmes de formation dans la république fédérale islamique des Comores." *Annuaire des Pays de l'Océan Indien*, 10 (1985): 119–125.

Chicot, Claude. *Éducation de base pour le développement rural aux Comores. Rapport de Mission*. Nairobi: Unicef, 1974.

Cogneau, Denis, & Alexander Moradi. *British and French educational legacies in Africa. Vox*, 2014, http://voxeu.org/article/british-and-french-educational-legacies-africa (accessed 14/02/2016).

Damir Ben Ali, G. Boulinier & P. Ottino. *Tradition d'une Lignée royale des Comores (L'inya Fwambaya de Ngazidja)*. Paris : L'Harmattan, 1985.

de la Roche, Jean. "Education in French Equatorial and French West Africa." *The Journal of Negro Education*, 15, no. 3 (1946): 396–409.

Eickelman, Dale F. "The Art of memory: Islamic education and its social reproduction." *Compara-tive Studies in Society and History*, 20, no. 4 (1978): 485–516.

Eisemon, Thomas Owen, and Ali Wasi. "Koranic schooling and its transformation in Coastal Kenya." *International Journal of Educational Development*, 7, no. 2 (1987): 89–98.

Furnivall, J. S. *Educational Progress in Southeast Asia*. New York: International Secretariat, Institute of Pacific Relations, 1943.

Gevrey, A. *Essai Sur Les Comores*. Pondichéry: Saligny, 1870.

Gou, Ali Mohamed. "La fondation des villes d'Anjouan selon le manuscrit de Mouchamou Ben Mohamed Ben Abdallah Ben Soiljhi," in Claude Allibert & Narivelo Rajaonarimanana, eds, *L'Extraordinaire et le Quotidien: Variations anthropologiques. Hommage au professeur Pierre Vérin*. Paris: Karthala, 2000.

Guillain, M. *Documents sur l'histoire, la géographie et le commerce de l'Afrique Orientale*. Paris: Arthus Bertrand, 1856.

Heggoy, Alf Andrew. "Education in French Algeria: an essay on cultural conflict." *Comparative Education Review*, 17, no. 2 (1973): 180–197.

Hendry, W. "Some aspects of education in Zanzibar." *Journal of the African Society*, 27, no. 108 (1928): 342–352.

Ibrahime, Mahmoud. *La Naissance de l'élite politique comorienne, 1945–1975*. Paris: L'Harmattan, 2000.

Kateb, Kamel. "Les séparations scolaires dans l'Algérie coloniale." *Insaniyat, Revue algérienne d'anthropologie et de sciences sociales*, 25–26 (2004): 65–100.

Lambek, Michael. "Certain knowledge, contestable authority: power and practice on the Islamic periphery." *American Ethnologist*, 17, no. 1 (1990): 23–40.

Loimeier, Roman. "'Je veux étudier sans mendier': the campaign against Q'uranic schools in Senegal," in Holger Weiss, ed., *Social Welfare in Muslim Societies*. Uppsala: Nordiska Afrikainstitutet, 2002.

Loimeier, Roman. *Between Social Skills and Marketable Skills: the Politics of Islamic Education in 20th Century Zanzibar*. Leiden: Brill, 2009.

Mercier-Tremblay, Céline. "Pédagogie de l'enseignement primaire nord-camerounais," in Renaud Santerre & Céline Mercier-Tremblay, eds, *La Quête du Savoir. Essais pour une anthropologie de l'éducation camerounaise*. Montreal: Presses de l'université de Montréal, 1982.

Merriam, Sharan B., & Young Sek Kim. "Non-Western perspectives on learning and knowing." *New Directions for Adult and Continuing Education*, no. 119 (2008): 71–81.

Millman, Brock. *British Somaliland: an Administrative history, 1920–1960*. London: Routledge, 2014.

Mohamed Said Assoumani. *L'enseignement Arabo-Islamique aux Comores*. Mémoire de Maîtrise de Lettres, Langues et Civilisations Etrangères Mention Arabe. Paris: Université Sorbonne Nouvelle, 2001.

Perrenoud, Philippe. *Stratification Socio-culturelle et Réussite Scolaire: les défaillances de l'explication causale*. Genève: Droz, 1970.

Raum, O. F. "Some aspects of indigenous education among the Chaga." *The Journal of the Royal Anthropological Institute of Great Britain and Ireland*, 68, no. 1 (1938): 209–221.

Rombi, Marie-Françoise, & Pierre Alexandre. "Les parlers comoriens. Caractéristiques differentielles. Position par rapport au swahili," in M. F. Rombi, ed., *Etudes sur le Bantu Oriental, Langues des Comores, de Tanzanie, de Somalie et du Kenya*. Paris-SELAF, LACITO documents Afrique, 9, 1982.

Schneider, Suzanne. "The other partition: religious and secular education in British Palestine," *Critical Studies in Education*, 55, no. 1 (2014): 32–43.

Toibibou Ali Mohamed. *La transmission de l'Islam aux Comores*. Paris: L'Harmattan, 2008.

UNESCO/UNICEF *Basic Education in Eastern Africa. Report on a seminar, Nairobi, Kenya, 19–23 August, 22–26 October, 1974*. Nairobi: UNESCO/UNICEF Co-Operation Programme, 1974.

Vérin, Pierre. "Le rapport Pechmarty sur les 'Ecoles coraniques' à la Grande Comore (1917)." *Etudes Océan Indien*, 16 (1993): 105–123.

Walker, Iain. "*Ntsambu*, the foul smell of home: Food, commensality and identity in the Comoros and in the diaspora." *Food and Foodways*, 20, no. 3–4 (2012): 187–210.

Watson, Keith. *Education in the Third World*. London: Croom Helm, 1982.

Wieschhoff, H. A. "Education in the Anglo-Egyptian Sudan and British East Africa." *The Journal of Negro Education*, 15, no. 3 (1946): 382–395.

Wodon, Quentin. *The Economics of Faith-Based Service Delivery: education and health in Sub-Saharan Africa*. New York: Palgrave Macmillan, 2015.

Wright, Henry, J. Knustad & R. Frey. *Rapport préliminaire*. Moroni: CNDRS, 1984.

Index

For Product Safety Concerns and Information please contact our
EU representative GPSR@taylorandfrancis.com Taylor & Francis
Verlag GmbH, Kaufingerstraße 24, 80331 München, Germany